;R/
;\

# A Case-Based Guide to Clinical Endocrinology

Terry F. Davies
Editor

# A Case-Based Guide
# to Clinical Endocrinology

Second Edition

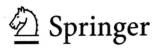 Springer

*Editor*
Terry F. Davies, MD, FRCP
Baumritter Professor of Medicine, Division of Endocrinology,
  Diabetes, and Bone Diseases
Icahn School of Medicine at Mount Sinai
New York, NY, USA

ISBN 978-1-4939-2058-7     ISBN 978-1-4939-2059-4 (eBook)
DOI 10.1007/978-1-4939-2059-4
Springer New York Heidelberg Dordrecht London

Library of Congress Control Number: 2015930737

Printed on acid-free paper

Springer is part of Springer Science+Business Media (www.springer.com)

# Preface

Where I come from in the North of England, a "second" refers to a piece of china with a fault in the decoration or a chip before entering the furnace. Buying "seconds" of very expensive china at low prices was, and is, a common practice of my middle class upbringing. So the term "second edition" does not do this volume justice in my own mind and it is unlikely to be gotten at a rock bottom price. I prefer to call it another volume. Of course there are a few reasons for another volume of Endocrinology Case Histories, but the most obvious is the fact that the earlier volume has created a demand. There was, at least to me, a surprisingly warm reception to the earlier case histories, and this was particularly evident in the download history. People still read a few paper books but the number reading digital versions is clearly exploding. One reason is the easy availability on an international scale. Another is that case histories are perfect for short commutes and the need for a quick revision. And let's not forget that the quality matters also. Having able and dedicated authors willing to submit their teaching cases and then holding their patience during the still long production period is the essential component of this book. I thank them all; many doing this a second time. The demands on medical practitioners continue to increase with no sign of relief and so our free time has become less and less and so has the willingness of many to contribute to such collections. This is a great shame because the multiplicity of authors makes for splendid reading; you never know what style is next and how the case will be revealed. I want to thank the Springer team, especially Richard Lansing and Maria Smilios, for encouraging the production of this collection. There is a lot of good and modern medicine to be learned here.

New York, NY, USA                                    Terry F. Davies

# Contents

**Part XII   Obesity**

# Contributors

**Sherley Abraham, M.D.** Division of Endocrinology and Metabolism, The Johns Hopkins University School of Medicine, Baltimore, MD, USA

**Abdulrahman Alkabbani, M.D.** Division of Endocrinology and Metabolism, Johns Hopkins Hospital, Baltimore, MD, USA

**C. Banti, M.D.** Endocrine Unit 2, University Hospital of Pisa, Pisa, Italy

**Giuseppe Barbesino, M.D.** Thyroid Unit, Massachusetts General Hospital, Boston, MA, USA

**Victor Bernet** Mayo Clinic, Jacksonville, FL, USA

**Conrad B. Blum, M.D.** Professor of Medicine at Columbia University Medical Center, Columbia University College of Physicians & Surgeons, New York, NY, USA

**Jessica Brzana, M.D.** Department of Medicine, Division of Endocrinology, Diabetes and Clinical Nutrition, Oregon Health & Science University, Portland, OR, USA

**Henry B. Burch, M.D.** Medical Corps, U.S. Army, Bethesda, MD, USA

Endocrinology Division, Uniformed Services University of the Health Sciences, Bethesda, MD, USA

**Kenneth D. Burman, M.D.** Endocrine Section, Medstar Washington Hospital Center, Washington, DC, USA

Department of Medicine, Georgetown University, Washington, DC, USA

**F. Cetani, M.D., Ph.D.** Endocrine Unit 2, University Hospital of Pisa, Pisa, Italy

**Silvia Chiavistelli, M.D.** Endocrine Unit 2, University Hospital of Pisa, Pisa, Italy

**Ana Maria Chindris** Mayo Clinic, Jacksonville, FL, USA

**Raffaella M. Colzani, M.D.** Mount Auburn Endocrinology, Waltham, MA, USA

**David S. Cooper, M.D.** Division of Endocrinology and Metabolism, The Johns Hopkins University School of Medicine, Baltimore, MD, USA

**Susana A. Ebner, M.D.** Department of Medicine, Division of Endocrinology, Columbia University Medical Center, New York, NY, USA

**Sergio Fazio, M.D., Ph.D.** William and Sonja Connor Chair of Preventive Cardiology, Professor of Medicine and Physiology & Pharmacology, Director, Center of Preventive Cardiology, Knight Cardiovascular Institute, Oregon Health and Science University, Portland, Oregon, USA

**Dorothy A. Fink, M.D.** Department of Medicine, Division of Endocrinology, Columbia University College of Physicians and Surgeons, New York, NY, USA

**Maria Fleseriu, M.D.** Department of Medicine, Division of Endocrinology, Diabetes and Clinical Nutrition, Oregon Health & Science University, Portland, OR, USA

Department of Neurological Surgery, Oregon Health & Science University, Portland, OR, USA

OHSU Northwest Pituitary Center, Portland, OR, USA

**David Frankfurter, M.D.** George Washington University School of Medicine and Health Sciences, Washington, DC, USA

**Walter Futterweit, M.D.** Division of Endocrinology, Icahn School of Medicine at Mount Sinai, New York, NY, USA

**Sandi-Jo Galati, M.D.** Division of Endocrinology, Diabetes and Bone Diseases, Department of Medicine, Icahn School of Medicine at Mount Sinai Hospital, New York, NY, USA

**Eliza B. Geer, M.D.** Division of Endocrinology, Diabetes and Bone Diseases, Department of Medicine, Icahn School of Medicine at Mount Sinai Hospital, New York, NY, USA

**Gillian M. Goddard, M.D.** Division of Endocrinology, Diabetes and Bone Diseases, Department of Medicine, Icahn School of Medicine at Mount Sinai Hospital, New York, NY, USA

**Rachna M. Goyal, M.D.** Division of Endocrinology, Washington Hospital Center, Washington, DC, USA

**Daniel Herron, M.D.** Professor of Surgery, Chief of Laparoscopic and Bariatric Surgery, Icahn School of Medicine at Mount Sinai, New York, NY, USA

**Jacqueline Jonklaas** Division of Endocrinology, Georgetown University, Washington, DC, USA

**Se Min Kim, M.D.** Mount Sinai Bone Program, Mount Sinai School of Medicine, New York, NY, USA

**Lawrence R. Krakoff, M.D.** Division of Endocrinology, Diabetes and Bone Diseases, Department of Medicine, Icahn School of Medicine at Mount Sinai Hospital, New York, NY, USA

Cardiovascular Institute, Mount Sinai Hospital, New York, NY, USA

**Sathya Krishnasamy, M.D.** Division of Endocrinology, Metabolism and Diabetes, University of Louisville, Louisville, KY, USA

**David W. Lam, M.D.** Division of Endocrinology, Diabetes, and Bone Diseases, Icahn School of Medicine at Mount Sinai, New York, NY, USA

**Derek LeRoith, M.D., Ph.D.** Division of Endocrinology, Diabetes, and Bone Diseases, Icahn School of Medicine at Mount Sinai, New York, NY, USA

**Alice C. Levine, M.D.** Division of Endocrinology, Diabetes and Bone Diseases, Department of Medicine, Icahn School of Medicine at Mount Sinai Hospital, New York, NY, USA

**Carol J. Levy, M.D., C.D.E.** Division of Endocrinology, Diabetes, and Metabolism, Mount Sinai School of Medicine, New York, NY, USA

**Jessica S. Lilley, M.D.** Assistant Professor of Pediatrics, Division of Pediatric Endocrinology, University of Mississippi School of Medicine, Jackson, MS, USA

**Ritu Madan, M.D.** National Institutes of Health/National Institute of Diabetes and Digestive and Kidney Diseases, Bethesda, MD, USA

**Michael Magnotti, M.D.** Diabetes, Endocrinology, Metabolism Specialties, Teaneck, NJ, USA

**Claudio Marcocci, M.D.** Department of Clinical and Experimental Medicine, University of Pisa and Endocrine Unit 2, University Hospital of Pisa, Pisa, Italy

**Nestoras Mathioudakis, M.D.** Division of Endocrinology and Metabolism, Johns Hopkins Hospital, Baltimore, MD, USA

**Shirley McCartney, Ph.D.** Department of Neurological Surgery, Oregon Health & Science University, Portland, OR, USA

**Antonella Meola, M.D.** Endcorine Unit 2, University Hospital of Pisa, Pisa, Italy

**Joshua D. Miller, M.D., M.P.H.** Department of Medicine, Division of Endocrinology and Metabolism, Stony Brook University Medical Center, Stony Brook, NY, USA

**Kim T. Nguyen, M.D.** Department of Medicine, Division of Endocrinology, Columbia University College of Physicians and Surgeons, New York, NY, USA

Division of Endocrinology at Columbia University/New York Presbyterian Hospital, New York, NY, USA

**Elizabeth N. Pearce, M.D., M.Sc.** Boston University School of Medicine, Boston, MA, USA

**Luca Persani, M.D., Ph.D.** Department of Clinical Sciences and Community Health, University of Milan, Milan, Italy

Division of Endocrine and Metabolic Diseases, Ospedale San Luca, Istituto Auxologico Italiano IRCCS, Milan, Italy

**Binh An P. Phan, M.D.** Division of Cardiology, University of California, San Francisco, CA, USA

**Rachel Pessah-Pollack, M.D.** Division of Endocrinology, Diabetes, and Bone Diseases, Icahn School of Medicine at Mount Sinai, New York, NY, USA

**Roberto Salvatori, M.D.** Division of Endocrinology and Metabolism, Johns Hopkins Hospital, Baltimore, MD, USA

**F. Saponaro, M.D.** Endocrine Unit 2, University Hospital of Pisa, Pisa, Italy

**Alex Stagnaro-Green, M.D., M.H.P.E** Professor of Medicine, Obstetrics & Gynecology and Medical Education, University of Illinois College of Medicine at Rockford, Rockford, IL, USA

**Nikolaos Stathatos, M.D.** Thyroid Unit, Massachusetts General Hospital, Harvard Medical School, Boston, MA, USA

**Neil J. Stone, M.D., M.A.C.P., F.A.H.A., F.A.C.C.** Bonow Professor of Medicine, Feinberg School of Medicine, Northwestern University, Suzanne and Milton Davidson Distinguished Physician and Medical Director, Vascular Center of the Bluhm Cardiovascular Institute of Northwestern Memorial Hospital, Chicago, Illinois

**Li Sun, M.D., Ph.D** Mount Sinai Bone Program, Mount Sinai School of Medicine, New York, NY, USA

**Joy Tsai, M.D.** Thyroid Unit, Massachusetts General Hospital, Harvard Medical School, Boston, MA, USA

**G. Viccica, M.D.** Endocrine Unit 2, University Hospital of Pisa, Pisa, Italy

**E. Vignali, M.D.** Endcorine Unit 2, University Hospital of Pisa, Pisa, Italy

**Jason A. Wexler, M.D.** Section of Endocrinology, MedStar Washington Hospital Center, Washington, DC, USA

Georgetown University Medical Center, Washington, DC, USA

**Stephen J. Winters, M.D.** Division of Endocrinology, Metabolism and Diabetes, University of Louisville, Louisville, KY, USA

**Robert T. Yanagisawa, M.D.** Division of Endocrinology, Diabetes, and Bone Diseases, Icahn School of Medicine at Mount Sinai, New York, NY, USA

**Christine G. Yedinak, D.N.P.** Department of Neurological Surgery, Oregon Health & Science University, Portland, OR, USA

**Tony Yuen, Ph.D.** Mount Sinai Bone Program, Mount Sinai School of Medicine, New York, NY, USA

**Mone Zaidi, M.D., Ph.D., F.R.C.P.** Mount Sinai Bone Program, Mount Sinai School of Medicine, New York, NY, USA

# Chapter 1
# Introduction

Maria Fleseriu

## Secretory Pituitary Adenomas

Pituitary adenomas can cause symptoms by hormonal hypersecretion. Hypersecretion of prolactin (PRL) is responsible for amenorrhea–galactorrhea in women and decreased libido in men, growth hormone (GH) for acromegaly, adrenocorticotropic hormone (ACTH) for Cushing's disease, and thyroid-stimulating hormone (TSH) for hyperthyroidism. Tumor mass-related effects such as headaches, visual field abnormalities, and depression of hormonal secretion (hypopituitarism) may also be present.

All patients who present with a pituitary tumor should be evaluated for gonadal, thyroid, and adrenal function as well as an assessment of PRL and GH. To detect the cause of hypersecretion and response to treatment, specific pituitary hormone stimulation and suppression tests are performed, in selected cases. To determine the presence, size and extent of the lesion magnetic resonance (MR) imaging (unless contraindicated) is the gold standard.

Pituitary tumor classification is based on cell cytoplasm staining properties as viewed by light microscopy and immunocytochemistry. Silent functioning adenomas (clinically nonfunctioning adenomas) also exhibit positive pituitary cell-type immunostaining. Most commonly, these include silent gonadotroph adenomas, silent corticotroph adenomas, and silent somatotroph adenomas.

M. Fleseriu, M.D., F.A.C.E. (✉)
Department of Medicine, Division of Endocrinology,
Diabetes and Clinical Nutrition, Oregon Health & Science University,
3181 SW Sam Jackson Park Road, Mail Code BTE28, Portland, OR 97239, USA

Department of Neurological Surgery, Oregon Health & Science University,
3303 SW Bond Ave, Mail Code CH8N, Portland, OR 97239, USA

OHSU Northwest Pituitary Center, 3303 SW Bond Ave, Mail Code CH8N,
Portland, OR 97239, USA
e-mail: fleseriu@ohsu.edu

© Springer Science+Business Media New York 2015
T.F. Davies (ed.), *A Case-Based Guide to Clinical Endocrinology*,
DOI 10.1007/978-1-4939-2059-4_1

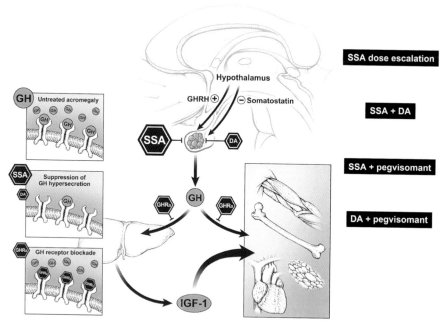

**Fig. 1.1** Adapted from *Neurosurg Focus* 29(4):E15, Fleseriu, M., Delashaw, J.B., and Cook, D.M. *Acromegaly: a review of current medical therapy and new drugs on the horizon,* page 3, Copyright (2010), with permission from Journal of Neurosurgery Publishing Group and American Association of Neurological Surgeons

In the last few decades, significant improvement in surgical technique (>99 % of cases performed via a transphenoidal route) has resulted in low mortality rates. Medical treatment with therapeutics such as dopamine agonists (DA), somatostatin analogs (SSA), GH-receptor antagonists, and glucocorticoid receptor (GR) antagonists has had a profound impact on the indications for radiotherapy. Generally, drugs are now utilized as a second-line treatment, (after surgery) or even as a first-line treatment (Fig. 1.1). Radiotherapy, in selected cases, using stereotactic techniques such as gamma-knife, has been relegated to a third-line treatment. Recently, temozolomide, an orally active alkylating agent used principally in the management of glioblastomas, was shown to be effective in controlling aggressive/invasive pituitary adenomas/carcinomas.

Pituitary tumor patients are best cared for by a multidisciplinary neuroendocrine team at a specialized center; one that includes neurosurgeons, endocrinologists, radiation oncologists, neuro-ophthalmologists, and otolaryngologists. No single treatment algorithm applies to all patients. Treatment should be individualized and include long-term follow-up. Treatment models for individual pituitary adenomas vary and are summarized above (Fig. 1.1).

## Prolactinomas

Prolactinomas are the most common type of hormone-secreting pituitary tumor. First-line therapy is with DAs. Surgery is generally reserved for patients who do not respond to medical therapy, with severe pituitary hemorrhage, are pregnant with progressive tumor enlargement or are not responding to DA therapy.

Treatment aims to normalize PRL levels, restore fertility in those of child-bearing age, decrease tumor mass, save or improve the residual pituitary function, and inhibit disease relapse. Dopamine agonists available in the United States (US) are bromocriptine and cabergoline.

Cabergoline is usually better tolerated (less headache, nausea, postural hypotension, and fatigue) and offers the convenience of twice-a-week administration; starting dose is usually 0.25 mg up to a maximum dose of 1 mg. Cabergoline appears to be more effective in lowering PRL levels within the first 2–3 weeks of treatment in about 90 % of patients and in restoring ovulation. The drug usually decreases the size of micro- and macroadenomas (several weeks to months to observe detectable decreases). In cases whereby the adenoma affects vision, improvement may be observed within days of starting treatment. If tumor response to drug is therapeutically good, medical therapy can be withdrawn after 3–5 years. Hyperprolactinemia will not recur in two-thirds of these patients.

The best treatment to restore fertility in women with a microadenoma is a DA. Cabergoline is less used in women attempting conception or in pregnancy. Bromocriptine does not appear to increase the risk of miscarriage or birth defects when discontinued early in pregnancy. Before attempting pregnancy, a detailed discussion with patients should include when to discontinue bromocriptine, the chances that the adenoma will grow during pregnancy and further treatment details as necessary. Microadenomas rarely increase in size during pregnancy. On the other hand, if the adenoma is large or is affecting vision, surgery is usually recommended before attempting to conceive.

## Acromegaly

Treatment of GH-secreting adenomas should include a comprehensive treatment strategy to alleviate pituitary tumor effects, normalize GH and insulin-like growth factor-1 (IGF-1) hypersecretion, improve associated comorbidities, and reverse the increase in mortality risk, all while preserving normal pituitary function. Surgery is the first-line treatment choice for acromegaly patients, with two caveats, an experienced surgeon is available and tumor is visible on MR imaging. If the tumor has invaded the cavernous sinus, or has been determined to be not completely resectable, medical therapy can be also offered as first-line treatment in addition to surgery. The treatment of patients with persistently active acromegaly has been facilitated over the past decade by the advent of highly specific and selective pharmacological agents that are sometimes used in combination. Radiation therapy is a potential adjuvant therapy, usually reserved for patients who have some remaining tumor postsurgery. These patients often concomitantly take medications to lower GH levels as there is usually a long waiting period before radiation is effective. Decrease in pituitary function (hypopituitarism) is a significant complication. Radiotherapy remains a third-line treatment option for acromegaly in the US.

Three classes of medical therapy are available to treat acromegaly, each with unique advantages and disadvantages. In patients with uncontrolled hormone levels after surgery, SSAs are the first-line treatment choice. Dopamine agonists and GH receptor antagonists are generally indicated after failure of SSAs or in combination with SSAs (Fig. 1.1).

## Somatostatin Analogues

There are three SSAs approved for use in the US: octreotide short release, octreotide long acting release (LAR) or Sandostatin LAR, and lanreotide ATG (Somatuline depot). It is difficult to appreciate the true efficacy of SSAs in achieving biochemical control due to varied clinical trial study entry criteria and "desirable" cut-off goals. Although early on a study data meta-analysis showed that overall GH and IGF-1 were normalized in 49–56 % and 48–66 % of patients, respectively. Other study results suggest symptom control in a large majority, with biochemical control only being achieved in approximately half of patients if "unselected" for responsiveness. Somatostatin analogues are generally safe and well tolerated. The most frequent adverse events of SSA treatment are abdominal symptoms, which usually improve over time glucose intolerance and gallbladder sludge/stones. The distinctions between different types of GH-secreting tumors (sparsely vs. densely granulated tumors), and presence of somatostatin receptor type 2a (SSTR2a) can impact response to therapy as well as prognosis; therefore, accurate classification is important.

It has been suggested that SSA treatment prior to surgery can reduce surgical risks and potentially improve surgical cure rates. Conversely, tumor debulking is often used with SSA therapy when GH is partially but not completely controlled with treatment. In these cases, debulking the tumor may allow SSA therapy to reduce GH and IGF-1 into the normal age-adjusted range.

A number of studies have reported tumor shrinkage in patients with acromegaly treated with SSA therapy, both adjunctive and primary. This shrinkage can be significant (20–80 % in about one-third of patients), however results are unpredictable.

## Dopamine Agonists

Dopamine agonists inhibit GH secretion in some acromegaly patients. The beneficial effects could occur even when pretreatment PRL levels are normal and/or there is no evidence of tumor PRL staining. A lower IGF-1 level at the start of treatment seems overall to be the best predictor of efficacy. Cabergoline is administered orally and is thus more convenient, although not as effective as other medical therapies.

## Growth Hormone Receptor Antagonists

The GH receptor antagonist, pegvisomant, (Somavert) directly inhibits the peripheral action of GH by interfering with functional dimerization of the two GH receptors subunits and thus blocks the signal for IGF-1 production. In early clinical trials, normalized IGF-1 levels were observed in approximately 90 % of patients, however, data from large observational studies has revealed a much lower IGF-1 normalization rate (70 % of patients), most probably due to inadequate dosage. Pegvisomant adverse events include disturbed liver function tests and injection site reactions. Tumor growth has not been proven to be a concern, but continued long-term surveillance of tumor volume is needed, especially in nonirradiated patients. It is recommended that pegvisomant be reserved for SSA nonresponders or patients intolerant of SSAs, patients whose diabetes is worsened by SSAs or considered in combination therapy.

For acromegaly patients who are poorly or non-responsive to, presently available single drug therapies, the use of combination drug therapy holds promise. However, currently the use of combination therapy is not approved by the Federal Drug Administration (FDA) in the US.

## Monitoring Therapy

General consensus is to lower the IGF-1 levels to within the reference range for the patient's age and gender and to lower the random serum GH levels to <1 ng/mL or <0.4 ng/mL (depending on the assay) after a glucose load (oral glucose tolerance test; OGTT). Pegvisomant is unique in that the drug does not lower GH levels (levels are raised, due to feed-back mechanics), thus making IGF-1 the only available marker for disease activity.

It is recommended that all patients undergo biochemical testing and pituitary MR imaging during long-term follow-up, irrespective of medical treatment.

## Drugs in Clinical Trial

The role of SSTRs and dopamine receptors (DR) as molecular targets for the treatment of pituitary adenomas is well established.

Pasireotide (SOM 230; Signifor) is a unique somatotropin release-inhibiting factor with a high binding affinity to SSTR subtypes 1, 2, 3, and 5 and up to a 40-fold greater affinity for $SSTR_5$ than octreotide. Phase III clinical trials results show that subjects treated with pasireotide LAR were significantly more likely to achieve disease control than those treated with octreotide LAR. Also, approximately 20 % of subjects uncontrolled on octreotide achieved full disease control after switching to pasireotide LAR. However, a higher degree and frequency of hyperglycemia has been observed and reported with pasireotide use. The long-term and future role of pasireotide in treating acromegaly remains to be determined.

Alternate drug delivery systems are an exciting and developing area of research. Octreolin, an investigational oral form of octreotide, is currently being studied in a pivotal phase III clinical trial to determine efficacy and safety in acromegaly patients who are currently receiving parenteral SSAs.

## Cushing's Disease

Cushing's disease (CD) is defined as hypercortisolism caused by an ACTH-secreting pituitary adenoma. While rare, the disease is associated with significant morbidity and mortality.

Treatment goals include the reversal of clinical features, normalization of cortisol levels, minimal morbidity, preservation of pituitary function, and long-term disease control without recurrence. In patients with macroadenomas, removal of the tumor mass is an additional treatment goal.

For most CD patients, primary treatment is transsphenoidal surgery to remove the pituitary adenoma. However, success rates are variable (reportedly, 65–90 % dependent on the surgeon's expertise) and recurrence rates are observed in more than 25 % of patients during long-term follow-up. Second-line therapy includes more radical surgery, radiation therapy (stereotactic radiosurgery), medical therapy, and lastly bilateral adrenalectomy.

While there are several potential CD therapeutic targets, clinical experience is lacking. Recently, however, prospective studies have demonstrated the potential of pituitary-directed medical interventions that target the underlying adenoma and block GRs. Medical therapies for CD patients are summarized below (Fig. 1.2).

### Pituitary-Targeted Therapy

Corticotroph adenomas frequently express both dopamine (D2) and somatostatin receptors (predominantly $SSTR_5$). Pituitary-targeted therapies may provide both antisecretory and an antiproliferative treatment results. Research into patterns of receptor expression in corticotroph adenomas may lead to increased understanding of tumor pathogenesis, and allow development of therapies specifically tailored to individual patients following surgical pathology analysis.

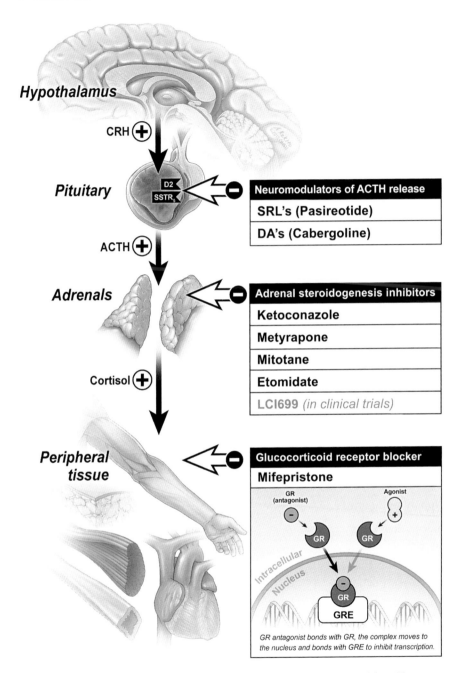

**Fig. 1.2** Potential targets and medical therapies in Cushing's disease. Reprinted from Neurosurg Clin N Am volume 23(4);653–668, Fleseriu, M., *Medical management of persistent and recurrent cushing disease*, page 657, Copyright (2012), with permission from Elsevier

## Somatostatin Analog: Pasireotide (Signifor)

Following promising results in a 15-day phase II clinical trial, a randomized, double-blind phase III trial of pasireotide was undertaken in adult subjects with de novo, persistent, or recurrent CD. Eligible subjects ($n = 162$) were randomized to receive 600 or 900 mcg of pasireotide twice daily: the majority of subjects had declines in urine free cortisol (UFC) levels at 6 months and 15 % and 26 % of subjects in the 600 mcg and 900 mcg groups, respectively, had normal UFC levels within the normal range without dose increases. Median percentage changes in UFC levels from baseline to 6 months in both groups were −47.9 %. Moreover, subjects who responded to treatment could generally be identified within the first 2 months of treatment. In those subjects with observable tumor on MR images, tumor volume changed by an average of −9.1 % and −43.8 % in the 600 mcg and 900 mcg groups, respectively. There were also significant improvements in the signs and symptoms hypercortisolism, reductions in systolic and diastolic blood pressure, triglycerides, low-density lipoprotein cholesterol, body weight, and health-related quality of life.

The safety and adverse event profiles of pasireotide in the phase III trial were similar to those observed with other SSAs with the exception of the degree and severity of hyperglycemia-related events. Nearly three quarters of the study subjects had hyperglycemia-related adverse events, and nearly half of those subjects who did not have diabetes at baseline developed diabetes. A published proposal for management of hyperglycemia in patients with CD treated with pasireotide recommends metformin as first-line medical treatment for CD patients who develop new or worsening hyperglycemia with pasireotide, with an adjunctive dipeptidyl peptidase 4 (DPP-4) inhibitor, sulfonylurea/glinide, and/or glucagon-like peptide-1 (GLP-1) analog, as required, to achieve glycemic control.

Pasireotide was recently approved in the US and Europe for the treatment of adult CD patients for whom pituitary surgery is not an option or who have failed surgery.

## Dopamine Agonists

Like SSTRs, DRs are widely expressed in normal neuroendocrine tissues and pituitary adenomas, including approximately 80 % of corticotroph adenomas. In a single-center study of ten subjects treated with cabergoline (1–3 mg/week for 3 months), a normalization rate of 40 % for UFC was observed. The long-term efficacy of cabergoline (up to 7 mg/week) in selected CD patients is about 30–40 %. The results of these small prospective and retrospective studies have shown promise for the use of cabergoline as medical therapy for CD, but no large-scale trials have been conducted.

## Retinoic Acid

Retinoic acid has been shown to be potentially useful in decreasing corticotroph secretion and proliferation in animal models, and more recently, in a small open-label prospective study in humans. Recent animal models indicate that inhibiting epidermal growth factor receptor (EGFR) signaling may be also a valuable strategy for treating CD. Further studies evaluating clinical efficacy and safety in patients with CD are needed.

## Adrenal-Targeted Therapeutics

Drugs inhibiting adrenocortical steroidogenesis include ketoconazole, mitotane, etomidate, and metyrapone. There is little prospective information on the long-term use of adrenal-targeted agents; however, small retrospective studies have revealed promising results. In general, use of adrenal targeted drugs requires careful clinical monitoring for adverse effects, including adrenal insufficiency (AI). Ketoconazole has been widely used to treat CD because it inhibits several steps in adrenal steroid synthesis and reduces UFC in the majority of patients. However, ketoconazole also inhibits androgen synthesis and is associated with liver toxicity in some patients. The availability of ketoconazole is also limited in many countries. Mitotane also inhibits several steps in steroidogenesis and at doses >4 g/day can be adrenolytic during long-term therapy. Mitotane is sequestered in adipose tissue and eliminated slowly, as such; pregnancy must be avoided for 5 years after discontinuation. Etomidate is the only adrenal steroidogenesis inhibitor compound available for intravenous administration, and as such is useful in situations where rapid control of hypercortisolism is required, or oral therapy is contraindicated. LCI699, a potent inhibitor of 11-$\beta$-hydroxylase and 18-hydroxylase (aldosterone synthase) has shown promising results in a small proof of concept study in CD subjects; LCI 699 is currently under investigation in larger study. No adrenal steroidogenesis inhibitors are approved in the US for treatment of CS.

## Glucocorticoid Receptor Blockers

### Mifepristone (Korlym)

Mifepristone directly blocks the cortisol glucocorticoid receptor (GR-II) and the progesterone receptor (PR). There are >50 case reports detailing mifepristone use and the multi-center, open-label, 6-month SEISMIC study conducted in the USA, included 50 subjects (43 with CD) treated with daily mifepristone 300–1,200 mg (mean of 900 mg) over 6 months. Overall, 60 % of the 29 subjects with glucose intolerance or diabetes were defined as responders (a $\geq$25 % reduction in glucose on a standard OGGT as measured from baseline to 24 weeks. Of the 12 subjects taking insulin at baseline, seven cut their daily dose by $\geq$50 %. There was a statistically significant reduction in mean HbA$_{1c}$, from 7.43 % to 6.29 %. Over half of the subjects experienced weight loss of $\geq$5 % when compared to baseline and 87 % of subjects experienced improvement in their individual clinical manifestations (as assessed by eight clinical parameters by a blinded data review board). Elevation in cortisol (up to sevenfold) and ACTH (up to twofold) was observed in all study subjects with CD, which returned to baseline after stopping drug. There were two cases of AI, and symptoms compatible with AI (e.g., weakness, nausea, fatigue, abdominal pain, emesis, and hypotension) were more frequent. Hypokalemia (as expected) was common but generally mild to moderate and associated with alkalosis and edema. All cases responded well to potassium replacement and spironolactone, albeit at high doses. An increase in endometrial thickness (due to antiprogestin effects) was observed in 38 % of the study's female population including five cases of vaginal bleeding. Overall, for most subjects, mifepristone had an acceptable benefit–risk profile and long-term studies are currently in progress. Monitoring side effects of hypokalemia and hypertension, as well as early recognition of clinical AI, is essential. As there is no biochemical marker to follow (cortisol values are not reliable), treatment efficacy and the potential for AI must be assessed through changes in clinical signs and symptoms and metabolic improvements. Mifepristone was approved in 2012 approved in the USA for treatment of hyperglycemia associated with Cushing's syndrome.

In conclusion, medical therapy for CD poses unique challenges for the patient and clinician alike. The biochemical control and tumor shrinkage results achieved in patients with prolactinomas and acromegaly have yet to be achieved in CD patients. Generally, patients with moderate to severe hypercortisolism require combination therapy to normalize cortisol production.

## Thyroid Stimulation Hormone-Secreting Pituitary Adenomas

Thyroid stimulation hormone-secreting pituitary adenomas (TSH-omas) are a rare cause of thyrotoxicosis. First-line therapy for TSH-omas is surgery, although medical therapy with SSAs is on the increase and has been shown to be effective in reducing TSH secretion in >90 % of patients with resultant normalization of free T4 and free T3 levels and a return to a euthyroid state.

## Summary

A substantial number of patients with pituitary adenomas require multimodal therapy; medical therapy, surgery, and rarely, pituitary radiation. The biologic make-up of pituitary adenomas varies considerably and as such any given patient with a pituitary adenoma requires lifelong regular monitoring for; hormone secretion, tumor recurrence, and development of any new pituitary hormone deficiency. If biochemical control is not achieved or the therapy is not well tolerated, a switch to a different medication or a combination therapy should be considered. Cost: benefit ratio for each therapy and the overall burden of uncontrolled disease and complications should also be taken into account. The treating clinician must be prepared to think in terms of today's therapy for patients, while maintaining an open view to the future. Guidelines for treatment of prolactinomas and acromegaly are available and provide insight.

Two cases of acromegaly and Cushing's follow. These cases are intended to emphasize and demonstrate that more than choosing the right diagnosis, the importance of selecting the right treatment is paramount. Above is a succinct review of medical therapy for secretory pituitary adenomas; while not comprehensive the suggested readings are intended to supplement the text.

# Further Reading

1. Biller BM, Grossman AB, Stewart PM, Melmed S, Bertagna X, Bertherat J, et al. Treatment of adrenocorticotropin-dependent Cushing's syndrome: a consensus statement. J Clin Endocrinol Metab. 2008;93:2454–62.
2. Colao A, Petersenn S, Newell-Price J, Findling JW, Gu F, Maldonado M, et al. A 12-month phase 3 study of pasireotide in Cushing's disease. N Engl J Med. 2012;366:914–24.
3. Cooper O, Melmed S. Subclinical hyperfunctioning pituitary adenomas: the silent tumors. Best Pract Res Clin Endocrinol Metab. 2012;26:447–60.
4. Fleseriu M. Medical management of persistent and recurrent cushing disease. Neurosurg Clin N Am. 2012;23:653–68.
5. Fleseriu M. The role of combination medical therapy in acromegaly: hope for the nonresponsive patient. Curr Opin Endocrinol Diabetes Obes. 2013;20:321–9.
6. Fleseriu M, Biller BM, Findling JW, Molitch ME, Schteingart DE, Gross C. Mifepristone, a glucocorticoid receptor antagonist, produces clinical and metabolic benefits in patients with Cushing's syndrome. J Clin Endocrinol Metab. 2012;97:2039–49.
7. Fleseriu M, Petersenn S. Medical management of Cushing's disease: what is the future? Pituitary. 2012;15:330–41.
8. Katznelson L, Atkinson JL, Cook DM, Ezzat SZ, Hamrahian AH, Miller KK. American Association of Clinical Endocrinologists medical guidelines for clinical practice for the diagnosis and treatment of acromegaly–2011 update. Endocr Pract. 2011;17 Suppl 4:1–44.
9. Laws ER, Vance ML, Jane Jr JA. TSH adenomas. Pituitary. 2006;9:313–5.
10. Melmed S, Casanueva FF, Hoffman AR, Kleinberg DL, Montori VM, Schlechte JA, et al. Diagnosis and treatment of hyperprolactinemia: an Endocrine Society clinical practice guideline. J Clin Endocrinol Metab. 2011;96:273–88.
11. Melmed S, Colao A, Barkan A, Molitch M, Grossman AB, Kleinberg D, et al. Guidelines for acromegaly management: an update. J Clin Endocrinol Metab. 2009;94:1509–17.
12. Molitch ME. Prolactinoma in pregnancy. Best Pract Res Clin Endocrinol Metab. 2011;25:885–96.

# Chapter 2
# Acromegaly, Awareness Is Paramount for Early Diagnosis: Highlights of Diagnosis and Treatment Challenges

**Jessica Brzana, Christine G. Yedinak, and Maria Fleseriu**

## Objectives

- To highlight clinical features of acromegaly at presentation, to facilitate early diagnosis.
- To review the multi-modal approach in the management of acromegaly: surgical indications and medical treatment.

J. Brzana, M.D.
Department of Medicine, Division of Endocrinology, Diabetes and Clinical Nutrition, Oregon Health & Science University, 3181 SW Sam Jackson Park Road, Mail Code BTE28, Portland, OR 97239, USA

C.G. Yedinak, D.N.P.
Department of Neurological Surgery, Oregon Health & Science University, 3303 SW Bond Ave, Mail Code CH8N Portland, OR 97239, USA

M. Fleseriu, M.D. (✉)
Department of Medicine, Division of Endocrinology, Diabetes and Clinical Nutrition, Oregon Health & Science University, 3181 SW Sam Jackson Park Road, Mail Code BTE28, Portland, OR 97239, USA

Department of Neurological Surgery, Oregon Health & Science University, 3303 SW Bond Ave, Mail Code CH8N, Portland, OR 97239, USA

OHSU Northwest Pituitary Center, 3303 SW Bond Ave, Mail Code CH8N, Portland, OR 97239, USA
e-mail: fleseriu@ohsu.edu

© Springer Science+Business Media New York 2015
T.F. Davies (ed.), *A Case-Based Guide to Clinical Endocrinology*,
DOI 10.1007/978-1-4939-2059-4_2

15

## Case Presentation

A 31-year-old male presented to a new neurologist for management of a long-standing "absence" seizure disorder with new monthly breakthrough seizures. Diagnosed at 12 years of age, seizures were reportedly poorly controlled until aged 19 years of age, when there was some improvement after treatment with Depakote. The patient reported migraine headaches with "visual symptoms" over several years and recent worsening, in addition to new diagnoses of renal calculi, sleep apnea, carpal tunnel syndrome, and hypertension prior to this presentation. He also noted a 2–3 year history of increasing fatigue, anxiety, worsening memory, profuse sweating, new onset of diffuse and generalized joint pains, and increased central adiposity. In the previous year, he had been troubled by the development of gynecomastia and had undergone breast reduction surgery. Furthermore, he had undergone lip-reductive cosmetic surgery in the same year due to the large size of his lips.

Brain magnetic resonance (MR) imaging at 19 years of age was apparently undertaken, however the patient was unaware of any abnormal findings and MR imaging had not been repeated since that time.

The neurologist, concerned about vision symptoms, selected to repeat evaluation elements and include brain imaging. MR imaging revealed an "incidental" hypoenhancing sellar lesion 2.5×2.6×2.3 cm in size with bilateral cavernous sinus invasion (Fig. 2.1) indicative of a pituitary macroadenoma. The lesion had compressed and induced superior displacement of the optic chiasm. The patient was subsequently referred to the multidisciplinary Oregon Health & Science University, Northwest Pituitary Center for further assessment and treatment. On evaluation, the patient noted that while he was tall at 6′8″ in height, other family members were also on average quite tall. During the initial clinic visit evaluation, he also admitted to some changes in facial features and rounding of the shape of his face as well as a significant increase in ring and shoe size. Further questioning revealed; oily skin, more abundant skin tags, profuse sweating, and the return of more frequent and more severe headaches. A physical exam revealed typical signs indicative of acromegaly: large hands and large wide feet, significant prognathia, frontal bossing, a large tongue, and several gaps between his teeth. Pulmonary and cardiac auscultations were unremarkable. Examination of his skin showed multiple skin tags in his axilla, which demonstrated acanthosis nigricans. Visual field (VF) testing by confrontation suggested bitemporal field deficits. Formal VF testing by a neuro-ophthalmologist confirmed the finding of bitemporal hemianopsia.

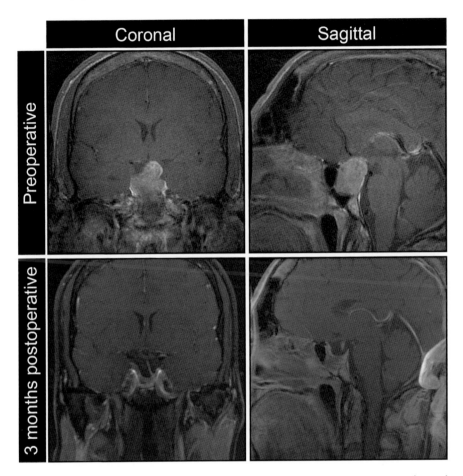

**Fig. 2.1** Contrast-enhanced T1-weighted coronal and sagittal MR images; preoperative and 3 months postoperative

## Why Does Acromegaly Fail to Be Diagnosed for Years?

Growth hormone (GH) is the most abundant of the pituitary hormones and GH secretory cells (somatotrophs) make up to 50 % of total anterior pituitary cells. GH hypersecretion is usually the result of somatotroph adenomas. Ectopic GH or GH-releasing hormone (GHrH) hypersecretion is very rare.

Clinical features of GH excess are usually progressive and insidious with a mean delay in diagnosis of 10 years or more. Mean age at diagnosis is on average 42 years, with both genders affected equally. Characteristic soft tissue proliferation with local bone overgrowth in the skull and mandible become clinically more striking over time, but often occur so gradually that they are unnoticed and unrecognized by family members and medical providers alike. Patients most commonly report growth of hands and feet and may present for orthodenture for bite abnormalities and increasing gaps between their teeth (diastema). Tufting of the distal phalanges, carpel tunnel syndrome, peripheral neuropathies, joint remodeling, and paresthesias occur. Once the epiphyses of the long bones are fused, linear growth is arrested. Spinal cord or nerve root compression from bony over growth, cardiomyopathy, and left ventricular mass enlargement leading to hypertension, cardiac arrhythmias, and valvular dysfunction are all possible. Facial features become course and the skin becomes thickened and oily with hypertrichosis and acne. Often profuse sweating associated with minimal or no physical activity is reported. Upper airway obstruction and sleep apnea commonly develop from soft tissue overgrowth. Patients report fatigue, weight gain, heat intolerance, and have often developed a decreased libido and impotence.

In the case we describe, the patient had several clear features of acromegaly that were possibly overlooked for more than 10 years. Furthermore, there was the unusual history of cosmetic procedures including a lip reduction and breast reduction surgery. A detailed history of developing symptoms such as profuse sweating, increased ring size and shoe size, and a diagnosis of obstructive sleep apnea in a tall, slim, young, and otherwise healthy patient should immediately prompt a hormonal evaluation. Unfortunately, in this case, hormonal evaluation was not undertaken when these features were developing. If a diagnosis had been made earlier, this patient would most likely have avoided the development of vision loss and joint damage and he may have avoided several cosmetic procedures. Additionally, early alterations from excess GH causes joint thickness, which can be reversed with treatment, whereas later boney complications are irreversible even with disease control and in the case of this patient may translate to permanent skeletal disabilities.

## How Was the Diagnosis of GH Excess (Acromegaly) Made?

Laboratory studies collected at the time of initial evaluation showed a marked elevation in the patient's IGF-1 levels; 1,569 ng/mL (upper limited of normal for equivalent age and sex 331 ng/mL, Table 2.1). An afternoon random GH level draw was 39.4 ng/mL (normal <5 ng/mL). Additional confirmatory testing drawn the following day (before any results available) showed that his GH level did not suppress after administration of an oral glucose load: his nadir GH level during the 2-h evaluation test was 20.9 ng/mL.

Age and gender matched IGF-1 levels are elevated in acromegaly patients and as such provides a useful screening test. A single random GH value is not a reliable screening method due to the pulsitivity of GH secretion by the pituitary. In addition to evaluating IGF-1, dynamic testing of GH is needed for confirmation of GH excess in most cases. Failure of GH to suppress after a 75 g oral glucose load to <1.0, or <0.4 ng/mL (as assessed by newer assays), confirms an acromegaly diagnosis. Nevertheless, there are acromegaly cases that present with an elevated IGF-1 and a

**Table 2.1** Patient laboratory results collected at various treatment endpoints

|  | Time (min) | GH (ng/mL) | IGF-1 (ng/mL; normal range) |
|---|---|---|---|
| Preoperative | Baseline[a] | 31 | 1,569 (53–131) |
|  | 30 | 27.5 |  |
|  | 60 | 26.5 |  |
|  | 90 | 23.8 |  |
|  | 120 | 20.9 |  |
| Postoperative | Baseline[a] | 2.4 | 415 (53–331) |
|  | 30 | 1.2 |  |
|  | 60 | 0.8 |  |
|  | 90 | 0.9 |  |
|  | 120 | 0.9 |  |
| SSA therapy | Mean 5 points GH profile | 1.6 | 385 (53–331) |
| Combination therapy |  | – | 131 (53–331) |

[a]Pre-glucose administration

suppressible GH after glucose administration. This test is less reliable in the setting of uncontrolled diabetes mellitus (DM), which is a frequent comorbidity in acromegaly patients. In the case we present, the patient had a significantly elevated IGF-1 level, which, in corroboration with his multiple clinical features and symptoms, secured a diagnosis of acromegaly. An oral glucose tolerance test (OGTT) substantiated these findings, but in retrospect, an OGTT was not absolutely necessary diagnostically in this particular patient.

## What Additional Evaluation Should Be Performed?

After having determined acromegaly as a diagnosis or when evaluating any patient found to have a pituitary macroadenoma, a full evaluation of pituitary function is recommended. It is important to also evaluate prolactin (PRL) levels when making a new acromegaly diagnosis. This patient's PRL was found to be mildly elevated at 29 ng/mL (normal range, 3–13 ng/mL). This was felt consistent with mass effect on the pituitary stalk from the adenoma with associated interruption of the normal tonic inhibition of PRL by dopamine.

Many GH secreting tumors also secrete PRL due to somatotroph and lactotroph cells having a common progenitor cell. It is therefore helpful to distinguish a pure somatotroph adenoma from a mammosomatotroph or a tumor with two distinct cell lines. Conversely, IGF-1 levels should also be measured in any patient presenting with evidence of a prolactinoma.

Additional biochemical assessments in the case we present included: a cortrosyn stimulation test to evaluate hypothalamic–pituitary–adrenal (HPA) axis function, which revealed a baseline cortisol of 4 mcg/dL and with stimulation up to 11 mcg/dL (stimulation to <18 mcg/dL is considered an inadequate adrenal response). His base-line ACTH level was low at 11 pg/mL thus, confirming a diagnosis of central adrenal insufficiency (AI). Thyroid function evaluation revealed a low Free T4 at 0.5 ng/dL (normal range, 0.6–1.2 ng/dL) with a corresponding normal range TSH of 2 mIU/L (normal range, 0.4–4.5 mIU/L), which was clearly inappropriate for the low free T4 and indicative of central hypothyroidism. Total serum testosterone drawn in the morning was in the low to normal range with inappropriately low to normal lutein-izing hormone and follicle-stimulating hormone. This biochemical evaluation was consistent with a diagnosis of probable central hypogonadism.

## How Is Acromegaly Treated?

Surgery is the first-line therapy for most patients with acromegaly. In the presence of a pituitary macroadenoma with optic chiasm displacement, a surgical approach for decompression and subsequent resection or at least tumor debulking is recom-mended. After initiation of replacement glucocorticoid (GC) therapy, the patient underwent semi urgent transsphenoidal surgery (TSS) due to his VF deficit. His pathology was positive for pituitary tumor cells that stained strongly (>90 %) for GH, and PRL was found in scattered cells in the sample (<10 %). Staining for other pituitary hormones was negative. The pathology report described cytokeratin stain-ing as occurring in round perinuclear structures called fibrous bodies and as such his tumor was classified as a sparsely granulated somatotroph adenoma (Fig. 2.2).

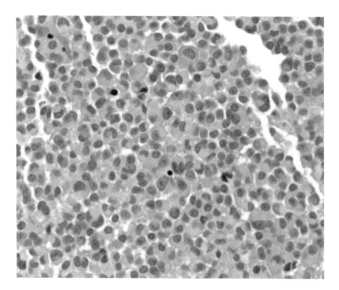

**Fig. 2.2** Immunostaining for tumor cell types (magnification ×400). Sparsely granulated ade-noma: cytokeratin immunostaining highlights fibrous bodies, a histological "dot–like" appearance, typically seen in these sparsely granulated tumors (cytokeratin-IHC stain)

In experienced hands, surgical remission from acromegaly can be achieved in 70–80 % of cases with microadenomas and <50 % of patients with macroadenomas at presentation. However, 40–60 % of patients surgically treated will, at some time, experience persistent or recurrent disease which requires addition of either medical or radiation therapy.

After surgery, despite a decrease in GH level within 24 h, normalization of IGF-1 level can take up to 3 months or more. Thus a diagnosis of remission vs. persistent disease should not be determined any earlier than 2–3 months postoperatively. It is apparent from several new epidemiologic studies that previous criteria for cure or remission were loosely defined. Based on new data associated with mortality rates in retrospective studies, new cut-offs have been defined: normal age and sex IGF-1 and GH suppression after a 75 g oral glucose load to <0.4 ng/mL (using newer assays).

In the case we present, the patient showed significant improvement in many of his symptoms including headache and fatigue; however, he continued to experience arthritic pain and sweating. His 3-month postoperative IGF-1 level remained elevated at 415 ng/mL (normal range, 53–331 ng/mL) although GH nadir was dramatically lower, albeit not normal (Table 2.1). Postoperative brain MR imaging at 3 months showed residual tumor (Fig. 2.1).

Repeat surgery could be indicated if there is residual tumor that is surgically accessible and there is a significant likelihood for surgical cure, or if there is persistent mass effect upon the optic chiasm. Further surgery was not indicated in this patient owing to residual tumor in the cavernous sinus, an area not surgically accessible. A decision was made that adjuvant medical therapy to achieve disease control was required.

Radiotherapy is considered a third-line treatment when medical therapy is not effective or not well tolerated and/or if the cost of long-term medical therapy is a concern. After radiation, medical therapy usually needs to be maintained until biochemical control is achieved and may be necessary for upwards of 5–10 years.

Somatostatin receptor analogues (SSAs) have been considered the cornerstone of medical therapy to treat acromegaly. Control of GH and IGF-1 excess has been reportedly achieved in approximately 50 % of patients who are naïve to medical therapy, and clinically significant tumor shrinkage (>20 %) has been reported in up to 75 % of patients treated with SSAs. Commercially available SSAs bind to tumor cell somatostatin receptors, most specifically somatostatin receptor subtype 2 (SSTR2a). Studies have shown correlation between tumors that stain for SSTR2a and the degree of responsiveness to SSA therapy; this highlights the importance and usefulness of a detailed immunohistochemical pathologic assessment of tumor tissue.

For most patients, Federal Drug Administration (FDA) approved and recommended starting SSA doses are 20 mg for octreotide LAR (long acting release) and 90 mg for lanreotide administered by injection every 28 days. Subsequent dose titrations, based on both biochemical and clinical response to therapy, are usually required. Currently, the maximum FDA approved dose is 30 mg for octreotide LAR and 120 mg for lanreotide, although octreotide LAR has been extensively used in doses up to 40 mg in clinical practice and clinical trials. Patients require close monitoring and dose optimization of SSA therapy should be performed at 3- to 4-month intervals. Additionally, it is important to monitor liver function tests, HbA$_{1c}$ and thyroid function.

In the case we present, the patient was initially treated with lanreotide at 90 mg subcutaneously every 28 days, and titrated after 4 months to 120 mg. He tolerated therapy well and experienced clinical improvement, although normalization of IGF-1 at 376 ng/mL (normal range; 53–331 ng/mL) and GH were not achieved.

It has been determined that while taking a SSA, the value of nadir GH after an OGGT is unreliable, we therefore recommend using random GH and if possible 5-point GH profiles for an integrated estimation of GH secretion. The patient's HbA$_{1c}$ increased from 4.9 to 5.9 on treatment.

## Treatment Options If Disease Is Uncontrolled Despite SSA Optimization

The goal of acromegaly therapy is to normalize GH levels, limit comorbidities, and reduce the known increased morbidity and mortality associated with persistent GH excess. Increased mortality associated with acromegaly is most often secondary to cardiovascular or pulmonary disease.

If disease control is not achieved with SSA therapy, options include switching to alternative therapy or combination therapy. It is well established that a combined treatment regimen of pegvisomant and SSA is effective for disease control in patients who are partially resistant to SSA monotherapy.

In this patient we selected combination therapy with a SSA and the GH receptor antagonist, pegvisomant.

Pegvisomant is a genetically engineered analog of GH, which inhibits GH action by preventing functional dimerization and IGF-1 production. In contrast with SSA, pegvisomant does not reduce GH secretion by the pituitary tumor, but effectively blocks the systemic effects of GH. In addition, it improves glucose tolerance and insulin sensitivity. Observational studies, which are closer to real life scenarios, have shown that pegvisomant is successful in lowering IGF-1 levels in approximately 70 % of cases. This is lower than initial studies where disease control was reported in more than 90 % of patients and is thought to be due to the use of lower treatment doses. There has been a concern that treatment with pegvisomant could cause residual tumor growth, but this risk does not seem to exceed that of other treatment modalities.

With the addition pegvisomant at 10 mg subcutaneous injection daily, in parallel with a reduction in lanreotide dose to 90 mg every 30 days, our patient was able to achieve a normal IGF-1 value for his age and gender of 131 ng/mL (normal range, 53–331 ng/mL). Once disease control was achieved, we continued to monitor his IGF-1 levels every 6 months as well as periodically assessment his HPA, HP-thyroid, HP-gonadal axes, and liver function tests (LFTs).

It is notable that elevated liver enzymes have been reported with the use of pegvisomant as mono and in combination therapy, however, our patient continued to have normal LFTs throughout treatment. In cases with uncommon but pronounced elevations in LFTs, pegvisomant treatment should be stopped. Other side effects such as mild erythemathous reactions at the injection site are commonly observed in the first months of treatment and quickly disappeared. The patient's $HbA_{1c}$ decreased to 5.4 on combination therapy.

Due to the known presence of residual tumor in the cavernous sinus, he was initially re-evaluated every 6 months with MR imaging, and subsequent yearly MR imaging studies were stable. Biochemical control was maintained on this combination therapy and there were no signs of tumor growth at last follow-up 3½ years after surgery.

Overall, combination therapy is generally well tolerated. By using combination therapy, lower doses of both agents with minimization of the side effects associated with higher doses and improved biochemical control can be achieved. The effects of combination therapy on tumor shrinkage require further study. Combination treatment has the potential to increase compliance and reduce cost as well as reduce impact of possible tumor rebound after stopping SSA.

## Complications

Acromegaly is associated with serious morbidity and mortality, if not well controlled. Increased risk of mortality associated with cardiovascular and cerebrovascular atherosclerosis is estimated at 36–62 % and respiratory diseases up to 25 % increase over the normal population. The classic comorbidities may have variable presentation; it is important that ongoing evaluation include assessment of each comorbidity to ensure they are directly addressed in patient management.

In the case we present, a sleep study was performed, which revealed sleep apnea syndrome, and a trial of nasal continuous positive airway pressure was initiated. A colonoscopy was performed and demonstrated multiple colon polyps, which were removed and found to be benign. An echocardiogram showed mild concentric left ventricular hypertrophy, but normal ejection fraction.

Cardiac disease and hypertension are present in more than 60 % of acromegaly patients. Several studies reported increased prevalence of traditional cardiovascular risk factors and early development of endothelial dysfunction and of structural vascular alterations, with subsequent increased risk of coronary artery disease. Furthermore, a large proportion of patients have "acromegalic cardiomyopathy," while valvulopathies and arrhythmias have also been reported and may contribute to the deterioration of cardiac function. The control of GH/IGF-I secretion seems to reverse some cardiovascular abnormalities and could restore normal life expectancy. Cardiovascular risk markers, including lipids, should be monitored and treated aggressively.

Sleep apnea syndrome is present in approximately 70 % of subjects with active acromegaly. Although sleep apnea may improve, it may persist despite biochemical control. Metabolic derangements associated with cardiovascular consequences are also common in acromegaly.

Pre-cancerous or malignant polyps may be found in the colon and given the increase in incidence of colon polyps and the data that malignancies appear to be more aggressive in patients with uncontrolled acromegaly; a screening colonoscopy should be performed.

Panhypopituitarism is likewise more common in this population and all pituitary deficiencies need be appropriately replaced. Regrettably, the musculoskeletal abnormalities are generally not reversible with treatment.

# Conclusion

The appropriate treatment approach for any patient should be optimized to take into consideration tumor size, location within the sella and surrounding structures, symptoms, comorbid conditions and patient preferences, and long-term cost.

Once acromegaly/GH excess is considered in the differential diagnosis, it is not difficult to confirm a diagnosis. An acromegaly patient who presents with a VF deficit should be a thing of the past and delayed diagnosis eradicated.

# Lessons Learned

- Acromegaly often presents with nonspecific symptoms and conditions. Clinical presentations like carpal tunnel syndrome, sleep apnea, and symptoms of headache, sweating, increase in ring and shoe size should raise suspicion for acromegaly.
- Elevated IGF-1 and abnormal GH suppression to glucose are appropriate screening tests, each respectively confirmatory of a diagnosis. It is essential to use an age and sex adjusted value for IGF-1. Similarly, is important to use a highly sensitive GH assay and to use criteria that reflects the capabilities of new more sensitive assays.
- Treatment of acromegaly is complex and in most cases requires a stepwise, multimodal approach to control disease progression. Therapeutic goals include suppressing GH hypersecretion, normalizing IGF-1 levels, reducing tumor mass, and alleviating comorbidities. Transsphenoidal surgery remains the first line of therapy in the majority of cases with medication reserved for persistent GH excess after surgery or as a primary therapy in selected cases.
- SSAs represent the mainstay of acromegaly medical therapy. In patients who are inadequately controlled with conventional SSA therapy alone, combination therapy with pegvisomant could provide significant additional biochemical control.

While combination therapy results in significantly reduced weekly pegvisomant doses compared to monotherapy, there is wide variability in pegvisomant doses required.
- The advantages and disadvantages of each treatment should be evaluated to provide individually tailored care. It is important to consider the long-term cost: benefit ratio of combination therapy and the overall burden of uncontrolled disease and complications.
- Early diagnosis and intervention represents an important factor toward reducing morbidity and mortality and preventing comorbidities.

## Questions

1. A 28-year-old female has been referred to endocrinology because of infertility and irregular menses. Biochemical evaluation reveals an IGF-1 level that is 3 times over ULN and post-glucose GH nadir measurements of 1.4 ng/mL. Which of the following is the most accurate interpretation of her assessment?

   (A) Patient has irregular menses due to intense exercise
   (B) IGF-1 and post-glucose GH nadir are above normal range for a 28-year-old woman and suggestive of acromegaly
   (C) IGF-1 is elevated, but post-glucose nadir levels are normal; thus the patient does not have acromegaly
   (D) She needs repeat testing after she is started on estrogen progesterone treatment to normalize her menses

2. A patient presented with several signs and symptoms suggestive of acromegaly. Biochemical evaluation revealed significantly elevated IGF-1 levels. The following are correct about IGF-1 levels in acromegaly, *except*:

   (A) Will not decrease in response to pegvisomant treatment because the drug blocks only growth hormone receptors
   (B) IGF1 levels correlate with disease severity
   (C) It is important to adjust IGF1 levels for age and sex
   (D) Will normalize with successful treatment

3. A 38-year-old male is receiving a growth hormone receptor antagonist, pegvisomant, after unsuccessful treatment with surgery, radiation, and somatostatin receptor ligands. Clinical studies showed biochemical control with pegvisomant in a high proportion of patients. Which of the following surrogate markers of disease activity should be monitored to best assess treatment response?

   (A) IGF-1 and GH
   (B) Neither IGF-1 or GH; clinical response will be sufficient
   (C) Only IGF-1; GH might be unreliable
   (D) Only tumor size by MRI

4. Pasireotide is a new somatostatin receptor ligand (somatostatin analogue) with higher affinity for somatostatin receptor type 5. Based on recent phase III clinical trials data on treatment with pasireotide in acromegaly, which of the following statements is incorrect?

(A) Patients on pasireotide LAR were more likely to experience hyperglycemia compared to octreotide LAR
(B) Pasireotide achieved additional biochemical control in patients not controlled on octreotide or lanreotide
(C) Pasireotide does not act at the tumor level; thus tumor shrinkage is not expected
(D) Monitoring pituitary function prior to initiation of therapy, as well as periodically during treatment, as clinically appropriate, is recommended

## Answers to Questions

1. (B)
2. (A)
3. (C)
3. (C)

## Suggested Reading

1. Carmichael JD, Bonert VS, Mirocha JM, Melmed S. The utility of oral glucose tolerance testing for diagnosis and assessment of treatment outcomes in 166 patients with acromegaly. J Clin Endocrinol Metab. 2009;94:523–7.
2. Fleseriu M. Clinical efficacy and safety results for dose escalation of somatostatin receptor ligands in patients with acromegaly: a literature review. Pituitary. 2011;14:184–93.
3. Fleseriu M. The role of combination medical therapy in acromegaly: hope for the nonresponsive patient. Curr Opin Endocrinol Diabetes Obes. 2013;20:321–9.
4. Giustina A, Chanson P, Bronstein MD, Klibanski A, Lamberts S, Casanueva FF, et al. A consensus on criteria for cure of acromegaly. J Clin Endocrinol Metab. 2010;95:3141–8.
5. Katznelson L. Approach to the patient with persistent acromegaly after pituitary surgery. J Clin Endocrinol Metab. 2010;95:4114–23.
6. Katznelson L, Atkinson JL, Cook DM, Ezzat SZ, Hamrahian AH, Miller KK. American Association of Clinical Endocrinologists medical guidelines for clinical practice for the diagnosis and treatment of acromegaly–2011 update. Endocr Pract. 2011;17 Suppl 4:1–44.
7. Mathioudakis N, Salvatori R. Management options for persistent postoperative acromegaly. Neurosurg Clin N Am. 2012;23:621–38.
8. Melmed S, Casanueva FF, Klibanski A, Bronstein MD, Chanson P, Lamberts SW, et al. A consensus on the diagnosis and treatment of acromegaly complications. Pituitary. 2013;16:294–302.
9. Melmed S, Colao A, Barkan A, Molitch M, Grossman AB, Kleinberg D, et al. Guidelines for acromegaly management: an update. J Clin Endocrinol Metab. 2009;94:1509–17.

# Chapter 3
# A Nontraumatic Hip Fracture in a Young Woman: Cushing's Disease—Consequences of a Late Diagnosis and Treatment Highlights

**Christine G. Yedinak, Jessica Brzana, Shirley McCartney, and Maria Fleseriu**

## Objectives

- To describe the late diagnosis of hypercortisolemia and associated severe clinical complications.
- To review the multimodal approach in the management of Cushing's disease after failed transsphenoidal surgery: surgical re-exploration and the role of medical treatment.

C.G. Yedinak, D.N.P. • S. McCartney, Ph.D.
Department of Neurological Surgery, Oregon Health & Science University,
3303 SW Bond Ave, Mail Code CH8N, Portland, OR 97239, USA
e-mail: yedinakc@ohsu.edu

J. Brzana, M.D.
Department of Medicine, Division of Endocrinology, Diabetes and Clinical Nutrition,
Oregon Health & Science University, 3181 SW Sam Jackson Park Road,
Mail Code BTE28, Portland, OR 97239, USA

M. Fleseriu, M.D. (✉)
Department of Medicine, Division of Endocrinology, Diabetes and Clinical Nutrition,
Oregon Health & Science University, 3181 SW Sam Jackson Park Road,
Mail Code BTE28, Portland, OR 97239, USA

Department of Neurological Surgery, Oregon Health & Science University,
3303 SW Bond Ave, Mail Code CH8N, Portland, OR 97239, USA

OHSU Northwest Pituitary Center, 3303 SW Bond Ave, Mail Code CH8N,
Portland, OR 97239, USA
e-mail: fleseriu@ohsu.edu

© Springer Science+Business Media New York 2015
T.F. Davies (ed.), *A Case-Based Guide to Clinical Endocrinology*,
DOI 10.1007/978-1-4939-2059-4_3

## Case Presentation

A 34 year-old woman initially presented to her primary care physician (PCP) for evaluation of acne, depression, and a reported centrally localized weight gain of 30 lbs incurred over a 2-year period. She was treated with antidepressants and subsequently followed for 5 years. Her symptoms progressed with the development of lower extremity edema and weakness in all extremities. Although menarche had occurred at 12 years of age, she had developed menstrual irregularities that had progressed to secondary amenorrhea. She was given a diagnosis in her early 20s of polycystic ovary syndrome (PCOS) and therapy with oral contraceptives and metformin was initiated.

Her weakness escalated and she experienced several ground level falls that resulted in a wrist fracture and left hip fracture on separate occasions. While x-ray studies at the time of her hip injury were unremarkable, repeat assessment confirmed a hip fracture that required internal fixation; poor healing complicated surgical course. After discharge, further evaluation demonstrated a new diagnosis of hypertension and elevated lipids and treatment with hydrochlorothiazide and a low fat diet were initiated. Her depression was worsening and now included fleeting suicidal ideation; additional symptoms included easy bruising, poor concentration, and night sweats. She began researching her symptoms on the Internet and other media and ultimately asked her primary care physician to test her for Cushing's syndrome (CS) and for a referral to a local endocrinologist for consultation. This consultation revealed two elevated 24-h urine free cortisol levels (UFC) of 180 and 200 mcg/24 h with elevated adrenocorticotropic hormone (ACTH), and a 4-mm pituitary adenoma; she subsequently underwent pituitary surgery. Therefore treatment was initiated 16 months after her hip fracture, but probably 7–10 years after her initial symptoms were compatible with a CS diagnosis. Surgical pathology was positive for pituitary adenoma, but no hormonal staining was performed at the time of this surgery.

She presented for evaluation at the Oregon Health & Science University, Northwest Pituitary Center 3 months after her first pituitary surgery. Her depression had worsened and on exam she was hypertensive (blood pressure was 160/90 mmHg), body mass index was 39, and she had central obesity and facial rounding with red–purple facial plethora. Additionally, she had striking alopecia and some evidence of proximal muscle weakness. Evaluation of her skin revealed many violaceous striae on her trunk and axilla as well as skin tags and acanthosis nigricans. Further biochemical work-up revealed two elevated 24-h UFC levels of 120 and 100 mcg/24 h (normal level <45 mcg/24 h): ACTH levels were likewise elevated on multiple occasions. A dexamethasone suppressed corticotropin-releasing hormone (CRH) test revealed that cortisol levels were elevated, 2.8 μg/dl 15 min after CRH stimulation.

## How Was the Diagnosis Made?

Cushing's syndrome (CS) results from prolonged exposure to excessive levels of circulating glucocorticoids (Table 3.1). Excluding exogenous sources of glucocorticoids, Cushing's disease (CD) is the most common etiology, whereby excessive

**Table 3.1** Many of the signs and symptoms of Cushing's syndrome logically exhibit the actions of glucocorticoid action

Cushing's syndrome signs and symptoms

| Common symptoms | Physical exam signs | Less common symptoms | Physical exam signs |
|---|---|---|---|
| – Weight gain | – Dorso cervical (Buffalo) hump<br>– Supra clavicular fat<br>– Central weight with extremity sparing | – Skin changes<br>– Difficulty with wound healing<br>– Increased infections<br>– Easy bruising | – Skin lesions and ulcerations, thin skin, telangiectasias, purpura<br>– Ecchymosis<br>– Violaceous abdominal/breast striae<br>– Hyperpigmentation/acanthosis nigricans<br>– Skin tags (acrochordons)<br>– Kyphosis<br>– Height loss |
| *Facial changes*<br>– Acne<br>– Rounding<br>– Red facial flushing | – Facial plethora<br>– Acne<br>– Moon facies (rounding) | – Vision changes<br>– Blurred vision | *Macroadenomas*<br>– Visual-field defects (often bitemporal) |
| – Excess hair growth on face, neck, chest, abdomen and thighs<br>– Swelling of feet/legs<br>– Overall weakness and fatigue<br>– Hip and shoulder weakness | – Hirsutism/breast, back, abdominal hair<br>– Alopecia/frontal balding in woman<br>– Edema/generalized/LE<br>– Loss of muscle mass<br>– Proximal muscle weakness | *Psychological problems*<br>– Irritability<br>– Poor concentration and short-term memory<br>– Anxiety<br>– Mood swings<br>– Sleep disturbance and insomnia | *Less common*<br>– Glucose intolerance or diabetes mellitus<br>– Hypertension<br>– Hyperlipidemia<br>– Osteopenia/osteoporosis |
| – Menses irregular/absent<br>– Decreased fertility and/or libido or impotence<br>– Breast discomfort and discharge | – Decreased testicular volume in men<br>– Galactorrhea | *In children*<br>– Growth retardation | |

amounts of circulating cortisol result from overproduction of ACTH from a cortico-troph pituitary tumor. Harvey Cushing was the first to describe CD in 1912 and the disease has remained a complex diagnostic entity.

The prevalence of CD is estimated at 2.4 cases per million with an incidence of 1.2–2.4 cases per million per year. Women are more commonly affected than men.

Although a patient may be phenotypically "cushingoid," the etiology of excess hypercortisolism varies. The most common cause, by far, is the use of exogenous steroids for the treatment of an underlying disease. When this and factious hyper-cortisolism are excluded, other sources of pseudo-Cushing's need evaluation includ-ing anorexia, malnutrition, poorly controlled diabetes mellitus (DM), and glucocorticoid resistance. Once these are eliminated other endogenous etiologies should be evaluated and are generally divided into ACTH-dependent and ACTH-independent causes. ACTH-dependent cases account for approximately 80 % of all cases: 80 % of these are the result of a corticotroph producing pituitary adenoma and represent CD, while roughly 20 % are due to ectopic ACTH production. ACTH-independent CS is largely associated with adrenal adenomas and autonomous corti-sol production.

Cortisol excess predisposes the individual to increased risk of cardiovascular disease and hypertension, impaired glucose tolerance and DM, impaired immune function, carotid intimal changes, clotting disorders, and osteoporosis with associ-ated morbidity and mortality risks.

## Screening and Confirmatory Tests for Hypercortisolemia

When CS is suspected, clinicians are frequently faced with a complex symptomatol-ogy and perplexing laboratory tests: any evaluation is compounded by the compli-cated physiology of cortisol and ACTH, which are increased in patients who are stressed. These patients without CS can have mildly elevated 24-h UFCs while con-versely, patients with mild CS may have normal 24-h cortisol production rate.

A 1 mg overnight dexamethasone suppression test and a midnight salivary cortisol level are good screening tests. Normal cut-off values for the overnight suppression test have decreased over time from an a.m. cortisol level of <5 to <1.8 µg/dl, which increases sensitivity and decreases specificity. 24-h UFC represent also an important screening method, but could be normal in cases of early disease or recurrence.

In the case we present, additional studies were performed to rule-out elevated cortisol levels associated with pseudo-Cushing's, caused by other underlying dis-eases such as active depression, alcoholism, obesity, and PCOS. A dexamethasone suppressed CRH test is most commonly used to distinguish CS from pseudo-Cushing's and in our case, cortisol levels were >1.4 µg/dl at 15 min after the admin-istration of intravenous CRH (the cut of indicative of CS). Some recent reports have recommended a cut-off for cortisol of >2.5 µg/dl (or >20 % over baseline) and an ACTH increase of >35–50 % at 15 min after CRH administration as a better discrimi-nator. It is important to remember that no one test is 100 % sensitive and/or specific to determine if a patient has true CS or pseudo-Cushing's; therefore, physicians must make every attempt to avoid a misdiagnosis. At our center, we follow a conservative approach and do not proceed to imaging (or surgery) unless we are confident of a biochemical diagnosis. This can justifiably cause frustration for patients who are often troubled by absence of an explanation for their symptoms. Conversely, as CS is a progressive disease, it is important to follow-up initial negative or borderline results in 6 or 12 months to make sure that no patient with CS is overlooked.

## Localization of ACTH Excess

Brain magnetic resonance (MR) imaging in most, but not all, cases of CD reveals evidence of a pituitary adenoma; residual tumor was apparent in the case we present and the patient was referred to a neurosurgeon for further transsphenoidal resection of a pituitary microadenoma. Three months postoperatively, MR imaging did show postoperative changes, but no tumor was identified.

Pituitary adenoma in a patient with CS could represent an incidentaloma, thus bilateral inferior petrosal sinus sampling (IPSS) is considered the gold standard to differentiate between pituitary and ectopic sources of ACTH. A ratio of petrosal sinus to peripheral vein serum ACTH levels of >2–3:1 μg/dl measured after CRH is injected into a catheter positioned in both inferior petrosal sinuses is indicative of CD. The sensitivity of this test in CD is reportedly 94 % with a specificity of 100 %. However, both false positive and false negatives have been reported and are complicated by technical and venous anomalies. Tumor lateralization is also aided by IPSS, but with less accuracy.

Confirmation of a diagnosis after an initial failed TSS is paramount. While we considered petrosal sinus sampling to confirm CD as opposed to ectopic ACTH production, repeated assessment of her outside surgical pathology by our pathologist established the presence of a corticotroph adenoma at the first surgery.

## Persistent Cushing's Disease

The consequences of persistent hypercortisolism are severe and include immuno-suppression, poor wound healing, diabetes, high blood pressure, cardiac insufficiency, severe osteoporosis, and increased mortality. Hence, early identification of patients at risk of treatment failure is exigent. Diagnosing persistent or recurrent CD is perhaps even more challenging than making the initial CD diagnosis. Several investigators have recommended serial measurement of serum cortisol in the days after pituitary surgery to identify patients with persistent CD.

All therapeutic options were discussed with this patient's case: medication, bilateral adrenalectomy (BLA), or repeat transsphenoidal surgery (TSS). Transsphenoidal surgery in the hands of an experienced surgeon has demonstrated remission rates of between 65 and 93 % when used as first-line therapy. However, even with immediate re-exploration, after nonremission, rates drop to about 50 %. Remission rates are lower for larger, invasive tumors. On this basis, medical therapy with ketoconazole was recommended for our patient. However, despite acknowledging low chances of remission, she opted for a second surgery and she was reluctant to use medical therapy even as a preoperative treatment. She underwent repeat TSS; however, despite resection by a very experienced surgeon, no adenoma tissue was identified.

## Management/Treatment of Cushing Syndrome After Failed Surgery

The goals for treatment of patients with CS are; reversal of clinical features, normalization of cortisol levels, and long-term control without recurrence. The primary modality for definitive treatment is TSS. Recurrence rates vary widely and may be as high as 26 % during long-term follow-up. If surgery is unsuccessful or hypercortisolism recurs, second-line treatment options include repeat surgery, medical therapy, radiation, BLA, or a combination of these options (Fig. 3.1). Bilateral adrenalectomy has been described as a definitive cure for CD when pituitary

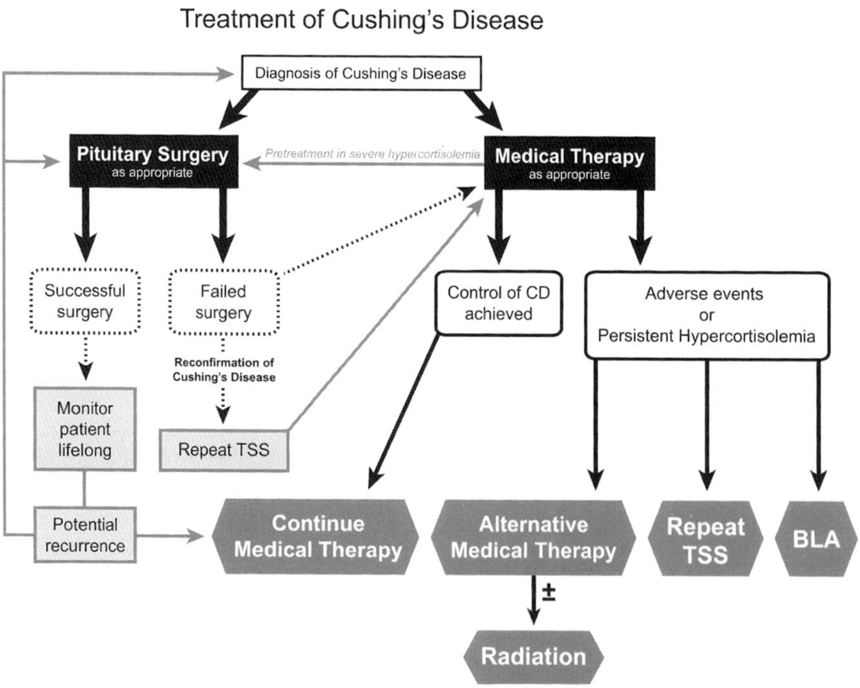

**Fig. 3.1** Cushing's disease treatment options. Reprinted from Neurosurg Clin N Am volume 23(4);653-668, Fleseriu, M., *Medical management of persistent and recurrent cushing disease*, page 655, Copyright (2012), with permission from Elsevier

adenomectomy fails to achieve remission. However, it falls far short of an ideal treatment. Tumor corticotroph progression has been reported in 39–47 % of patients within a median follow-up of 4.6 years but predictive factors have remained elusive. High ACTH levels associated with tumor progression can be accompanied by the development of marked skin hyperpigmentation tumor enlargement and visual field deficits. In one CD study, 50 % of patients continued to report persistent adverse symptoms despite BLA. Early identification of corticotroph tumor progression is possible with close monitoring with MR imaging and ACTH levels and further surgical resection and/or radiation therapy is usually indicated.

Radiation therapy and stereotactic radiosurgery for residual or recurrent tumors can be an effective alternative or additional treatment. However, tumors may be difficult to identify on MR images and the addition of medical therapies may be necessary for up to 60 months. It has been reported that 83 % of patients achieved remission following such treatment. Post-treatment complications are not insignificant and include hypopituitarism, cognitive deficits, visual deficits and neuropathy, radiation-induced necrosis and neoplasms, and cerebrovascular accidents.

## Postoperative Evaluation for Remission Versus Persistence of the Disease

Our patient's postoperative blood cortisol levels at midnight and 6 AM (after glucocorticoids were held ×2 h) were measured at 12 and 13 mcg/dl and she did not develop symptoms of adrenal insufficiency (AI) without glucocorticoids. Postoperatively, she also developed diabetes insipidus and hypothyroidism and required additional therapy with desmopressin and levothyroxine. Her symptoms of hypercortisolism persisted including irregular menses, weight gain, weakness, and depression. Further testing revealed persistently elevated 24-h UFCs (100 and 85 mcg/24 h, normal <45 mcg/24 h) elevated midnight cortisol levels at 8.2 nmol/l (cut-off <4.3 nmol/l) and elevated ACTH (>50 pg/ml, cut-off <46 pg/ml).

At this time, medical therapy was pursued to control her hypercortisolemia since she was reluctant to consider BLA. Radiation treatment was also discussed, but in the absence of a target tumor seen on MR images, desire for fertility and patient reluctance, this was postponed as a possible third-line therapy.

The initial agent was ketoconazole. While not approved in the USA for hypercortisolemia, it is a well-known off-label treatment option in the absence of appropriate alternative treatments. Ketoconazole acts to impair steroid hormone synthesis by blocking adrenal 11 beta-hydroxylase. She was started on a dose of 200 mg three times a day, which was increased to 400 mg twice a day. During therapy she had close monitoring of her liver function studies for elevations in liver enzymes as well as monitoring for signs of AI. While she had improvement in her cortisol measurements, she did not have normalization of her cortisol and her liver enzymes increased (Fig. 3.2). Her $HbA_{1c}$ improved from 6.8 to 5.8 and she continued treatment with metformin 500 mg orally twice a day. Her liver panel normalized after stopping ketoconazole.

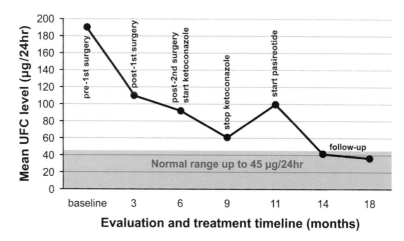

**Fig. 3.2** Case study patient evaluation and treatment timeline; mean urine free cortisol (μg/24 h) vs. time (months)

The addition of cabergoline was attempted, however, the patient did not tolerate the drug even at lower doses and experienced profound nausea and dizziness; cabergoline was stopped in less than a month.

Alternative medical agents were eventually considered. Mifepristone (Korlym), a steroid that binds competitively to glucocorticoid and progesterone receptors, blocks the action of cortisol at the level of the cortisol receptor and has been approved by the US Federal Drug Administration (FDA) for treatment of CS associated with hyperglycemia. On therapy, patients are monitored by following alterations in their clinical parameters such as improvement in diabetes, blood pressure, and weight. Cortisol levels rise as a result of the blockade and cannot be monitored while on this therapy and patients are at risk of developing AI despite high cortisol serum levels. Additionally, patients can develop hypokalemia and require additional therapy with potassium supplementation and/or spironolactone. There are many drug–drug interactions that need to be taken into account with this therapy. Due to mifepristone effects on progesterone receptors, women with intact uterus are also at risk for abnormal endometrial thickening and vaginal bleeding. This patient had a history of amenorrhea and intermittent unexplained vaginal bleeding, which is a contraindication for the use of mifepristone. She was subsequently treated with pasireotide (Signifor), a somatostatin receptor ligand, which has a high affinity for SSTR5. It has inhibitory effects on ACTH secretion in the corticotrophic cells and has been shown to normalize cortisol levels in up to 50 % of patients with mild CD. The main side effect with this therapy is hyperglycemia. Other adverse effects are similar to the other somatostatin analogues. Pasireotide was recently FDA approved for use in CD in the USA. After starting pasireotide at doses of 600 mcg subcutaneously twice daily, her UFC normalized (Fig. 3.2). Treatment was well tolerated overall, electrocardiogram was normal and no QTc prolongation was evident. Her liver panel remained normal and her menstrual cycle returned and normalized.

Patients with normal baseline HbA$_{1c}$ or pre diabetes may develop pasireotide associated hyperglycemia. Studies to elucidate the mechanism using healthy volunteers suggest that despite intact postprandial glucagon secretion there is reduced secretion of glucagon-like peptide (GLP)-1, glucose-dependent insulinotropic polypeptide, and insulin. Therefore patients treated with pasireotide need to be closely monitored for the development of glucose intolerance and medical therapy initiated as per standard guidelines for the treatment of DM with individual adaptation to this specific mechanism. The staged treatment intensification with a dipeptidyl peptidase-4 inhibitor and preferential use of GLP-1 based-medications and insulin may be required. Further studies are needed to optimize glycemic control while on this agent.

Her fasting glucose rose to 138 mg/dl in the first week after starting treatment and Hba$_{1c}$ from 5.8 % at baseline to 7 % after 8 weeks of treatment. The patient was switched from metformin to janumet (50 mg sitagliptin/500 mg metformin hydrochloride) twice daily, which controlled her blood sugars and her HbA$_{1c}$ decreased to 6.2 % after another 3 months. Despite the complication of hyperglycemia, the patient's cortisol studies showed normalization of UFC levels along with marked improvement of the many CD features.

## Conclusions

Recognition of CS and the identification of the underlying cause are often challenging. Patients with unexplained clinical findings suggestive of CS should undergo a careful evaluation for hypercortisolism. If the presence of hypercortisolism is confirmed, the cause should be investigated. Cushing's disease is the most likely diagnosis after ruling out exogenous CS. To date, evidence-based guidelines for screening criteria are missing. The Endocrine Society clinical practice guidelines recommend testing for CS in patients with multiple signs and symptoms compatible with the syndrome. In addition to the treatment guidelines, patients in high-risk groups such as those with poorly controlled diabetes, hypertension, and early-onset osteoporosis (particularly with fractures) have been shown to have a high prevalence of subclinical CS. The issue of cost-effectiveness of screening high-risk patients is still unresolved.

In the presence of clinical suspicion, the clinician should balance the history, physical, and laboratory findings and arrive at the best possible diagnosis. A period of watchful waiting is often required; in patients with CD the disease will progress while for those with pseudo-Cushing's it will not.

Once diagnosed, the first-line treatment for CD is surgery to remove the tumor. However, because surgery is not effective in all patients with CD, additional treatment is needed and can include repeat surgery medical therapy, BLA, and radiation therapy.

## Lessons Learned

- A history of a nontraumatic fracture in a young premenopausal female should prompt work-up of secondary causes including CS.
- After transsphenoidal surgery for CD, patients should undergo immediate postoperative evaluation of HPA axis and evaluation for persistence or recurrence of CD. Further treatment should be initiated as soon as possible.
- It is important to reconfirm the diagnosis of CD after failed surgery if pathology was negative for ACTH staining corticotroph adenoma.
- Medical therapy could offer remission of hypercortisolism after failed surgery. Ketoconazole has been extensively used for CS, but no prospective studies are available and patients have to be very closely followed due to a risk of liver failure. Cabergoline has also been shown to be effective in normalizing cortisol levels in some patients but is limited by adverse effects at higher doses. Pasireotide is a FDA drug approved for CD, but was proven efficacious in about half of the cases with mild CS and is associated with hyperglycemia in the majority of patients. Both mifepristone, FDA approved for hyperglycemia in CS, and pasireotide have a place in therapy, but require appropriate patient selection and close monitoring.

## Questions

1. Screening for Cushing's syndrome in all patients should include which one of the following options:

   (A) MRI of the pituitary
   (B) Adrenal CT
   (C) 24 h urine free cortisol
   (D) Bilateral inferior petrosal sinus sampling

2. A 50-year-old male with marked Cushingoid features has a clearly elevated serum cortisol that fails to suppress on the low-dose dexamethasone suppression test. His urine free cortisol has also been elevated twice, up to 3 times over upper limit of normal. Plasma ACTH also elevated. MRI showed a 2 mm pituitary heterogenous area and a decision to undergo transsphenoidal surgery was made. The surgeon removed a lesion that was diagnosed on pathology to be Rathke's cleft cyst. Biochemical evaluation 4 weeks postoperatively showed persistent hypercortisolemia (UFC >1.7 ULN) What is the next step in the evaluation and treatment of this patient?

   (A) Repeat pituitary surgery to look for the ACTH secreting tumor
   (B) Bilateral adrenalectomy
   (C) Bilateral inferior petrosal sinus sampling
   (D) Fractionated radiotherapy
   (E) Repeat biochemical evaluation at 6 weeks postoperatively to detect possible remission

3. Which is the most common scenario where medical therapy for Cushing's disease has been prospectively studied?

   (A) Primary medical treatment
   (B) Preoperatively
   (C) There are no prospective studies on medical therapy in Cushing's disease
   (D) Postoperatively in patients without biochemical normalization

4. Pasireotide is a multiligand somatostatin receptor ligand that has been recently approved for treatment of Cushing's disease. Biochemical normalization rates in patients with Cushing's disease may depend on a variety of factors. Which single factor has clearly been identified so far to influence response to treatment based on phase III trial results?

   (A) Duration of treatment over 1 year
   (B) Tumor size before surgery
   (C) Degree of cortisol elevation at baseline before starting treatment
   (D) Dose of the drug

5. Mifepristone is a glucocorticoid receptor blocker that has been approved for treatment of hyperglycemia in patients with Cushing's syndrome. Which of the following statement is incorrect?

   (A) Diabetes improvement was significant in most patients studied in the phase III trial
   (B) Cortisol is the best marker to follow response to this treatment
   (C) This medication cannot be used in women desiring pregnancy
   (D) Hypokalemia can be frequently seen and needs close monitoring

## Answers to Questions

1. (C)
2. (C)
3. (D)
4. (C)
5. (B)

## Suggested Reading

1. Arnaldi G, Angeli A, Atkinson AB, Bertagna X, Cavagnini F, Chrousos GP, et al. Diagnosis and complications of Cushing's syndrome: a consensus statement. J Clin Endocrinol Metab. 2003;88:5593–602.
2. Biller BM, Grossman AB, Stewart PM, Melmed S, Bertagna X, Bertherat J, et al. Treatment of adrenocorticotropin-dependent Cushing's syndrome: a consensus statement. J Clin Endocrinol Metab. 2008;93:2454–62.

3. Boscaro M, Arnaldi G. Approach to the patient with possible Cushing's syndrome. J Clin Endocrinol Metab. 2009;94:3121–31.

4. Colao A, De Block C, Gaztambide MS, Kumar S, Seufert J, Casanueva FF. Managing hyperglycemia in patients with Cushing's disease treated with pasireotide: medical expert recommendations. Pituitary. 2014;17(2):180–6.

5. Colao A, Petersenn S, Newell-Price J, Findling JW, Gu F, Maldonado M, et al. A 12-month phase 3 study of pasireotide in Cushing's disease. N Engl J Med. 2012;366:914–24.

6. Fleseriu M. Medical management of persistent and recurrent cushing disease. Neurosurg Clin N Am. 2012;23:653–68.

7. Fleseriu M, Biller BM, Findling JW, Molitch ME, Schteingart DE, Gross C. Mifepristone, a glucocorticoid receptor antagonist, produces clinical and metabolic benefits in patients with Cushing's syndrome. J Clin Endocrinol Metab. 2012;97:2039–49.

8. Fleseriu M, Petersenn S. Medical management of Cushing's disease: what is the future? Pituitary. 2012;15:330–41.

9. Guignat L, Bertherat J. The diagnosis of Cushing's syndrome: an Endocrine Society Clinical Practice Guideline: commentary from a European perspective. Eur J Endocrinol. 2010;163: 9–13.

10. Nieman LK, Biller BM, Findling JW, Newell-Price J, Savage MO, Stewart PM, et al. The diagnosis of Cushing's syndrome: an Endocrine Society Clinical Practice Guideline. J Clin Endocrinol Metab. 2008;93:1526–40.

# Chapter 4
# Idiopathic Granulomatous Hypophysitis Masquerading as a Pituitary Adenoma: Are There Reliable Diagnostic Criteria?

Christine G. Yedinak, Shirley McCartney, and Maria Fleseriu

## Objectives

- To review the clinical presentation of granulomatous hypophysitis (GrH) masquerading as a pituitary macroadenoma.
- To discuss the differential diagnosis of hypophysitis.
- To understand treatment options for GrH at initial presentation and recommendations for long-term management.

## Case Presentation

A 73-year-old Caucasian woman presented with a year-long history of hyponatremia of "unclear" origin. She had been diagnosed with syndrome of inappropriate antidiuretic hormone secretion (SIADH) based on sodium levels of 124–128 mmol/L on different occasions. She was treated initially with fluid restrictions for >10 months with no symptomatic improvement and persistence of chronic hyponatremia.

C.G. Yedinak, D.N.P. • S. McCartney, Ph.D.
Department of Neurological Surgery, Oregon Health & Science University,
3303 SW Bond Ave, Mail Code CH8N, Portland, OR 97239, USA
e-mail: yedinak@ohsu.edu; mccartns@ohsu.edu

M. Fleseriu, M.D. (✉)
Department of Medicine, Division of Endocrinology, Diabetes and Clinical Nutrition,
Oregon Health & Science University, 3181 SW Sam Jackson Park Road, Mail Code BTE28,
Portland, OR 97239, USA

Department of Neurological Surgery, Oregon Health & Science University,
3303 SW Bond Ave, Mail Code CH8N, Portland, OR 97239, USA

OHSU Northwest Pituitary Center, 3303 SW Bond Ave, Mail Code CH8N, Portland, OR 97239,
USA
e-mail: fleseriu@ohsu.edu

© Springer Science+Business Media New York 2015
T.F. Davies (ed.), *A Case-Based Guide to Clinical Endocrinology*,
DOI 10.1007/978-1-4939-2059-4_4

Other etiologies for hyponatremia were not entertained at that time. Following an Emergency Department (ED) presentation, she was found to be adrenally insufficient and started on prednisone at a dose of 5 mg daily. As per her medical record, hypothyroidism was "ruled out" during that admission based on a normal thyroid stimulating hormone (TSH) level. Medical history was otherwise significant for ulcerative colitis, basal cell carcinoma, familial essential tremor, and mitral valve prolapse.

Several weeks later, the patient again presented to the ED with a severe throbbing headache. There were no aggravating or relieving factors and the headache was not associated with vomiting, fever, or any other neurologic symptoms. During evaluation by a neurologist, brain computerized tomography (CT) was performed. This revealed a sellar mass, which was better delineated in a follow-up magnetic resonance (MR) imaging, showing a 1.2 cm sellar mass abutting the optic chiasm (Fig. 4.1) and diagnosed as a pituitary adenoma. She was referred to the Oregon Health & Science University, Northwest Pituitary Center, for surgery and endocrine work-up.

On review of symptoms she reported fatigue, nausea, which improved after starting steroids, brittle fingernails, edema in the legs, weakness in all extremities, memory deficits, sleep disturbances, and a history of chronic bronchitis with persistent shortness of breath.

Her family history was significant for heart disease in her mother, brother, aunt, uncles, and grandfather and tuberculosis in a great aunt.

In addition to treatment with prednisone daily at 5 mg (she was subsequently switched to hydrocortisone (HC) at a dose of 20 mg daily), medications included Azmacort, Nasonex, albuterol, a statin plus Zetia and niacin, Vivelle-Dot estrogen replacement, calcium, and multivitamins.

On physical exam she was normotensive, blood pressure was 136/69 mmHg, pulse 80, respirations 16, weight 156 lbs, and height 5'8". Head, ears, eyes, nose, and throat (HEENT) exam revealed a temporal visual field (VF) deficit in the right eye and a formal VF exam indicated right temporal field restriction (Fig. 4.2). The remainder of her HEENT exam was unremarkable with extraocular movements and cranial nerves grossly intact. Pituitary function testing was performed including cortrosyn stimulation testing for adrenal insufficiency (AI); after holding HC for 24 h, AI was confirmed (Table 4.1). A diagnosis of central hypothyroidism with low free T4 and inappropriately low TSH was evident and treatment with levothyroxine was initiated. Growth hormone (GH) deficiency was suspected based on low insulin growth factor-1 (IGF-1); prolactin (PRL) was low. Based on a presumed diagnosis of nonfunctioning pituitary adenoma, the patient underwent transsphenoidal surgery (TSS) for optic chiasm decompression. In retrospect, a few MR imaging features were possibly suggestive of hypophysitis such as mild stalk thickening, sellar mass with cystic areas, and a vague ring enhancement; these are not very specific and her atypical clinical presentation in addition to VF loss warranted optic chiasmal decompression and at least a biopsy for final diagnosis. Classic features of MR imaging in hypophysitis include the presence of a "dural tail" (enhanced tissue along the dura mater), the absence of mucosal thickening in the sphenoid sinus, isointensity with gray matter on T1-weighted images, and marked homogeneous or heterogeneous enhancement by gadolinium (Table 4.2).

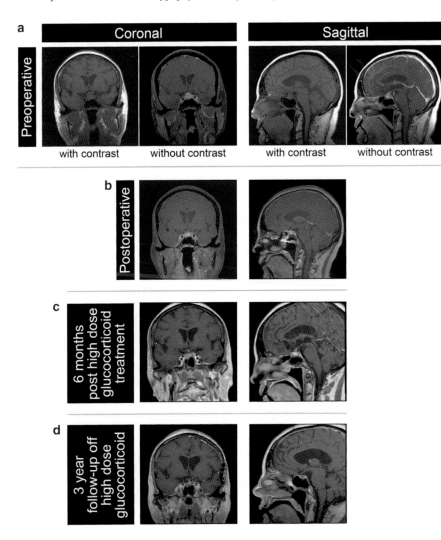

**Fig. 4.1** T1-weighted coronal and sagittal MR images show diffusive enlargement and enhancement of the pituitary gland. The gland pyramidal in shape extending to hypophyseal stalk from the sellar base. Images also note the presence of enhanced mucosa in the bilateral sphenoid sinus and enhanced meninges around the sella. Images: preoperative (**a**), postoperative (**b**), 6 months post-high-dose GC treatment (**c**), 3-year follow-up off high-dose GC (**d**)

## How Was the Diagnosis of Granulomatous Hypophysitis Made?

Pathology revealed necrotizing granulomas with giant cells and marked lympho-plasmacytic infiltration (Fig. 4.3). Rare acini of anterior pituitary parenchyma were also identified. Stains for microorganisms, bacilli, and fungi (Steiner, acid-fast bacilli, and Gomori methenamine silver) were negative and CD1a staining was also

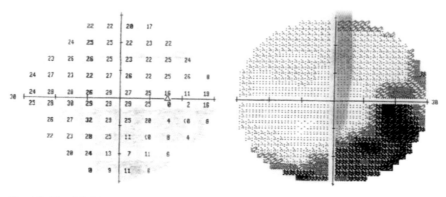

**Fig. 4.2** Visual field exam indicating right temporal field restriction

**Table 4.1** Results from laboratory test analysis

| Laboratory test (unit) | Reference range | Preoperative | 4 weeks postoperative |
|---|---|---|---|
| Glucose (mg/dL) | 65–110 | 115 | 52 |
| BUN (mg/dL) | 6–20 | 13 | 16 |
| Creatine (plasma mg/dL) | 0.6–1.1 | 0.9 | 1.2 |
| Total protein (g/dL) | 6.1–7.9 | | |
| Albumin (g/dL) | 3.5–4.7 | 4 | |
| Calcium (mg/dL) | 8.5–10.5 | 9.7 | 9.8 |
| Sodium (mmol/L) | 136–145 | 140 | 145 |
| Potassium (mmol/L) | 3.5–5.1 | 3.7 | 4.1 |
| Chloride (mmol/L) | 98–107 | 104 | 103 |
| Total $CO_2$ (mmol/L) | 23–29 | 23 | 29 |
| Alanine aminotransferase (U/L) | 13–48 | 64 | |
| Bilirubin (direct mg/dL) | Low: <0.4 | | |
| Adrenocorticotropic hormone (plasma pg/mL) | Low: <46 | <5 (L) | <5 (L) |
| Serum cortisol (total µg/dL) baseline | 5.0–23.0 µg/dL | <1 (L) | 1.2 |
| Serum cortisol (total µg/dL) post-stimulation | >18 µg/dL | 2.1 (L) | 3.0 |
| Prolactin (ng/mL) | 3–29 ng/mL | <1 | <1 |
| Lutenizing hormone (mIU/mL) | | <1 | |
| Thyroid stimulating hormone (µIU/mL) | 0.28–5.00 | 0.08 (L) | 0.010 (L) |
| Free T4 (ng/dL) | 0.7–1.8 | 0.4 (L) | 1.7 on replacement |
| Follicle stimulating hormone (mIU/mL) | | <1 | |
| IGF-1 | 64–188 ng/mL | 66 | 27 |

(L) = low

**Table 4.2** Imaging technique findings: lymphocytic hypophysitis vs. pituitary adenoma

| Imaging technique | Finding | Lymphocytic hypophysitis | Pituitary adenoma |
|---|---|---|---|
| Sellar X-ray | Sellar floor | – Intact<br>– Uniformly flat | – Not intact<br>– Unilateral depression |
| Pituitary MR | Pituitary | – Enlargement<br>– Symmetrical sovrasellar expansion | – Unilateral endosellar mass (microadenoma) or inhomogeneously expanding mass<br>– Asymmetrical sovrasellar extension |
| | Chiasm | – Compression<br>– Displacement | – No compression (microadenoma)<br>– No displacement (microadenoma) |
| | Stalk | – Thickened<br>– Not deviated | – Not thickened<br>– Contralateral deviation |
| After gadolinium | Pituitary mass enhancement | – Intense<br>– Homogeneous | – Slight, delayed<br>– Inhomogeneous (focal) |
| | "Dural tail" | – Appearance | – Lacking |
| | "Bright spot" of neurohypophysis | – Loss (if DI is associated) | – Persistence |

negative (Fig. 4.4). Reticulin staining revealed intact acinar structures, synaptophysin highlighted the native gland, and human GH was focally positive. Staining for PRL and adrenocorticotropic hormone (ACTH) was negative. There was no evidence of a tumor and no vasculitis was present in the specimen. In view of these findings, a diagnosis of granulomatous hypophysitis (GrH) with a component of lymphocytic hypophysitis (LH) was made.

Hypophysitis is classified into primary and secondary forms and further classified by histological appearance (Fig. 4.5). Primary hypophysitis can be autoimmune, granulomatous, necrotizing, or xanthomatous. It can also be secondary to local lesions such as germinomas, craniopharyngiomas, Rathke's Cleft cyst, and pituitary adenomas or secondary to systemic diseases. Recently, two other novel entities of hypophysitis have been described: drug-induced hypophysitis related to anti-CTLA-4 antibody therapy and hypophysitis due to IgG4-related disease. The incidence and prevalence of hypophysitis is unknown and population-based data are scarce.

Granulomatous hypophysitis is a rare entity (approximately 40 cases have been reported) and presents commonly with an enlargement of the pituitary gland, mimicking an adenoma. M. Simmonds, in 1917, first described four cases after review of pituitaries from 2,000 autopsies. Pathogenesis is unknown and males and females are affected equally. Diagnosis is made postoperatively by histopathology. Adrenal insufficiency has rarely been reported in GrH. On imaging, the gland is seen to be diffusely enlarged with a thickened stalk seen infrequently and not easily distinguishable from a pituitary adenoma on clinical/imaging data.

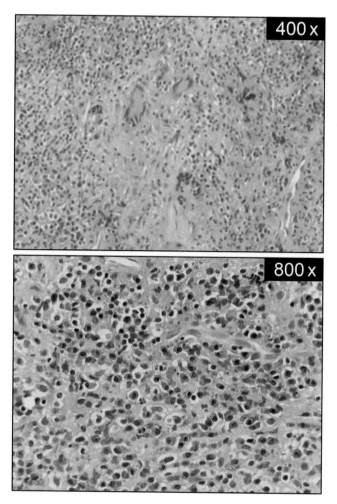

**Fig. 4.3** Hematoxylin and eosin stained biopsy sections showing focal replacement of pituitary architecture by a lymphocytic infiltrate (400× magnification), and non-caseating epithelioid cell granulomas with multinucleated giant cells (800× magnification), and areas of fibrosis

Clinical presentation in most cases often includes features such as headache, with fewer cases presenting as hypopituitarism. In the case we report, the patient presented with hypopituitarism with AI and hypothyroidism that was misinterpreted as SIADH for almost a year. Although AI was clinically apparent, during this time she was most likely also hypothyroid, which may have inadvertently prevented an adrenal crisis while she was not receiving glucocorticoid (GC) replacement therapy. Visual field defects, ophthalmoplegia, nausea and/or vomiting, diabetes insipidus, hyperprolactinemia, asthenia, and fatigue are also common presentations. It is notable that in hypophysitis, PRL may be high secondary to stalk involvement or conversely low. Undetectable PRL is indicative of long-term or permanent panhypopituitarism.

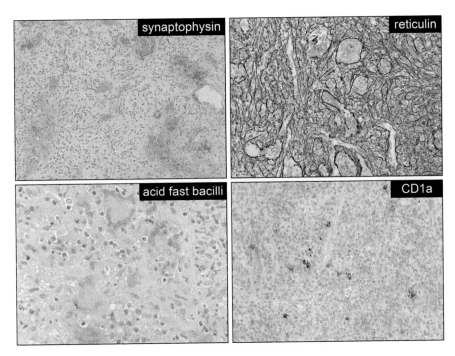

**Fig. 4.4** Immunochistochemistry: synaptophysin (positive) is the most reliable and best broad spectrum marker for neuroendocrine cells and reticulin shows intact pituitary acinar structures. Sections were negative for acid-fast bacilli and CD1a

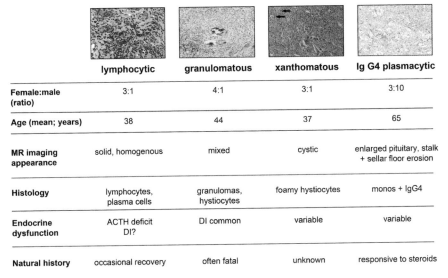

| | lymphocytic | granulomatous | xanthomatous | Ig G4 plasmacytic |
|---|---|---|---|---|
| **Female:male (ratio)** | 3:1 | 4:1 | 3:1 | 3:10 |
| **Age (mean; years)** | 38 | 44 | 37 | 65 |
| **MR imaging appearance** | solid, homogenous | mixed | cystic | enlarged pituitary, stalk + sellar floor erosion |
| **Histology** | lymphocytes, plasma cells | granulomas, hystiocytes | foamy hystiocytes | monos + IgG4 |
| **Endocrine dysfunction** | ACTH deficit DI? | DI common | variable | variable |
| **Natural history** | occasional recovery | often fatal | unknown | responsive to steroids |

**Fig. 4.5** Histological, demographic, MR imaging appearance, natural history, and endocrine dysfunction classification of hypophysitis

Necrotizing hypophysitis, as in the case we present, is the least common variant: it is unknown if this is a separate disease entity or a variant of other types of hypophysitis. Histologically, diffuse necrosis is found surrounded by dense infiltration with lymphocytes, plasma cells, and a few eosinophils with considerable fibrosis.

Lymphocytic hypophysitis is considered the most common of all the hypophysitis and was first described in a deceased female 14 months postpartum. Autopsy showed a diffusely infiltrated anterior pituitary, Hashimoto's thyroiditis, and atrophic adrenals. Only 18 % of cases have been reported in males with a large predominance (81 %) of cases being reported in women during late pregnancy or postpartum.

Clinically, LH, the most frequent type, and GrH are differentiated mainly by the temporal association of LH with peripartum. In LH, occasional spontaneous remission also occurs and an increased association with other autoimmune disease is described. However, LH and GrH can coexist and are possibly part of the same continuum with GrH ultimately progressing to LH.

Pituitary granulomas are rare specific lesions seen in sarcoidosis, tuberculosis, Langerhans histiocytosis (*Histiocytosis-X*), giant cell granulomatous hypophysitis, xanthomatous hypophysitis, and Wegener's granulomatosis or rarely in LH. Histologically, GrH is characterized by necrotizing granulomas that are formed by collection of histiocytes, multinucleated giant cell, and variable numbers of lymphocytes and plasma cells. In the case we present, both granulomatous and lymphocytic inflammation were evidenced by well-defined epitheloid granulomas, lymphocytic infiltration, and histiocytes on histopathological examination.

Sarcoidosis is known to involve the central nervous system in about 10 % of cases. Sellar involvement can be complicated by aseptic meningitis and cranial nerve palsies. In our patient, there was no evidence of neurosarcoidosis and angiotensin-converting enzyme (ACE) level was normal.

No other evidence of autoimmune disorders was found besides ulcerative colitis: anti-neutrophil cytoplasmic antibodies, lupus, thyroid peroxidase, and thyroglobulin antibodies were all negative, erythrocyte sedimentation rate was normal, and a chest X-ray was unremarkable. Wegener granulomatosis was not compatible either with negative antibodies and there was no reported vasculitis. Thus, a diagnosis of an idiopathic or primary GrH was made.

Preoperative diagnosis of GrH is rare and requires histologic confirmation. A careful evaluation of the clinical, biochemical, and radiological characteristics is imperative for accurate diagnosis and proper management to ensure optimal outcome. Acute presentations of pituitary-based pathology can include previously unrecognized but enlarging tumors, apoplectic hemorrhage and necrosis, and LH. GrH can have an insidious clinical presentation with the risk of unrecognized AI leading to misdiagnosis and possible catastrophic outcome.

This case illustrates that hypophysitis should not be ignored in the differential diagnosis when a pituitary mass presents with double vision associated with single oculomotorius or abducens nerve neuropathy, hypopituitarism with hyperprolactinemia, hypoprolactinemia, and/or meningitis-like symptoms.

# When Is Additional Treatment Postoperatively for GrH Needed?

Postoperatively, the patient reported resolution of right VF deficit and no symptoms or clinical evidence of DI or SIADH. Although DI is a frequent presentation in most cases of hypophysitis, the absence of DI does not exclude this diagnosis. Postoperative MR imaging showed optic chiasm decompression (Fig. 4.1). Formal VF was normal. She did have persistent AI and GCs were continued at replacement doses during a postoperative work-up for an etiology of GrH such as sarcoidosis and tuberculosis. However, she presented to the ED 4 weeks postoperatively with report of an acute deterioration and superior VF cuts with "graying vision" in her right eye, fatigue, and weakness. Imaging at the time indicated no change, but ophthalmologic exam indicated afferent pupillary defect and loss of color vision in the right eye but no VF deficit. She was treated with a prednisone burst of 60 mg daily tapering slowly over the following 2 months and maintained on prednisone 10 mg daily thereafter for a further 6 months. In the interim, she was also treated with Fosamax for osteoporosis prevention. After tapering to physiologic doses of GC, her VF remained normal, MR imaging remained unchanged, and her subjective visual symptoms improved.

# Recurrences Are Not Uncommon

After 24 months, she again experienced VF changes with acute diplopia, sixth nerve palsy, and new inferotemporal defect in the left eye on formal ophthalmolgic VF testing. The VF deficit resolved again with a second burst of high-dose prednisone for 6 months. MR imaging showed significant improvement after treatment, which persisted for 3 years (Fig. 4.1).

Recurrence has been documented in several cases of hypophysitis requiring further treatment. GrH has been unresponsive or only partially responsive to high-dose steroids in some cases. Conversely, visual changes resolved and mass size on MR images decreased in response to steroids at each event in our patient. Therefore, we consider a trial of high-dose steroids efficacious for the treatment of GrH. It is expected that panhypopituitarism would not resolve with this approach.

# Treatment

The natural history of inflammatory hypophysitis, including GrH, remains elusive and treatment is controversial. High-dose steroid therapy or anti-inflammatory and immunosuppressive (methotrexate, cyclosporine A, azathioprine) treatments have been reported with variable outcomes both as preoperative medical management and postoperative therapy.

Conservative management using clinical observation has also been advocated as the primary therapeutic option in hypophysitis variants other than GrH. Spontaneous remission has not been reported in cases of GrH. Transsphenoidal surgery is, however, both diagnostic and therapeutic and, therefore, should be performed in cases with progressive optic chiasmal compression, and when a definitive diagnosis is required for atypical presentation.

In this case, the patient required surgery to decompress the optic chiasm and surgical pathology elucidated the definitive diagnosis. Two separate prolonged courses of high-dose GC were fortunately successful in restoration of normal vision.

In conclusion, the diagnosis and treatment of hypophysitis for successful outcomes remains challenging, but is possible. Sophisticated imaging and histologic evaluation is required as well as skilled surgical excision. Symptomatic and ophthalmologic relief can be achieved with high-dose steroids, as in this patient, but is not successful in all cases. Close long-term follow-up and the timely initiation of appropriate treatment (repeat high-dose steroids, repeat surgery for optic chiasm decompression, and possibly radiation therapy) are required.

## Lessons Learned

- In the presence of hyponatremia, AI and hypothyroidism have to be ruled out before a diagnosis of SIADH is made. A normal TSH does not rule out central hypothyroidism.
- Not all sellar masses are pituitary adenomas. Despite the accuracy of current diagnostic tools, non-adenomatous lesions of the pituitary represent a challenge for the practicing physician.
- There are multiple forms of hypophysitis with variable anatomical and clinical presentations and precise diagnosis is challenging without biopsy, although this is not indicated in all cases. The incidence and prevalence of hypophysitis is unknown and population-based data are scarce.
- A pituitary lesion in a woman around the time of pregnancy, a rapidly progressive pituitary lesion, pituitary function that is discordant with the size of the lesion, and the presence of AI in the absence of other pituitary deficits are suggestive of a diagnosis of LH. Granulomatous hypophysitis is rarer, but should be considered in the differential diagnosis of a pituitary adenoma.
- New entities of hypophysitis (IgG-4 hypophysitis and drug-induced hypophysitis) have been discovered in relation to novel drug therapies and autoimmune diseases.
- Treatment goals include mass reduction, preservation of pituitary function, and replacement of pituitary deficits. High-dose GCs were effective in this case to reduce mass size and improve visual disturbances, but may need to be repeated. Fortunately, disease relapse was also responsive to GC therapy, but sometimes a multi-modal adjuvant treatment is needed.
- Long-term follow-up is mandatory to monitor for the development of other pituitary deficits and/or disease relapse.

## Questions

1. A 24-year-old female presents with new onset diabetes insipidus and was started on DDAVP. On further evaluation, she also has been found to have adrenal insufficiency. Pituitary function is otherwise normal. MRI shows significant stalk thickening. She has no significant past medical history and she delivered a healthy baby 3 months ago. Which is the most likely diagnosis in this young woman:

    (A) Lymphocytic hypophysitis
    (B) Pituitary adenoma
    (C) Granulomatous hypophysitis
    (D) Sarcoidosis

2. Pituitary lesions' characteristics on a dynamic MRI with gadolinium can establish with certitude a diagnosis of hypophysitis.

    (A) True
    (B) False

3. Which is the most common anterior pituitary dysfunction associated with hypophysitis?

    (A) Central hypothyroidism
    (B) Growth hormone deficiency
    (C) Adrenal insufficiency
    (D) Diabetes insipidus

4. Which of the following statements regarding therapy for hypophysitis is incorrect?

    (A) High-dose steroid therapy or anti-inflammatory and immunosuppressive (methotrexate, cyclosporine A, azathioprine) treatments have been used with variable outcomes in granulomatous hypophysitis
    (B) Conservative management using clinical observation has been advocated as the primary therapeutic option in lymphocytic hypophysitis
    (C) Spontaneous remission is very frequent in patients with granulomatous hypophysitis
    (D) Transsphenoidal surgery should be performed in cases with progressive optic chiasmal compression, and when a definitive diagnosis is required for atypical presentation

## Answers to Questions

1. (A)
2. (B)
3. (C)
4. (C)

# Suggested Reading

1. Bellastella A, Bizzarro A, Coronella C, Bellastella G, Sinisi AA, De Bellis A. Lymphocytic hypophysitis: a rare or underestimated disease? Eur J Endocrinol. 2003;149:363–76.
2. Carmichael JD. Update on the diagnosis and management of hypophysitis. Curr Opin Endocrinol Diabetes Obes. 2012;19:314–21.
3. Caturegli P, Newschaffer C, Olivi A, Pomper MG, Burger PC, Rose NR. Autoimmune hypophysitis. Endocr Rev. 2005;26:599–614.
4. Dillard T, Yedinak CG, Alumkal J, Fleseriu M. Anti-CTLA-4 antibody therapy associated autoimmune hypophysitis: serious immune related adverse events across a spectrum of cancer subtypes. Pituitary. 2010;13:29–38.
5. Freda PU, Beckers AM, Katznelson L, Molitch ME, Montori VM, Post KD, et al. Pituitary incidentaloma: an endocrine society clinical practice guideline. J Clin Endocrinol Metab. 2011;96:894–904.
6. Gutenberg A, Hans V, Puchner MJ, Kreutzer J, Bruck W, Caturegli P, et al. Primary hypophysitis: clinical-pathological correlations. Eur J Endocrinol. 2006;155:101–7.
7. Laws ER, Vance ML, Jane Jr JA. Hypophysitis. Pituitary. 2006;9:331–3.
8. Leporati P, Landek-Salgado MA, Lupi I, Chiovato L, Caturegli P. IgG4-related hypophysitis: a new addition to the hypophysitis spectrum. J Clin Endocrinol Metab. 2011;96:1971–80.
9. Leung GK, Lopes MB, Thorner MO, Vance ML, Laws Jr ER. Primary hypophysitis: a single-center experience in 16 cases. J Neurosurg. 2004;101:262–71.

# Part II
# Thyroid Overactivity

# Chapter 5
# Introduction

David S. Cooper

## Abbreviations

| | |
|---|---|
| ACTH | Adrenocorticotropic hormone |
| BMI | Body mass index |
| CRP | C-reactive protein |
| CT | Computed tomography |
| CTX | C-terminal telopeptide of type 1 collagen |
| ESR | Erythrocyte sedimentation rate |
| FDA | Food and Drug Administration |
| FSH | Follicle-stimulating hormone |
| FTI | Free thyroxine index |
| GH | Growth hormone |
| hCG | Human chorionic gonadotropin |
| IGF-1 | Insulin-like growth factor-1 |
| L5 | Lumbar vertebrae 5 |
| LH | Lutenizing hormone |
| MRI | Magnetic resonance imaging |
| PRL | Prolactin |
| RTH | Resistance to thyroid hormone |
| SHBG | Sex hormone binding globulin |
| SPECT | Single-photon emission computed tomography |
| T3 | Triiodothyronine |
| T4 | Thyroxine |
| TBG | Thyroxine-binding globulin |

D.S. Cooper, M.D. (✉)
Division of Endocrinology and Metabolism, The Johns Hopkins University School of Medicine, 1830 E. Monument St., Suite 333, Baltimore, MD, USA
e-mail: dscooper@jhmi.edu

© Springer Science+Business Media New York 2015
T.F. Davies (ed.), *A Case-Based Guide to Clinical Endocrinology*,
DOI 10.1007/978-1-4939-2059-4_5

TRH     Thyrotropin-releasing hormone
TSH     Thyroid-stimulating hormone
TSI     Thyroid stimulating immunoglobulin


## Introduction

Thyrotoxicosis is a syndrome caused by tissue exposure to excessive circulating amounts of thyroid hormone. Purists restrict the term "hyperthyroidism" to those disease entities in which the thyroid gland actively produces and secretes excessive hormones. They reserve the term "thyrotoxicosis" to refer generally to any condition in which an excessive amount of thyroid hormone is present, whether it is derived from excessive secretion by the gland (e.g., Graves' disease), from leakage from a damaged gland (e.g., various forms of thyroiditis), or is exogenous (e.g., iatrogenic or factitious thyrotoxicosis). However, many if not most clinicians use the terms "hyperthyroidism" and "thyrotoxicosis" interchangeably. In population based cross-sectional studies, hyperthyroidism is present in approximately 0.5–1 % of individuals. It is frequently "subclinical," meaning that thyroid hormone levels are within their reference ranges but circulating serum thyrotropin (TSH) is subnormal or undetectable.

As thyrotoxicosis is a syndrome, it has many potential etiologies. Graves' disease is the most common cause of hyperthyroidism in young and middle-aged people. It is caused by circulating antiTSH receptor antibodies (so-called thyroid-stimulating antibody or thyroid-stimulating immunoglobulin). Hyperthyroidism can also arise from autonomous function within the gland, due to activating mutations in the TSH receptor or the G protein signal transduction pathway. This produces solitary or multiple autonomously functioning thyroid nodules. The resulting "toxic multinodular goiter" is a common etiology of hyperthyroidism in older persons. Uncommon or rare causes of hyperthyroidism include ectopic thyroid tissue (struma ovarii), functioning metastases from follicular thyroid cancer, TSH secreting pituitary tumors, and hCG-mediated hyperthyroidism in patients with hyperemesis gravidarum or choriocarcinoma.

Thyrotoxicosis may develop due to destruction of thyroid follicles, leading to leakage of thyroid hormone into the bloodstream as part of the various forms of thyroiditis. These include subacute thyroiditis, a viral infection of the thyroid, "silent" thyroiditis, an autoimmune disease that has a predilection for the postpartum period, as well as thyroiditis associated with amiodarone administration.

Symptoms of thyrotoxicosis are well known to all clinicians and include palpitations, tremor, weight loss despite a normal caloric intake, anxiety, insomnia, heat sensitivity, muscle weakness, and irregular or absent menses in women. There is a relatively poor correlation between the symptoms of thyrotoxicosis and the degree of biochemical abnormality. For reasons that are not well understood, older patients may have few or no symptoms or signs of hyperthyroidism, but may present solely with atrial fibrillation or with unexplained weight loss. "Apathetic thyrotoxicosis" is a term that has been used to describe such elderly asymptomatic thyrotoxic patients.

Drugs are increasingly common causes of hyperthyroidism. Inorganic iodine can produce hyperthyroidism, especially in patients with an underlying nodular goiter (the Jod–Basedow phenomenon). Amiodarone is perhaps the most notorious cause of drug-induced thyrotoxicosis, occurring in 3–10 % of individuals exposed to the drug, depending on background iodine intake. Hyperthyroidism due to interferon alfa and other immune mediators is being recognized with greater frequency. Interestingly, all of these drugs (iodine, amiodarone, and interferon alfa) can also produce hypothyroidism depending on the patient and the presence of underlying thyroid disease.

The diagnosis of thyrotoxicosis rests with finding elevated levels of free thyroxine (T4) and/or total or free triiodothyronine (T3) in conjunction with a suppressed serum TSH level. In the very rare patients with TSH secreting tumors or resistance to thyroid hormone, the serum TSH will be inappropriately normal or elevated. Measurement of the 24-h radioiodine uptake may be helpful, as it is elevated in most conventional causes of hyperthyroidism, and low in thyroiditis of any cause and in cases of exogenous thyrotoxicosis. In struma ovarii, caused by ectopic thyroid tissue in an ovarian teratoma, the radioiodine uptake is low over the neck, but is elevated over the lesion in the pelvis.

The treatment of thyrotoxicosis depends on the underlying etiology, of course, but patient age, reproductive status, personal preferences, and a host of other factors go into making the final decision. In general, antithyroid drug therapy, radioiodine, and surgery are the "cornerstones" of treatment. Beta adrenergic blocking agents, glucocorticoids, lithium, potassium iodide, and other drugs may be used in special circumstances.

In the following section, three unusual cases of thyrotoxicosis will be discussed that illustrate some of the diagnostic and therapeutic difficulties that are often encountered in the clinic. First, a case of a man with a TSH-secreting pituitary tumor that went undiagnosed for over 15 years is presented, that only came to light when the patient presented in atrial flutter. Next, we present a woman with struma ovarii, who had persistent thyrotoxicosis after mistakenly undergoing a thyroidectomy. Finally, a patient with a mysterious form of thyrotoxicosis that perplexed two experienced endocrinologists is presented, that fortunately had a happy ending.

# Chapter 6
# TSH-Secreting Pituitary Adenoma

**Abdulrahman Alkabbani, Roberto Salvatori, and David S. Cooper**

## Objectives

TSH-producing pituitary adenoma is a rare cause of thyrotoxicosis, and the rarest of all types of secretory pituitary adenomas. We present a case of a 55-year-old man who, after 6 years of therapy for presumed hypothyroidism, was diagnosed with a TSH-producing pituitary adenoma. He was lost to follow-up after that, to present again with thyrotoxicosis and atrial flutter 10 years later. We review the presentation, evaluation, treatment, and differential diagnosis of TSH-producing adenomas.

## Case Presentation

A 55-year-old man presented to his local emergency department a month after the progressive worsening of palpitations, anxiety, insomnia, and heat intolerance.

Sixteen years prior to his current presentation, he started complaining of episodic paresthesias in his extremities. Thyroid function testing revealed an elevated TSH of 7.3 mIU/L (0.3–6) and a total T4 of 7.3 µg/dL (4.5–12.5). He was started on levothyroxine therapy, 75 mcg daily. Four weeks later, the dose was increased to 88 mcg daily because of a persistently elevated TSH (7.6 mIU/L) with normal total T4 (8.3 µg/dL). In the interim, while being investigated for multiple sclerosis, an MRI of the brain showed white matter changes in keeping with the diagnosis.

A. Alkabbani, M.D. • R. Salvatori, M.D.
Division of Endocrinology and Metabolism, Johns Hopkins Hospital, Baltimore, MD, USA

D.S. Cooper, M.D. (✉)
Division of Endocrinology and Metabolism, The Johns Hopkins University School of Medicine, 1830 E. Monument St., Suite 333, Baltimore, MD, USA
e-mail: dscooper@jhmi.edu

© Springer Science+Business Media New York 2015
T.F. Davies (ed.), *A Case-Based Guide to Clinical Endocrinology*,
DOI 10.1007/978-1-4939-2059-4_6

Incidentally, the pituitary gland showed "mild diffuse enlargement." The patient responded well to pulse glucocorticoid therapy, and 4 months later, he was referred by his neurologist to endocrinology for evaluation of hypothyroidism. He denied symptoms suggestive of hypothyroidism, and his clinical examination revealed a normal sized thyroid gland, but he was noted to be tachycardic (heart rate 100–120 beats per minute). Still on 88 mcg of levothyroxine, his laboratory tests showed a TSH 3.6 mIU/L, T4 9.9 µg/dL, and a free thyroxine index (FTI) of 3.9 (1–4.3), all within normal limits. Both antimicrosomal and antithyroglobulin antibody titers were negative so he was referred back to his primary care physician to continue the care of the presumed hypothyroidism. In addition, he continued to receive occasional glucocorticoid pulse therapy for multiple sclerosis flair-ups.

Five years later, his levothyroxine dose was increased to 100 mcg daily by his primary care physician because of an elevated TSH, 12.4 mIU/L, although his FT4 remained just below the upper limit of the normal range, 1.57 ng/dL (0.62–1.61). A month later, his dose was further increased to 112 mcg daily due to persistently elevated TSH. Two months later, his TSH was 13.2 mIU/L, and for the first time, his FT4 1.69 ng/dL, and FT3 4.40 pg/mL (2.3–4.2) were both elevated. This result prompted a pituitary MRI and another referral to endocrinology. The MRI showed a left-sided 12 mm pituitary macroadenoma, almost abutting the optic chiasm. He was clinically asymptomatic, but his thyroid showed asymmetric enlargement and he continued to be tachycardic. His endocrinologist discontinued the levothyroxine therapy and discussed the need for surgery to remove the presumed TSH-producing adenoma. The patient, however, was reluctant and decided to defer surgery, but then was lost to follow-up for 10 years.

At the current emergency department visit, he was found to be in atrial flutter with a heart rate of 140 beats per minute. Thyroid function tests showed a TSH of 15.7 mIU/L (0.4–4.5), free T4 of 2.8 ng/dL (0.8–1.8), and total T3 of 248 ng/dL (80–200).

The patient was admitted to the hospital, and started on propranolol and methimazole in addition to anticoagulation. Further tests showed prolactin 10.9 ng/mL (2–18), cortisol 23.8 µg/dL (4–22), ACTH 23 pg/mL (10–60), FSH 2.7 IU/L (1.0–18.0), LH 1.4 IU/L (1.8–8.6), IGF-1 126 ng/mL (50–317). Alpha subunit was 2.5 ng/mL (<0.5). An MRI of the pituitary showed a hypoenhancing sellar mass measuring 2.5 cm in the greatest dimension with mild left optic chiasmal displacement (Fig. 6.1).

Other evaluations during his hospitalization revealed evidence of cardiomyopathy that was attributed to chronic tachycardia, and he underwent a successful ablation procedure restoring sinus rhythm. He was discharged home on carvedilol 12.5 mg twice daily, methimazole 20 mg three times daily, ramipril 2.5 mg daily, zolpidem and alprazolam as needed.

One month later, he presented to the endocrinology clinic with a TSH of 7.5 mIU/L, FT4 1.7 ng/dL, and total T3 206 ng/dL. Total testosterone was 581 ng/dL (250–1,100) and free testosterone was 52.3 pg/mL (35–155). The methimazole dose was increased to 30 mg three times daily and he was referred to us for further management and surgical intervention.

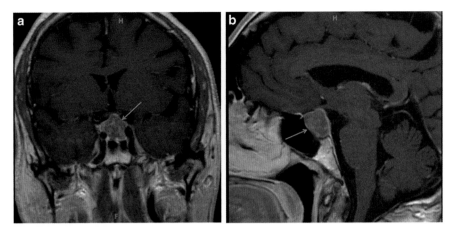

**Fig. 6.1** Pituitary macroadenoma (*arrows*) abutting the optic chiasm superiorly on contrast-enhanced coronal (**a**) and sagital (**b**) MRIs

On his first presentation to our center, the patient described improvement in his thyrotoxic symptoms after 2 months of treatment with methimazole and beta blockers. He denied headaches, peripheral vision disturbances, weight loss, tremors, excessive sweating, or hyperdefecation. He also denied polyuria and polydipsia, change in shoe or ring size, or coarsening of his facial features. His libido remained intact and he denied galactorrhea or gynecomastia.

His past history was significant for multiple sclerosis and psoriasis, in addition to the pituitary adenoma. He had no family history of pituitary disease, but there was suspicion of thyroid disease in his father.

On examination his blood pressure was 126/72, heart rate 80 beats per minute and in sinus rhythm, temperature 97.2 °C, and his weight was 200 pounds. There was no lid lag or exophthalmos. His thyroid gland was normal in size and there were no nodules. Chest was clear to auscultation. Cardiovascular exam showed normal first and second heart sounds with no murmurs. The abdominal exam was unremarkable. There was no peripheral edema or tremor. His cranial nerve exam was intact, along with normal power and reflexes in his extremities. Psoriatic lesions on the extensor surfaces of his lower extremities were noted but the skin examination was intact otherwise.

Laboratory studies performed at the time (2 months after his diagnosis and initiation of therapy) showed a TSH of 68.59 mIU/L with a free T4 of 0.5 ng/dL. A formal visual field exam was normal. His methimazole dose was cut from 90 mg/day to 40 mg/day, but TSH continued to rise, reaching >150 mIU/L with FT4 0.2 ng/dL 2 weeks later, so methimazole was stopped. A month off methimazole, TSH was 18 mIU/L, FT4 1.7 ng/dL, Total T3 214 ng/dL, and thus he was restarted on 10 mg daily. Two months later, TSH was 57.7 mIU/L and FT4 1.1 ng/dL. The patient underwent transsphenoidal adenomectomy and pathology confirmed a pituitary adenoma. The immunohistochemistry was negative for ACTH, but focally positive for GH and prolactin. TSH staining was not performed.

On the first day after surgery, his TSH fell to 6.47 mIU/L. One month after surgery, his TSH was 2.95 mIU/L, FT4 0.6 ng/dL, and total T3 58 ng/dL. Prolactin was 4.2 ng/dL and morning cortisol was 17.7 μg/dL. Two months after surgery, TSH was 2.0 mIU/L, FT4 1.1 ng/dL and total T3 83 ng/dL. Other pituitary axes were within normal limits, but his total testosterone was 204 ng/dL, and is currently being watched for possible spontaneous recovery.

## How the Diagnosis Was Made

The lack of suppressible TSH despite escalating levothyroxine therapy is certainly unusual in primary hypothyroidism. Nevertheless, the patient did not manifest frankly elevated thyroid hormone levels until a few years after his "hypothyroidism" diagnosis. This peculiar situation may be explained by the well described variation in the biological activity of the secreted TSH molecules, where despite being measurably elevated by TSH immunoassays, they may not have enough biological activity to produce high levels of thyroid hormones in vivo (see below). It is likely that as the tumor grew over time, it was able to produce more bioactive TSH, leading to frank elevation in thyroid hormones, which eventually lead to the correct diagnosis 6 years later. Retrospectively, his negative thyroid antibodies at the time of the "hypothyroidism" diagnosis are supportive of the hypothesis that he did not have primary hypothyroidism, but rather the elevated serum TSH levels due to the TSH-producing adenoma. Unfortunately, he was lost to follow-up for many years to later present with thyrotoxic symptoms and atrial flutter.

At the time of his latest presentation, both serum TSH and thyroid hormone levels were elevated suggesting secondary hyperthyroidism. With the elevated alpha subunit and the MRI evidence of an enlarging macroadenoma, it was clear that this was a TSH-producing adenoma.

An important and characteristic feature of adenoma thyrotrophs is their relative insensitivity to the negative feedback of thyroid hormones, leading to the hypersecretion of TSH despite the hyperthyroidism that was seen in this case. However, there is still integrity of the negative feedback of thyroid hormone, evidenced by the sharp rise of serum TSH levels when the patient was rendered hypothyroid on high-dose methimazole therapy.

## Lessons Learned

TSH-secreting pituitary adenomas are considered the least common of all types of pituitary adenomas, accounting for 0.6–1.5 % of them. Thyrotrophs, which represent 5 % of adenohypophyseal cells, originate from the same common progenitor cell that expresses Pit-1 transcription factor along with somatotrophs (growth hormone-secreting cells) and lactotrophs (prolactin-secreting cells). Therefore, TSH-producing adenomas cosecreting GH or PRL are seen in up to one fourth of patients [1].

The majority (75 %) of TSH-producing adenomas are macroadenomas (measuring >10 mm) at the time of diagnosis, with no gender difference. The mean age at presentation is 45 years, with a wide age range (8–84). Those tumors are almost always benign but can be locally invasive, especially in patients with non-intact thyroid glands [2].

Patients typically present with overt thyrotoxicosis and diffuse goiters mimicking Graves' disease, while others present with manifestations of a mass effect related to the pituitary tumor, resulting in headaches, visual field compromise, and/or loss of other anterior pituitary functions. In most patients, thyrotoxic symptoms are mild to moderate in severity [1]. Severe cardiovascular symptoms like atrial fibrillation or decompensated heart failure are less commonly reported compared to primary thyrotoxicosis. Nevertheless, similar to our patient, atrial fibrillation had been reported as the presenting symptom [3].

In most patients, a latency of a few years separates the onset of thyrotoxic symptoms from the establishment of the correct diagnosis; $6 \pm 2$ years in patients with intact thyroid glands, and $12 \pm 3$ years in patients who underwent unnecessary thyroidectomy or radioactive iodine ablation due to the erroneous diagnosis of Graves' disease [4]. This latency seems to be shorter ($4 \pm 6$ years) in more recent large series [5]. About one-third of patients with TSH-producing adenoma undergo unnecessary thyroidectomy or thyroid ablation due to misdiagnosis [6].

On clinical examination, up to 93 % of patients have diffuse or multinodular goiters due to chronic thyrotropin stimulation [1]. Other features of Graves' disease like exophthalmos, pretibial myxedema, and positive antithyroid autoantibodies are absent. Nevertheless, cases of TSH-producing adenomas in patients with autoimmune thyroid disease including Graves' disease and Hashimoto's thyroiditis have been reported, with the clue to diagnosis of the latter being the lack of suppressibility of serum TSH by escalating thyroxine hormone replacement doses [7].

Laboratory investigations in patients with TSH-producing adenomas typically show elevated thyroid hormone levels with elevated, inappropriately normal, or incompletely suppressed TSH level (range from 0.4 to 393 mIU/L) [2]. This wide range of serum TSH levels despite frankly elevated thyroid hormone levels has been attributed to variations of the biologic activity of the secreted TSH molecules. It is important to stress that about 30 % of patients with TSH-producing adenomas present with serum TSH level in the normal range, which highlights the importance of measuring serum FT4 level in all patients with suspected thyrotoxicosis (and all patients with known pituitary disease).

The picture can be less obvious in patients previously treated with thyroid radioablation or thyroidectomy, since they do not have elevated serum thyroid hormone levels. In such patients, TSH levels tend to be much higher than in patients with intact thyroid glands. This observation highlights a peculiar feature of the tumoral thyrotrophs: that they are relatively resistant to the suppressive effect of elevated thyroxine, but retain sensitivity to the lack of thyroid hormones.

Most TSH-secreting adenomas produce high levels of alpha-subunit and an alpha-subunit/TSH molar ratio greater than 1 is described in about 82 % of cases. This is not true, however, for microadenomas where normal serum levels of alpha-subunit is the rule [5]. Elevated alpha-subunit levels should be interpreted with care in post-menopausal women or men with primary hypogonadism, given that alpha-subunit levels are higher in these circumstances.

Several dynamic tests have been used to distinguish TSH-producing adenomas from other potential diagnoses, particularly in patients whose imaging studies are not revealing or those who present with microadenomas. Most TSH-producing adenomas (about 80 %) do not respond to intravenous TRH stimulation by doubling the basal serum level of TSH. In addition, the T3 suppression test fails to suppress serum TSH levels in patients with TSH-producing adenomas after 10 days of receiving high doses of T3, typically 80–100 mcg/day [6]. TRH is not available in the USA, and T3 suppression testing in patients with history of coronary artery disease or tachyarrhythmia is contraindicated.

MRI with gadolinium is the most commonly used imaging modality for diagnosis. Most TSH-producing tumors are macroadenomas, and in two-thirds of patients, the tumor invades the surrounding structures, including the cavernous sinuses, or extends superiorly compressing the optic chiasm [6].

Once the diagnosis is established, treatment is directed towards restoring euthyroid state and eliminating the local mass effects of the pituitary tumor. Surgical resection via transsphenoidal or transcranial approach is the mainstay of therapy. "Cooling off" the thyrotoxic state preoperatively is required in symptomatic patients, using beta blockers, antithyroid medications, or somatostatin analogs.

Because of the invasive nature of these tumors, and the fact that most are macroadenomas at the time of diagnosis, complete surgical resection may not always be possible. Medical therapy plays an important role in these situations. Surgical cure rates vary widely depending on criteria used to define cure, and the percentage of macro- and microadenomas in each series. Those criteria include reestablishment the euthyroid state, achievement of undetectable TSH 1 week after surgery, normalization of alpha-subunit or the alpha-subunit/TSH molar ratio, or suppression of serum TSH following T3 administration [4]. Post-operative evaluation for partial or complete hypopituitarism is essential.

Due to the expression of somatostatin receptors in TSH-producing adenomas, the preferred medical therapy is treatment with long-acting somatostatin analogs like octreotide or lanreotide. These agents have been shown to reduce serum TSH and alpha-subunit levels in almost all cases, in addition to shrinking tumor size. They are typically used in patients not cured by pituitary surgery, or those who are awaiting the effect of radiation therapy. Primary therapy with somatostatin analogs is restricted to specific situations only, as when surgery is contraindicated. Dopamine agonists have also been used, especially in mixed TSH/prolactin secreting tumors [8]. Radiotherapy, conventional fractionated or gamma knife, is indicated when surgery is contraindicated, as an adjuvant to surgery when remission is not achieved after surgery, or in rare cases of resistance to medical therapy.

Due to the rarity of this condition compared to primary thyrotoxicosis, it is not uncommon for some patients presenting with diffuse goiter and overt thyrotoxicosis to be misdiagnosed as having Graves' disease, and many undergo radioactive iodine ablation or thyroidectomy before the correct diagnosis is eventually made. The importance of recognizing this pitfall is the deleterious effect shown in some studies, where thyroid ablation or resection may change the behavior of the adenoma into a more aggressive tumor with a tendency for local invasion [2]. This is similar to the development of Nelson's syndrome following bilateral adrenalectomy to treat Cushing's disease.

## Differential Diagnosis

1. Graves' disease: with the highly sensitive TSH immunoassays used nowadays, it is easier to distinguish Graves' disease from a TSH-producing adenoma, since serum TSH levels as low as 0.4 mIU/L have been reported in cases of TSH-producing adenoma (TSH-oma), which would have been below the detection level of older TSH assays. Therefore, the lack of complete suppression of TSH when thyroid hormones are elevated should be an important clue to differentiating Graves' disease from a TSH-producing adenoma.
2. Resistance to thyroid hormone (RTH): Differentiating TSH-omas from resistance to thyroid hormone can be challenging, as both can present with elevated serum TSH and free thyroid hormone levels [9]. Key differences are that RTH is often a familial condition, is not associated with an elevated alpha-subunit, and peripheral markers of elevated thyroid hormone, such as sex hormone-binding globulin (SHBG) and carboxy-terminal collagen crosslinks (CTX), are not elevated. Dynamic testing with TRH stimulation or T3 suppression lead to elevation and suppression of serum TSH, respectively, in the case of RTH, but not TSH-omas. Finally, RTH is not associated with pituitary adenomas, but pituitary incidentalomas are not an uncommon finding in the general population, making such imaging findings nondefinitive.
3. Euthyroid hyperthyroxinemia: Elevated thyroxine-binding globulin (TBG) levels (e.g., due to pregnancy, estrogen therapy or liver disease) can cause elevation of total thyroid hormone levels. Serum TSH is typically normal in these cases, and normal free thyroid hormone levels are the key to establishing the diagnosis. Other conditions that increase protein binding, such as that seen in familial dysalbuminemic hyperthyroxinemia, can lead to a similar picture although in that case, the free T4 can be artifactually elevated, leading to further diagnostic confusion.

## Questions

1. A 45-year-old woman with history of Graves' disease with documented post ablative hypothyroidism is well controlled on L-thyroxine. She was noted to have elevated TSH despite escalating her L-thyroxine dose, which ultimately lead to symptomatic hyperthyroxinemia. Further testing revealed an elevated level of alpha-subunit but her pituitary MRI showed a normal gland. T3 suppression test was negative (TSH failed to suppress).

What is the most likely diagnosis?

A. Resistance to thyroid hormone
B. Ectopic TSH-producing adenoma
C. Poor compliance to L-thyroxine
D. Hashimoto's thyroiditis

2. A 50-year-old man developed palpitations, sweating, and weight loss. On examination, he appeared to be anxious and had a diffuse goiter. Laboratory tests showed TSH: 0.4 mIU/L (0.5–5), FT4: 2.8 ng/dL (0.8–1.7). Family history was positive for autoimmune thyroid disease. A diagnosis of Graves' disease was made and he underwent radioiodine therapy. Two months later he developed hypothyroidism, and was started on L-thyroxine therapy, and was lost to follow up. Nine months later, he presented with bitemporal visual field defects, and an urgent MRI revealed a large 4 cm pituitary macroadenoma invading the cavernous sinuses and compressing the optic chiasm.

What is the likely etiology that explains the aggressive behavior of his tumor?

A. Pituitary carcinoma
B. Craniopharyngioma
C. TSH-producing adenoma
D. TSH/GH-producing adenoma

3. A 60-year-old man with coronary artery disease presents with tachycardia. His TSH and FT4 were found to be elevated. A pituitary MRI showed a microadenoma. Alpha-subunit level was normal.

What is the best test to distinguish a TSH-producing adenoma from thyroid hormone resistance syndrome?

A. Total T3
B. T3 suppression test
C. SHBG

## Answers to Questions

1. B: Resistance to thyroid hormone is not associated with an elevated alpha-subunit level. In addition, T3 suppression testing results in suppression of serum TSH level in patients with resistance to thyroid hormone, but not in TSH-omas, thus answer A is incorrect. Poor compliance to L-thyroxine and Hashimoto's thyroiditis are also not associated with elevated level of alpha-subunit and should respond to a T3 suppression test, therefore answers C and D are incorrect. Finally, since the biochemical picture is suggestive of a TSH-producing adenoma but no tumor was identified on the pituitary MRI, one must think of an ectopic pituitary tumor and look for it in its most common location, the pharynx.

The reason behind that is that the pituitary gland develops embryologically from Rathke's pouch which originates from the primitive oral cavity. Ectopic TSH-producing adenomas have been reported with masses discovered in the nasopharynx.

2. C: The clue to the correct diagnosis in this case is the lack of complete suppression of TSH when thyroid hormones are elevated. This is never seen in primary hyperthyroidism and should raise the suspicion of a secondary cause of the patient's hyperthyroidism. Unfortunately, the patient was incorrectly diagnosed with Graves' disease and underwent radioiodine therapy. The resultant primary hypothyroidism is known to alter the behavior of TSH-producing adenomas causing them to behave more aggressively with marked elevation of serum TSH levels and local tumor invasion, as a result of the lack of the negative feedback of thyroid hormones. Answer C is correct. There is no distant metastasis to suggest a pituitary carcinoma in this patient, thus answer A is incorrect. Craniopharyngioma can cause secondary hypothyroidism with low TSH, but that is associated with low FT4 as well, thus answer B is incorrect. Finally, there is no evidence to suggest that plurihormonal tumors cosecreting TSH and GH are more aggressive that tumors that secrete TSH alone, therefore answer D is incorrect.

3. C: The T3 suppression test can help distinguish RTH from TSH-omas but administering high levels of T3 over 10 days can be risky in patients with coronary artery disease, thus answer B is incorrect. Total T3 does not help discrimiate the two diagnoses from each other, thus answer A is not correct. SHBG is a peripheral marker of elevated thyroid hormone actions, and thus is high in TSH-omas but not in RTH, therefore answer C is correct. Tachycardia has no discriminating value as it could be a manifestation of hyperthyroidism secondary to TSH-omas, or a finding in generalized RTH, as it is mediated by the thyroxine receptor alpha (TRα) isoform in the heart, which is not affected by the TRβ mutations that characterize RTH. Finally, it is important to note that alpha-subunit is usually normal in TSH-producing microadenomas, but elevated in macroadenomas.

# References

1. Beck-Peccoz P, Persani L, Mannavola D, Campi I. Pituitary tumours: TSH-secreting adenomas. Best Pract Res Clin Endocrinol Metab. 2009;23:597–606.
2. Rouach V, Greenman Y. Thyrotropin-secreting pituitary tumors. In: Melmed S, editor. The pituitary. Burlington: Academic Press; 2011. p. 619–36.
3. George JT, Thow JC, Matthews B, Pye MP, Jayagopal V. Atrial fibrillation associated with a thyroid stimulating hormone-secreting adenoma of the pituitary gland leading to a presentation of acute cardiac decompensation: a case report. J Med Case Rep. 2008;2:67.
4. Brucker-Davis F, Oldfield EH, Skarulis MC, Doppman JL, Weintraub BD. Thyrotropin-secreting pituitary tumors: diagnostic criteria, thyroid hormone sensitivity, and treatment outcome in 25 patients followed at the national institutes of health. J Clin Endocrinol Metab. 1999;84:476–86.
5. Socin HV, Chanson P, Delemer B, et al. The changing spectrum of TSH-secreting pituitary adenomas: diagnosis and management in 43 patients. Eur J Endocrinol. 2003;148:433–42.

6. Beck-Peccoz P, Brucker-Davis F, Persani L, Smallridge RC, Weintraub BD. Thyrotropin-secreting pituitary tumors. Endocr Rev. 1996;17:610–38.
7. Losa M, Mortini P, Minelli R, Giovanelli M. Coexistence of TSH-secreting pituitary adenoma and autoimmune hypothyroidism. J Endocrinol Invest. 2006;29:555–9.
8. Colao A, Pivonello R, Di Somma C, Savastano S, Grasso LF, Lombardi G. Medical therapy of pituitary adenomas: effects on tumor shrinkage. Rev Endocr Metab Disord. 2009;10:111–23.
9. Dumitrescu AM, Refetoff S. The syndromes of reduced sensitivity to thyroid hormone. Biochim Biophys Acta. 2013;1830(7):3987–4003.

# Chapter 7
# Struma Ovarii

**Sherley Abraham and David S. Cooper**

## Objectives

Struma ovarii is a rare cause of hyperthyroidism. We report a case of a 52-year-old woman with the typical signs and symptoms of hyperthyroidism, in whom the diagnosis of struma ovarii was missed. We discuss the approaches leading to the correct diagnosis and we review the management of the disease.

## Case Presentation

A 52-year-old secretary presented to our Center for evaluation of persistent hyperthyroidism despite having had a total thyroidectomy. Two years earlier she went to a new primary care physician and was noted to have slightly depressed TSH of 0.27 mU/l, but denied any specific symptoms of thyrotoxicosis. She was evaluated by an Endocrinologist and underwent a 24-h radioiodine uptake and scan which showed symmetric low uptake over the thyroid with 1 % uptake in 24 h (normal 10–35 %). She was initially treated with Methimazole which she did not tolerate due to gastrointestinal symptoms. She was switched to Propylthiouracil and reported similar side effects. She had a history of coronary artery disease with stent placements, and her medical regimen included beta blockers. Due to a history of sialadenitis, she did not pursue radioiodine treatment.

S. Abraham, M.D.
Division of Endocrinology and Metabolism, The Johns Hopkins University School of Medicine, Baltimore, MD, USA

D.S. Cooper, M.D. (✉)
Division of Endocrinology and Metabolism, The Johns Hopkins University School of Medicine, 1830 E. Monument St., Suite 333, Baltimore, MD, USA
e-mail: dscooper@jhmi.edu

© Springer Science+Business Media New York 2015
T.F. Davies (ed.), *A Case-Based Guide to Clinical Endocrinology*,
DOI 10.1007/978-1-4939-2059-4_7

She underwent total thyroidectomy and final pathology showed chronic thyroid-itis with focal nodular hyperplasia and focal Hurthle cell change. Postoperatively, she was placed on thyroxine 75 mcg daily. After 3 weeks, her serum TSH was <0.02 mU/l and a free T4 was 1.99 ng/dl. The dose of thyroxine was reduced to 50 mcg daily, but her serum TSH remained suppressed, and the patient reported symptoms of insomnia, nausea, diarrhea, and irritability. The thyroxine was subse-quently discontinued. Four months after the total thyroidectomy, on no thyroid hor-mone replacement, laboratory testing showed a serum TSH of 0.02 mU/l (0.34–5.6), a Free T4 of 2.0 ng/dl (0.6–1.12), and a Total T3 of 237 ng/ml (60–181). A thyroid ultrasound showed no identifiable thyroid tissue and no lymphadenopathy.

The patient was then evaluated at our Center 5 months after surgery and reported that if she was late in taking her dose of beta blocker, she experienced palpitations, but denied any other symptoms of thyroid hormone excess. She denied any anterior neck symptoms and denied visual complaints. Her family history included a mater-nal aunt with Graves' disease with eye involvement, treated with radioactive iodine. Medications included metoprolol, atorvastatin, fenofibrate, aspirin, and a multivita-min. Physical examination showed a blood pressure 141/69 mmHg, a pulse of 74 beats per minute and regular, height 67 in., weight 276 pounds, temperature 97.3 °F. Neck exam showed a midline thyroidectomy scar that was well healed with no palpable thyroid tissue and no cervical lymphadenopathy. Her laboratory evalu-ation showed a serum TSH of <0.02 mU/l, a Free T4 of 2.1 ng/dl (0.7–1.8), a Total T3 of 183 ng/dl, Thyroid Stimulating Immunoglobulin (TSI) 28 % (<140), Thyroglobulin 264 ng/ml (1.1–35). She was restarted on low divided dose methima-zole 5 mg twice a day because of her prior gastrointestinal symptoms, and the beta blocker was continued.

She underwent an I-123 Whole Body Scan with SPECT/CT imaging, which showed intense iodine uptake within the pelvis from an irregular lobulated mass in the region of the uterus, measuring approximately $12 \times 10 \times 10$ cm. There was no evidence of radiotracer uptake in the region of the thyroid bed or along the expected course of an ectopic lingual or mediastinal thyroid (Fig. 7.1). She underwent a pel-vic MRI, which showed heterogeneous mass measuring $11.0 \times 10.6 \times 8.8$ cm, that was cystic and solid enhancing septations and fat, consistent with a teratoma broadly abutting the uterus and the rectum, with significant mass effect. The mass was thought to be of left ovarian origin as there was only visualization of the right ovary, and there was significant vascular supply and drainage from left ovarian vessels. There was also effacement of the fat plane between uterus and the mass, suspicious enhancing bone lesions in the left sacrum and L5, and prominent bilateral external iliac and right pelvic lymph nodes (Fig. 7.2).

She was referred to the Gynecologic Oncology Clinic, and the methimazole dose was titrated until the free T4 and total T3 were within the normal range. Five months after her presentation, she underwent exploratory laparotomy, total abdominal hysterectomy, bilateral salpingo-oophorectomy, right and left pelvic node sampling. The surgical pathology showed a 13 cm struma ovarii (Figs. 7.3 and 7.4). The lesion was proliferative, with follicular crowding and nuclear atypia, which are indetermi-nate microscopic features, but insufficient to establish a diagnosis of carcinoma.

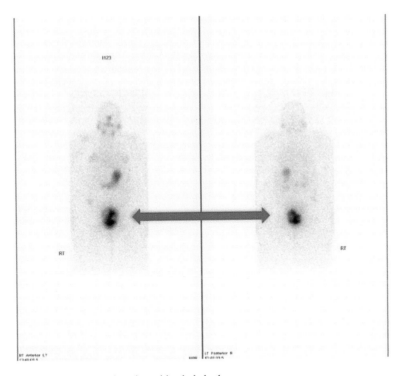

**Fig. 7.1** Radioiodine I-123 imaging with whole body scan

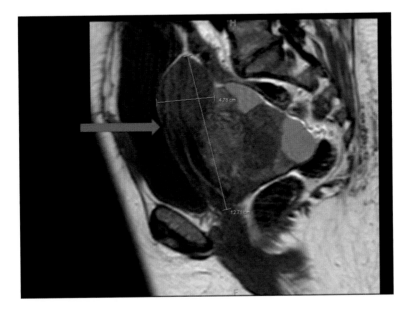

**Fig. 7.2** MRI of pelvic mass

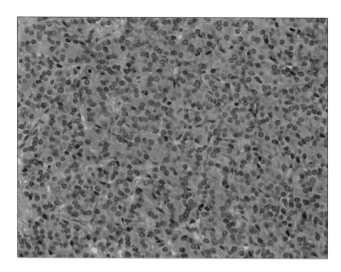

**Fig. 7.3** Ovarian tumor containing thyroid tissue as the predominant cell type, which typically occurs as part of a teratoma

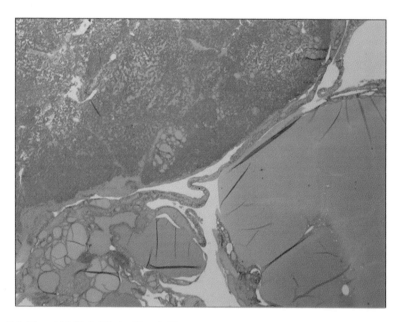

**Fig. 7.4** Thyroid follicle filled with colloid

Three lymph nodes were negative for tumor. Postoperatively, the patient was placed on thyroxine, which was titrated to a dose of 125 mcg×7.5 tablets per week. Her laboratory tests showed an undetectable serum thyroglobulin level while on this replacement dose. Four months after surgery, she underwent Thyrogen-stimulated testing which showed a thyroglobulin of 0.9 ng/ml, and a whole body scan showed two foci of increased radiotracer localization within the thyroid bed, compatible with residual thyroid tissue. There was no evidence of uptake in the extrathyroidal neck or at distant sites, and no evidence of uptake within the pelvis outside the bladder.

## Background

"Struma" is the Latin term for a "swelling in the neck," and struma ovarii was first described in 1895 by Vol Kalden [1]. It is a rare ovarian tumor defined by the presence of thyroid tissue as a major cellular component, and most commonly occurs as part of a teratoma. In a pathologic study from two major academic centers, out of 1,390 ovarian tumors, 167 were teratomas [2]. Less than 1 % contained foci of thyroid tissue or were struma ovarii. Struma ovarii is most commonly diagnosed between the ages of 40 and 60 years [3]. Pathologically, the thyroid epithelium in the teratoma may be organized in a solid, embryonal or pseudotubular pattern, rather than forming thyroid follicles, and thyroglobulin staining may be required to identify the cells as thyroidal in origin [3].

The clinical presentation may include symptoms ranging from thyrotoxic complaints, a pelvic mass, or ascites [4]. If there is autonomous production of thyroid hormone by the struma ovarii, this would lead to TSH suppression and absence of function by the normal thyroid gland [2]. The diagnosis may be suspected in a woman with hyperthyroidism who has no goiter and minimal or absent thyroidal uptake of radioiodine. In such cases, the far more likely causes remain exogenous thyroid hormone use and various forms of thyroiditis. The diagnosis is made, as in our case, by radioiodine imaging of the pelvis. Rarely, women with struma ovarii and hyperthyroidism also have a goiter, which may be due the coexistence of Graves' disease and struma ovarii, in which thyroid-stimulating immunoglobulins stimulate the thyroid tissue in the ovary as well as the neck, or the presence of toxic nodular goiter, in which there is also radioiodine uptake over the ovary and the neck [5].

An antithyroid drug, preferably methimazole, is given for 4–6 weeks prior to surgery, depending on the severity of the thyrotoxicosis and underlying risk factors (older age, underlying cardiovascular disease, etc.). As in this case, beta blocking drugs may also be used for symptomatic relief and for heart rate control. In cases of benign struma ovarii causing hyperthyroidism, after resection, the cervical thyroid gland that was previously suppressed may resume normal function [2].

Surgical removal is the treatment for struma ovarii, even in a patient with coexisting Graves' disease or toxic nodular goiter, due to the risk of carcinoma. The pathologic criteria for carcinoma in struma ovarii include tumor invasion, metastases, or recurrence, or the typical cytopathologic features of papillary thyroid cancer. A pathologic study evaluated 54 patients with ovarian tumors due to struma ovarii and 13 (24 %) were found to be carcinomas, 11 with features of papillary carcinoma and 2 with features of follicular carcinoma [6]. Cancer is more likely in larger tumors and was present in 75 % of tumors >16 cm, and rarely in tumors <5 cm [6].

In cases of malignant struma ovarii, there is no standard treatment protocol. Generally, treatment includes oophorectomy and total thyroidectomy. Following surgery, a radioiodine scan is performed, after Thyrogen stimulation or thyroxine withdrawal, although there has been no consensus recommendation. If there is abnormal radioiodine uptake in the abdomen or possible metastases, high-dose radioiodine is administered [3, 7–9].

The follow-up involves monitoring for recurrence, including radioiodine whole body scan and at least 10 years of surveillance with serum thyroglobulin [3, 7–9]. An increase in serum thyroglobulin may prompt a repeat radioiodine scan [3]. Aside from recurrences of malignant struma ovarii in the abdomen, there have also been reports of recurrences at distant sites, including the bones, brain, and lung [8]. After surgical resection of the struma ovarii and total thyroidectomy, patients will require lifelong thyroxine replacement. The dose should be titrated to a goal TSH in the low normal to slightly suppressed range, although no specific cutoffs have been established [7].

The overall prognosis for benign struma is excellent. In malignant cases, surgery and I-131 treatment is often curative. The clinical behavior of thyroid-type lesions arising in struma ovarii cannot necessarily be predicted on the basis of microscopic features. Highly differentiated proliferations lacking fully developed features of carcinoma can recur. Smaller lesions qualifying for a diagnosis of carcinoma based on histologic criteria used for thyroid gland tumors can demonstrate clinically benign behavior and not recur [10]. If recurrences are detected, repeat radioiodine ablation may be indicated. In a pathologic study of 88 patients with malignant struma ovarii, the clinical factors associated with recurrence or extraovarian spread included adhesions, peritoneal fluid >1 l, ovarian tissue on membrane surfaces, papillary histology, or a struma component ≥12 cm [11]. The overall survival rate in this study was 89 % at 10 years, and 84 % at 25 years [11].

## How the Diagnosis Was Made

This patient demonstrated clinical symptoms and laboratory evidence of persistent hyperthyroidism 4 months after total thyroidectomy, while she was off any known thyroxine supplementation. In this case, the elevated thyroglobulin level indicated that the hyperthyroidism was caused by an endogenous source, which was ectopic thyroid tissue. The radioiodine whole body scan revealed increased radiotracer localization in the pelvis. This was further evaluated by MRI, which characterized the pelvic mass. Surgical resection was indicated as there is a risk for malignancy, and the final pathology confirmed benign struma ovarii.

## Lessons Learned

- Struma Ovarii can present with the typical symptoms of hyperthyroidism, and a radioiodine whole body scan may help localize abnormal uptake in the body.
- Prior to surgical treatment, hyperthyroidism from struma ovarii may be treated with antithyroid drugs and beta blockers.
- Patients may undergo unilateral oophorectomy, or hysterectomy and bilateral salpingo-oopherectomy if there is concern about malignancy
- If thyroid cancer is present, radioiodine treatment may be used after the thyroid has also been removed.
- Monitoring includes serum thyroglobulin testing and radioiodine whole body scanning.

## Questions

1. What is the most likely reason for thyrotoxicosis in a patient without a goiter and low uptake on radioiodine imaging?

   A. Thyroiditis
   B. Thyroxine intake
   C. Ectopic thyroid tissue in neck
   D. Struma Ovarii
   E. A or B

2. After thyroidectomy, which laboratory test is the most useful in determining thyrotoxicosis from endogenous thyroid tissue versus exogenous thyroxine intake?

   A. Thyroglobulin
   B. TSH
   C. Free T4
   D. Thyroid-stimulating immunoglobulin (TSI)

3. Which imaging study would be most helpful in locating ectopic thyroid tissue?

   A. Radioiodine I-123 imaging with neck imaging
   B. Radioiodine I-123 imaging with whole body scan
   C. MRI
   D. Ultrasound

## Answers to Questions

1. E: In cases of hyperthyroidism with low radioiodine uptake, the causes are far more likely to be thyroxine intake or various forms of thyroiditis.

2. A: Thyroglobulin is made by thyroid tissue located in the neck or ectopic thyroid tissue. TSH (answer B) and Free T4 (answer C) are affected by thyroid function and thyroxine intake. Elevated TSI (answer D) may indicate Graves' disease, but would not suggest ectopic thyroid tissue.
3. B: The radioiodine imaging with whole body scan will help locate ectopic thyroid tissue in the body. Limiting the scan to the neck (answer A) may miss cases of struma ovarii in the pelvis. Further imaging with ultrasound (answer D) or MRI (answer C) may then be directed to the areas of increased radiotracer localization.

# References

1. Yannopoulos D, Yannopoulos K, Ossowski R. Malignant struma ovarii. Pathol Annu. 1976;11:403–13.
2. Dunzendorfer T, deLas Morenas A, Kalir T, Levin RM. Struma ovarii and hyperthyroidism. Thyroid. 1999;9(5):499–502.
3. Makani S, Kim W, Gaba AR. Struma ovarii with a focus of papillary thyroid cancer: a case report and review of the literature. Gynecol Oncol. 2004;94(3):835–9.
4. Roth LM, Talerman A. The enigma of struma ovarii. Pathology. 2007;39(1):139–46.
5. Chiofalo MG, Misso C, Insabato L, Lastoria S, Pezzullo L. Hyperthyroidism due to coexistence of graves' disease and struma ovarii. Endocr Pract. 2007;13(3):274–6.
6. Devaney K, Snyder R, Norris HJ, Tavassoli FA. Proliferative and histologically malignant struma ovarii: a clinicopathologic study of 54 cases. Int J Gynecol Pathol. 1993;12(4):333–43.
7. McGill JF, Sturgeon C, Angelos P. Metastatic struma ovarii treated with total thyroidectomy and radioiodine ablation. Endocr Pract. 2009;15(2):167–73.
8. Jean S, Tanyi JL, Montone K, McGrath C, Lage-Alvarez MM, Chu CS. Papillary thyroid cancer arising in struma ovarii. J Obstet Gynaecol. 2012;32(3):222–6.
9. DeSimone CP, Lele SM, Modesitt SC. Malignant struma ovarii: a case report and analysis of cases reported in the literature with focus on survival and I131 therapy. Gynecol Oncol. 2003;89(3):543–8.
10. Shaco-Levy R, Peng RY, Snyder MJ, et al. Malignant struma ovarii: a blinded study of 86 cases assessing which histologic features correlate with aggressive clinical behavior. Arch Pathol Lab Med. 2012;136(2):172–8.
11. Robboy SJ, Shaco-Levy R, Peng RY, et al. Malignant struma ovarii: an analysis of 88 cases, including 27 with extraovarian spread. Int J Gynecol Pathol. 2009;28(5):405–22.

# Chapter 8
# Exogenous Thyrotoxicosis

**Nestoras Mathioudakis and David S. Cooper**

## Objectives

Ingestion of excessive amounts of thyroid hormone, whether intentionally or unintentionally, results in exogenous thyrotoxicosis. Surreptitious ingestion of thyroid hormone for the purpose of feigning hyperthyroidism is more precisely termed factitious thyrotoxicosis. Less commonly, however, exogenous thyrotoxicosis may result from *inadvertent* ingestion of thyroid hormone. This can be a challenging diagnosis to establish and requires a high index of clinical suspicion. Here, we report the case of a 33-year-old woman with an 18 month history of progressive, severe hyperthyroidism who had unknowingly been consuming thyroid hormone contained in an herbal weight-loss supplement. We review the etiologies, evaluation, and treatment of exogenous thyrotoxicosis.

## Case Presentation

A 33-year-old woman with no history of thyroid disease was referred for evaluation of hyperthyroidism of unclear etiology. The patient had seen two prior endocrinologists and no explanation had been found for her progressive hyperthyroidism. She had presented 18 months earlier with anxiety, diaphoresis, tremor, weight loss, and tachycardia, especially while exercising. These symptoms began 18 months after

N. Mathioudakis, M.D.
Division of Endocrinology and Metabolism, Johns Hopkins Hospital, Baltimore, MD, USA

D.S. Cooper, M.D. (✉)
Division of Endocrinology and Metabolism, The Johns Hopkins University School
of Medicine, 1830 E. Monument St., Suite 333, Baltimore, MD, USA
e-mail: dscooper@jhmi.edu

© Springer Science+Business Media New York 2015
T.F. Davies (ed.), *A Case-Based Guide to Clinical Endocrinology*,
DOI 10.1007/978-1-4939-2059-4_8

the birth of her second child. She had no complaints of anterior neck discomfort and had not had any recent illness. Thyroid function tests drawn at the onset of these symptoms revealed a thyroid-stimulating hormone (TSH) 0.03 mU/L (normal, 0.40–4.50), free thyroxine (T4) 1.24 ng/dL (normal, 0.8–1.8), and triiodothyronine (T3) 180 ng/dL (normal, 60–181). A technetium scan showed diminished thyroid uptake, suggestive of thyroiditis.

Over the course of the next 6 months, the patient progressed to overt hyperthyroidism, with a TSH <0.01 mU/L (normal, 0.40–4.50), free T4 2.1 ng/dL (normal, 0.8–1.8), and T3 356 ng/dL (normal, 60–181). A radioiodine uptake was 4.9 % at 24 h (normal, 18–35 %), with a heterogeneous pattern seen in both lobes. A thyroid sonogram showed a normal gland with a tiny cyst in the left lobe. To exclude the possibility that iodine contamination contributed to the low 24-h radioiodine uptake, a 24-h urine iodine level was obtained and measured 313 mcg (normal, 100–460).

Eighteen months after the onset of symptoms, the hyperthyroidism had become more severe with a free T3 > 2,000 pg/dL (normal, 230–420), free T4 6.4 ng/dL (normal, 0.8–1.8), and TSH < 0.01 mU/L (normal, 0.40–4.50). A repeat 24-h radioiodine uptake was 2.5 % (normal, 18–35 %) and scan of the patient's body including the thorax, abdomen, and pelvis showed no tracer uptake. Antithyroglobulin, antithyroperoxidase, and thyroid stimulating immunoglobulin levels were negative. The serum thyroglobulin was 1.4 ng/mL (normal, 2.0–35.0). Despite the lack of evidence of endogenous hyperthyroidism by imaging and laboratory studies, a second endocrinologist started the patient on methimazole 10 mg twice daily. This was ineffective at normalizing thyroid function, so the patient was referred to our endocrine clinic for further evaluation.

The patient had recently been diagnosed with depression in the setting of a marital separation. Her prescribed medications included methimazole 20 mg daily, fluoxetine, and an oral contraceptive pill. She denied taking any exogenous thyroid hormone preparations, but admitted to taking Redline, an herbal supplement advertised on the internet as a "multisystem rapid fat loss catalyst." It contains a number of stimulants including caffeine, synephrine, yohimbine, and other compounds. Previously, the patient had taken another weight loss supplement, Hydroxycut. Thyroid hormone is not listed as an ingredient in either of these supplements.

On physical examination, the blood pressure was 134/86, pulse was 133, weight 117 pounds. The patient was slightly hyperkinetic and anxious. There was no proptosis, lid lag, or conjunctival injection. The thyroid gland was not palpable. Lungs, heart, and abdomen were unremarkable. There was a fine tremor of the outstretched hands. Deep tendon reflexes were brisk. The skin was warm and moist.

The patient was strongly urged to discontinue Redline and any other herbal supplements she might be taking. She was also advised to stop the methimazole. Eight weeks later, the patient was euthyroid with a TSH 0.79 mU/L (normal, 0.40–4.50), free T4 0.96 ng/dL (normal, 0.8–1.8), and T3 141 ng/dL (97–219). The patient gained three pounds and her hyperthyroid symptoms resolved.

# Background

Exogenous thyrotoxicosis can be intentional or inadvertent (Table 8.1). The most common and easily recognizable etiology is iatrogenic thyrotoxicosis. An excessive dose of thyroxine may intentionally be prescribed to suppress TSH secretion in the management of thyroid cancer or goiter. In some cases, patients insist on supraphysiologic doses of thyroxine to maintain energy or lose weight, frequently dismissing healthcare providers who do not accommodate their request. This condition has been termed "thyrotoxicosis insistiates" [1].

The intentional and surreptitious ingestion of thyroid hormone to feign the diagnosis of hyperthyroidism is factitious thyrotoxicosis. A form of Munchausen's syndrome, this psychiatric disorder is motivated by the patient's desire to assume the sick role for emotional gain [2]. This is most commonly observed in young or middle-aged women with a history of childhood emotional deprivation and/or current sexual or relationship problems; in some cases, the patient may carry a diagnosis of borderline personality disorder or post-traumatic stress disorder [3]. Other suggestive historical features may include a connection to the healthcare profession, lack of appropriate concern for health problems, or a past history of feigning illness [2]. On the other hand, thyroid hormone abuse may also be observed in individuals without an underlying psychiatric disorder, usually for the purpose of weight loss [4]. In these cases, the patient's motivation is not to feign a medical condition, but rather to derive perceived benefits of hyperthyroidism (weight loss, increased energy, etc.) [4].

As challenging as it may be to diagnose factitious thyrotoxicosis, it can be even more difficult to identify cases of inadvertent thyrotoxicosis. In some cases, the problem may be as simple as a pharmacy or patient medication error. For patients already prescribed thyroid hormone, it may be helpful to verify that they are taking the prescribed dose by having them bring in their medications for review and/or

**Table 8.1** Examples of clinical situations resulting in exogenous thyrotoxicosis

| Intentional | Inadvertent |
| --- | --- |
| 1. Iatrogenic<br>(a) Suppressive thyroxine dose in thyroid cancer<br>(b) Excessive thyroxine dose to shrink goiter<br>(c) Patient's insistence on higher thyroid hormone dose<br>2. Factitious<br>(a) Surreptitious ingestion of thyroid hormone to feign hyperthyroidism<br>3. Thyroid hormone abuse<br>(a) Supplements or thyroid hormone/extracts usually taken for the purpose of weight loss, without willful intention to feign hyperthyroidism | 1. Medication error (i.e., patient or pharmacy)<br>2. Accidental ingestion of another person's or (rarely) pet's thyroxine dose in place of the patient's dose<br>3. Accidental overdose (i.e., children)<br>4. Meat contamination with thyroid hormone ("hamburger thyrotoxicosis")<br>5. Ingestion of herbal/weight loss supplements but unaware that thyroid hormone is an unspecified ingredient |

contacting their pharmacy. One unusual cause of medication error is inadvertent ingestion of a pet's thyroxine dose in place of prescribed thyroxine [5]. Accidental thyroxine poisoning has occurred in young children with access to the medication [6, 7]. Rarely, outbreaks of thyrotoxicosis have occurred following consumption of ground beef contaminated with bovine thyroid gland (so-called hamburger thyrotoxicosis) [8].

In recent years, there have been increasing reports of accidental overdose of thyroid hormone caused by weight-reducing herbal medications containing thyroid hormone as a hidden ingredient [9, 10]. The use of herbal or natural supplements is widespread in the USA and these products are not regulated by the FDA. Surprisingly, as many as 7 % of such supplements contain undisclosed substances [9]. It has been estimated that half of patients do not disclose their use of supplements to physicians [9]. Some easily accessible nonprescription supplements taken for the purposes weight loss, energy, or "thyroid support" have been found to contain clinically significant amounts of T3 and T4 [9–11]. Therefore, the use such supplements poses a serious risk of hyperthyroidism-related cardiovascular complications. In some instances, supplements adulterated with thyroid hormone may have a beta-blocker added to mask hyperadrenergic symptoms, which could make recognition of the thyrotoxic patient even more difficult [9]. In patients with underlying thyroid disease, exogenous thyrotoxicosis can complicate the clinical picture and lead to a delay in diagnosis [10].

## How the Diagnosis Was Made

The patient described in the case above presented with classic features of hyperthyroidism. Given the absence of a goiter or exophthalmos, a nontender thyroid gland, and low radioiodine uptake, the initial suspicion was that she had painless thyroiditis. The onset of symptoms 18 months after the delivery of her child made postpartum thyroiditis less probable, as this typically occurs at a shorter interval (2–12 months) after delivery.

At the outset, conservative management was recommended with the expectation that the hyperthyroid phase of thyroiditis would resolve within 3–4 months; instead, the hyperthyroidism persisted and progressed over the subsequent 18 months. Repeat radioiodine uptake was persistently low. The differential diagnosis for thyrotoxicosis associated with decreased radioiodine uptake includes various forms of thyroiditis, exogenous thyrotoxicosis, and excess iodine intake (radiographic contrast, amiodarone, iodine supplementation). Table 8.2 summarizes features that distinguish exogenous thyrotoxicosis from these other causes. Struma ovarii was another etiology considered in her case, but this was excluded by absence of ectopic uptake on whole body scan. With a normal urine iodine level, iodine contamination was ruled out as a cause of low radioiodine uptake. The patient was not taking any medications known to cause thyroiditis. The absence of thyroid autoantibodies provided further evidence against underlying thyroid disease.

**Table 8.2** Distinguishing exogenous thyrotoxicosis from other causes of thyrotoxicosis associated with decreased radioiodine uptake

| Factor | Exogenous thyrotoxicosis | Other causes of thyrotoxicosis associated with decreased radioiodine uptake |
|---|---|---|
| Thyroid function tests | Low TSH, high free T4, high T3 | Low TSH, high free T4, high T3 |
| Ratio of T3/T4 | Suggested by high T3/T4 ratio (>19), but not excluded by low T3/T4 ratio (<16) [12] | T3/T4 ratio usually <16 [12] |
| Thyroid autoantibodies | Absent, unless underlying thyroid disease | May be positive in painless or postpartum thyroiditis |
| Physical examination | Normal or nonpalpable, nontender thyroid; absence of exophthalmos or other stigmata of Graves' disease | Thyroid may be enlarged or tender to palpation in some types of thyroiditis |
| Inflammatory markers | Normal | Elevated ESR, CRP, leukocytosis, in subacute thyroiditis |
| Duration of thyrotoxicosis | Variable, depending on duration of exogenous thyroid hormone intake | Usually 3–4 months in thyroiditis |
| 24-h radioiodine uptake | Low (usually <1 %); may be higher in patients with underlying autonomy (toxic nodules) | Low (usually <1 %) |
| Serum thyroglobulin | Low, but not necessarily undetectable | Normal or high (may be low in presence of antithyroglobulin antibodies) |
| Urine iodine | Normal | Very high in cases of excess iodine (i.e., radiographic contrast, amiodarone, iodine supplementation) |
| Fecal thyroid hormone measurement | High | Normal |

Since an 18 month phase of hyperthyroidism in the context of thyroiditis would be untenable, the differential diagnosis was narrowed down to exogenous thyrotoxicosis. This was corroborated by the patient's very low serum thyroglobulin level. Thyroglobulin can be a helpful diagnostic clue in this setting because it is typically low (though not necessarily undetectable) in exogenous thyrotoxicosis, whereas it is high in thyroiditis and endogenous hyperthyroidism [1]. It should be noted that serum thyroglobulin levels may not be suppressed to undetectable levels in all cases of exogenous thyrotoxicosis, particularly in those with adenomatous goiter or persistent thyroid cancer [10]. Regrettably, a thyroglobulin level was not obtained early in this patient's course, and this may have contributed to the long delay in diagnosis.

In addition, the markedly elevated T3 and T4 concentrations in this case suggested that the patient was either consuming thyroid extract or a combination of synthetic T4/T3. A high total T3/total T4 ratio (>19) in conjunction with low radioiodine uptake is a pattern unique to exogenous thyrotoxicosis resulting from combination T4/T3 ingestion. By contrast, thyroiditis typically results in a lower total T3/total T4 ratio (typically <16) [12]. In clinical practice, the T3/T4 ratio is typically used to distinguish between endogenous hyperthyroidism (i.e., Graves' disease or toxic adenoma) and destructive thyroiditis, but it has a limited role in distinguishing thyroiditis from exogenous thyrotoxicosis [12]. This is because patients taking pure thyroxine have elevations in both T3 and T4 with a ratio that may overlap with that observed in thyroiditis [12]. In other words, only a high T3/T4 ratio has discriminative value in this context.

In this case, the patient explicitly denied taking exogenous thyroid hormone. With the exception of recent depression in the setting of marital problems, she had no history of a personality disorder or connection to the medical profession, and she seemed truly bothered by her symptoms. When it was discovered that she was taking an herbal weight-loss supplement, the ingredients were carefully scrutinized. Although the Redline capsules were not subjected to laboratory analysis for detection of thyroid hormones, the prompt resolution of thyrotoxicosis with discontinuation of this supplement suggests that it was indeed the culprit. Another method that could have aided in the evaluation is measurement of fecal thyroxine content, which may be markedly elevated in cases of exogenous thyrotoxicosis due to thyroxine ingestion [13].

## Treatment

Typically, the only treatment required in exogenous thyrotoxicosis is discontinuation or reduction in the dose of thyroid hormone. L-thyroxine has a half-life of 7 days, so it takes approximately 5 weeks for the drug to be cleared. Liothyronine is cleared more rapidly, with a serum half-life of approximately 1 day. Patients who are very symptomatic may require beta-adrenergic blockade while awaiting resolution of thyrotoxicosis. In cases of massive overdose of thyroid hormone, management may consist of induced emesis, gastric lavage, and intragastric installation of charcoal [14]. Cholestyramine can also be given as intestinal binder of T4 and T3, thereby interrupting the normal enterohepatic circulation of the two hormones [14]. Plasmapheresis and exchange transfusion have been used to treat massive thyroid hormone overdose [14]. Fortunately, most patients, especially children, have few signs and symptoms of hyperthyroidism following accidental poisoning, and conservative management is usually satisfactory [14].

## Lessons Learned

1. Exogenous thyrotoxicosis is not always intentional.
2. Thyroid hormone may be an undisclosed ingredient in many herbal supplements advertised as weight loss, energy, or "thyroid support" agents.

3. Diagnostic clues to exogenous thyrotoxicosis include the absence of a goiter or exophthalmos, a nontender thyroid gland, low radioiodine uptake (after exclusion of iodine contamination), low serum thyroglobulin, and high fecal thyroxine content.
4. The hyperthyroid phase in thyroiditis does not typically last longer than several months; therefore, in cases where thyrotoxicosis persists for a longer duration, the differential diagnosis should be expanded to include exogenous thyrotoxicosis.
5. A careful review of medications, including non-prescription over-the-counter or herbal supplements, should be undertaken when exogenous thyrotoxicosis is suspected.
6. A high T3/T4 (>19) ratio in the setting of a low radioiodine uptake favors exogenous thyrotoxicosis over thyroiditis as the etiology.

## Questions

1. A 52-year-old woman with no prior history of thyroid disease is referred to you for unexplained hyperthyroidism of 1 year duration. On physical examination, there is no exophthalmos and the thyroid is small and nontender. Which of the following tests would be most helpful test in differentiating painless thyroiditis from exogenous thyrotoxicosis?

   A. Antithyroperoxidase antibody, antithyroglobulin antibody, and serum thyroglobulin
   B. Radioiodine uptake and scan
   C. T3/T4 ratio
   D. Erythrocyte sedimentation rate

2. A 28-year-old woman with a history of Hashimoto's thyroiditis returns for follow-up. She had been prescribed levothyroxine 112 mcg daily for several years and had consistently normal thyroid function tests during regular visits. She noticed that her hair was coarse and falling out in the shower, and wondered whether the levothyroxine "was working." She did some research on the internet and found an herbal supplement that claimed to provide more "natural" thyroid hormone support. She decided to stop the levothyroxine and has been taking three tablets of this herbal supplement twice daily for the last 3 months. You investigate the "thyroid support" supplement and do not see thyroid hormone listed as an ingredient. When you examine her, she appears hyperkinetic and anxious. She has lost 12 pounds since last visit and her BMI is 17 kg/m². Her pulse is 118, blood pressure 138/72. She has a nonpalpable, nontender thyroid gland. TSH is <0.01 mU/L (normal, 0.40–4.50), free T4 2.5 ng/dL (normal, 0.8–1.8), and T3 300 ng/dL (normal, 60–181). Which of the following is the preferred treatment strategy?

A. Refer her to a psychiatrist to evaluate for factitious disorder.
B. Advise her to reduce the dose of her supplement to three tablets once daily and recheck thyroid function tests in 6 weeks.
C. Obtain a serum thyroglobulin level and fecal thyroxine measurements.
D. Tell the patient she most likely has painless thyroiditis and arrange for an I-123 uptake and scan.
E. Advise the patient to stop the "thyroid support" supplement. Inform her that these products are not regulated by the FDA and may contain undisclosed amounts of thyroid hormone, placing her at risk of complications related to thyrotoxicosis.

3. A 68 year old woman with papillary thyroid cancer returns to see you with her husband, who is also your patient. The patient has a history of atrial fibrillation and osteoporosis. She underwent total thyroidectomy followed by radioactive iodine remnant ablation 15 years earlier and has been in remission from her thyroid cancer since. You have been aiming to maintain her serum TSH level in the normal range, and she has been well-controlled on a stable dose of L-thyroxine for years. She was recently hospitalized for an episode of atrial fibrillation with rapid ventricular response and was noted to have a TSH<0.01 mU/L (normal, 0.40–4.50), free T4 2.9 ng/dL (0.8–1.8). The hospital team reduced her dose of levothyroxine from 150 mcg to 50 mcg daily. Thyroid function studies at the time of her visit with you show a TSH of 10.4 mU/L (normal, 0.40–4.50), free T4 0.7 ng/dL (normal, 0.8–1.8). She reports that she had been taking the medication as you prescribed. In fact, she has all of her medications organized in a pill box at home. She denies taking any herbal or over-the-counter supplements. Which of the following is the preferred treatment strategy?

A. Arrange for thyrogen-mediated thyroglobulin and whole body scan to exclude recurrent thyroid cancer.
B. Obtain a serum thyroglobulin level.
C. Contact the patient's pharmacy to verify recent medications dispensed. Ask the patient to bring in the bottles of all the medications she is taking and inquire about any over-the-counter or herbal supplements.
D. Order a 24-h urine iodine level.
E. Check a free and total T3 level.

## Answers to Questions

1. A: Laboratory tests in patients with exogenous thyrotoxicosis mimic those of thyrotoxicosis caused by thyroiditis. Both conditions show low radioiodine uptake, so answer choice B is incorrect. The total T3/total T4 ratio can sometimes be helpful to distinguish between thyroiditis and exogenous thyrotoxicosis. In the former, it is usually low (<16), while in the latter it can overlap with

the pattern seen in endogenous hyperthyroidism (>19). However, in cases of exogenous T4 ingestion alone (i.e., without T3), the T3/T4 ratio may not distinguish between thyroiditis and exogenous thyrotoxicosis. In this context, the T3/T4 ratio has discriminative value only when very high, as this would be unusual for thyroiditis. Therefore, answer choice C is not correct. Thyroid autoantibodies are positive in a majority of individuals with painless or post-partum thyroiditis; these levels are typically positive early in the course of painless thyroiditis and usually remain elevated even after normalization of thyroid function. The thyroglobulin level will best distinguish between thyroid-itis and exogenous thyrotoxicosis. In the former, it will be high, and in the latter it will be low. It is important to know the thyroid autoantibody status of the patient when interpreting the serum thyroglobulin level as it may be falsely low in the setting of positive antithyroglobulin antibodies. Thus, answer choice A is correct.

2. E: The patient has disclosed that she is taking thyroid hormone to you; therefore, the diagnosis is not factitious thyrotoxicosis, so answer choice A is incorrect. The "thyroid support" supplement almost certainly contains an undisclosed amount of T3 and T4. Since the amount of these compounds is uncertain, it would be difficult for the physician to safely adjust the dose of this compound to achieve euthyroidism, so answer choice B is incorrect. Answer choice C would be a possible choice to evaluate for factitious thyrotoxicosis, but the patient does not have this condition. Rather, this clinical picture is better described as unintentional thyroid hormone abuse. Painless thyroiditis is less likely than thyroid hormone abuse in this clinical scenario, so answer choice D is incorrect. The correct answer is E. The patient should be urged to stop the herbal supplement.

3. C: This is most likely a case of iatrogenic thyrotoxicosis due to a medication error. The fact that the patient's husband is also your patient raises the possibil-ity that she may have inadvertently taken his higher thyroxine dose in place of hers. This resulted in thyrotoxicosis, which likely contributed to the episode of atrial fibrillation w/rapid ventricular response. Careful review of her medica-tions to verify that the she was taking the correct dose is the first-step in man-agement. It may be helpful to contact the pharmacy to verify that the correct dose was recently dispensed. Although thyrotoxicosis can be observed in some cases of metastatic thyroid cancer, this would be less likely given the patient's long duration of remission, so answer choices A and B are incorrect. The patient is status post total thyroidectomy. Urinary iodine would be used to exclude iodine contamination obscuring the interpretation of a radioiodine uptake and scan, which is not directly applicable to this case. Since the patient does not have a thyroid gland, there is no concern for T3-toxicosis, unless there is suspi-cion that she is taking a supplement containing T3. Given her long history of stable thyroid function on levothyroxine, this is highly unlikely, so answer choice E is incorrect.

# References

1. Mittra ES, Niederkohr RD, Rodriguez C, El-Maghraby T, McDougall IR. Uncommon causes of thyrotoxicosis. J Nucl Med. 2008;49:265–78.
2. Wise MG, Ford CV. Factitious disorders. Prim Care. 1999;26:315–26.
3. McMullumsmith C, Ford C. Simulated illness: the factitious disorders and malingering. Psychiatr Clin N Am. 2011;34:621–41.
4. Braunstein GD, Koblin R, Sugawara M, Pekary AE, Hershman JM. Unintentional thyrotoxicosis factitia due to a diet pill. West J Med. 1986;145:388–91.
5. Feit S, Feit H. Thyrotoxicosis factitia veterinarius. Ann Intern Med. 1997;127:168.
6. Gorman RL, Chamberlain JM, Rose SR, Oderda GM. Massive levothyroxine overdose: high anxiety–low toxicity. Pediatrics. 1988;82:666–9.
7. Shilo L, Kovatz S, Hadari R, Weiss E, Nabriski D, Shenkman L. Massive thyroid hormone overdose: kinetics, clinical manifestations and management. Isr Med Assoc J. 2002;4:298–9.
8. Hedberg CW, Fishbein DB, Janssen RS, et al. An outbreak of thyrotoxicosis caused by the consumption of bovine thyroid gland in ground beef. N Engl J Med. 1987;316:993–8.
9. Poon WT, Ng SW, Lai CK, Chan YW, Mak WL. Factitious thyrotoxicosis and herbal dietary supplement for weight reduction. Clin Toxicol. 2008;46:290–2.
10. Ohye H, Fukata S, Kanoh M, et al. Thyrotoxicosis caused by weight-reducing herbal medicines. Arch Intern Med. 2005;165:831–4.
11. Kang GY, Parks J, Fileta BB, Chang AS, Abdel-Rahim, M, Burch, HB, Bernet V. Thyroxine and triiodothyronine content in commercially available thyroid health supplements. Poster session presented at: 81st Annual Meeting of the American Thyroid Association, Indian Wells, CA, 26–30 October 2011
12. Mortoglou A, Candiloros H. The serum triiodothyronine to thyroxine (T3/T4) ratio in various thyroid disorders and after Levothyroxine replacement therapy. Hormones. 2004;3:120–6.
13. Bouillon R, Verresen L, Staels F, Bex M, De Vos P, De Roo M. The measurement of fecal thyroxine in the diagnosis of thyrotoxicosis factitia. Thyroid. 1993;3:101–3.
14. Ho J, Jackson R, Johnson D. Massive levothyroxine ingestion in a pediatric patient: case report and discussion. CJEM. 2011;13:165–8.

# Part III
# Thyroid Underactivity

# Chapter 9
# Introduction

Giuseppe Barbesino

Thyroid hormones are unique in that they are formed from the coupling and iodination of a nonessential amino acid, tyrosine. The thyroid almost exclusively produces thyroxine (T4), a precursor of the active hormone, triiodothyronine (T3). T3 is largely derived from deiodination of T4 in peripheral tissues, a still partially understood method for regionally regulating T3 levels. The thyroid also secretes a small amount of T3, but the physiological relevance of this is unclear. Upon binding with its ubiquitous nuclear receptors, T3 facilitates or activates transcription of a great variety of genes throughout almost all organ systems [1]. It is therefore not surprising that lack of thyroid hormones affects several physiologic pathways. Since T4, (after being deiodinated in the tyrotroph to T3) is largely predominant in the regulation of TSH production at the pituitary-hypothalamic levels and since TSH is the only natural regulator of T4 production, serum TSH levels are very tightly correlated to serum T4 levels. However changes in T4 result in TSH changes on a logarithmic scale. As a consequence, when the hypothalamic-pituitary-thyroid axis feedback mechanism is preserved, thyroid function can be effectively tested through TSH measurements.

## Thyroid Underactivity

Thyroid underactivity or hypothyroidism is defined as the condition deriving by insufficient thyroid hormone levels in the circulation. In primary hypothyroidism, the defect is at the thyroid gland level. In primary hypothyroidism, free T4 levels are low, while the intact pituitary responds with elevated TSH levels. Elevated TSH

G. Barbesino, M.D. (✉)
Thyroid Unit, Massachusetts General Hospital, Harvard Medical School,
ACC730S, 15 Parkman St., Boston, MA 02114, USA
e-mail: gbarbesino@partners.org

© Springer Science+Business Media New York 2015
T.F. Davies (ed.), *A Case-Based Guide to Clinical Endocrinology*,
DOI 10.1007/978-1-4939-2059-4_9

**Table 9.1** A concise list of symptoms of hypothyroidism

| Organ system | Manifestations |
|---|---|
| Cardiovascular | Bradycardia, heart failure, pericardial effusion |
| CNS | Depression, fatigue, cognitive dysfunction, myxedema coma |
| Hematopoietic | Macrocytic anemia, target cells |
| Metabolic | Hyperlipidemia, weight gain |
| Musculoskeletal | Arthralgias, myositis |
| Gastrointestinal | Constipation |
| Renal | Hyponatremia |
| Reproductive | Polymenorrhea, galactorrhea, erectile dysfunction, infertility |
| Skin and appendages | Alopecia, coarse hair, dry and discolored skin, myxedema |

levels, with normal free T4 levels, define subclinical primary hypothyroidism. Patients with elevated TSH (usually >10 mIU/L) and low FT4 are said to have overt hypothyroidism. In central hypothyroidism, the defect is at the hypothalamus-pituitary level and results in low free T4 levels, with low or inappropriately normal TSH levels. In both conditions, T3 levels are often normal and are therefore of little help in the diagnosis. The symptoms of hypothyroidism vary greatly depending on the severity of the insufficiency, the rate of drop in thyroid hormones, the age of the patient and poorly understood individual factors. As mentioned before, most, if not all, organ systems are affected. Table 9.1 shows a concise list of most commonly described symptoms of hypothyroidism.

## Causes of Hypothyroidism

World-wide, iodine deficiency remains the most significant cause of hypothyroidism. Thyroid autoimmune disease (Hashimoto's thyroiditis) [2] is the most common cause of spontaneous primary hypothyroidism in regions with normal or even moderately low iodine intake. The degree of hypothyroidism is most often mild (subclinical) and slowly progressive in Hashimoto's thyroiditis, but all degrees of hypothyroidism can be seen and sudden onset is sometimes seen. Many patients with Hashimoto's thyroiditis have a rubbery goiter, diffusely hypoechoic and vascular on neck ultrasound. In some cases, the thyroid becomes completely atrophic and cannot be palpated. Thyroid peroxidase antibody tests are almost universally positive in Hashimoto's thyroiditis. Almost all other forms of primary hypothyroidism are iatrogenic, caused by either thyroid surgery, or radioactive iodine treatment of hyperthyroidism. Inflammatory or toxic forms of hypothyroidism can occur as a consequence of medications (amiodarone) or viral insults (subacute thyroiditis) and may result in transient forms of primary hypothyroidism. Central hypothyroidism is vastly less common than primary and usually occurs in the setting of multiple pituitary hormone insufficiencies.

## Management of Hypothyroidism

Hypothyroidism is usually diagnosed by finding of an elevated serum TSH [3]. In many laboratories, "reflex" serum T4 or freeT4 levels confirm the diagnosis. A normal TSH does not rule-out central hypothyroidism, but normal FT4 does. All patients with overt hypothyroidism and with central hypothyroidism should receive treatment with thyroid hormone. The benefit of treating asymptomatic patients with subclinical hypothyroidism remains uncertain and may be limited to patients of younger age, especially women in the childbearing age [4]. The goal of hypothyroidism treatment is restoration of normal TSH levels and resolution of symptoms. Synthetic L-thyroxine is the most appropriate treatment for most patients with hypothyroidism. Athyreotic patients will require 1.6 mcg/kg BW/day to achieve complete thyroid replacement, but patients with subclinical hypothyroidism typically need lower doses due the contribution of their residual thyroid function. T4/T3 combination therapy has been studied, based on the finding that thyroid hormone production includes a small amount of T3 and on data indicating a slightly lower FT3 in many patients treated with T4, when compared with euthyroid patients with similar TSH levels. There is also the desire to help those patients whose symptoms are not resolved when normal TSH levels are re-established with T4 alone. The available studies have not confirmed a statistically significant beneficial effect of combined therapy. However the understanding of these issues is limited and therefore we administer combination to the occasional patient on an empiric basis.

Treatment with thyroid hormone is usually very well tolerated and very efficient in restoring euthyroidism. In select cases, such as cardiac or elderly patients, replacement should be initiated with smaller doses. The fact that by measuring TSH and T4 we actually measure the medication, rather than relying on an indirect measure of its effect, allows for very precise titration and quick recognition of instances of malabsoprtion or noncompliance [5].

## References

1. Kopp P. Thyroid hormone synthesis. In: Braverman L, editor. Werner & Ingbar's the thyroid. 9th ed. Philadelphia, PA: Lippincott Williams & Wilkins; 2005. p. 52–76.
2. Dayan CM, Daniels GH. Chronic autoimmune thyroiditis. N Engl J Med. 1996;335(2): 99–107.
3. Garber JR, Cobin RH, Gharib H, Hennessey JV, Klein I, Mechanick JI, et al. Clinical practice guidelines for hypothyroidism in adults: co-sponsored by American Association of Clinical Endocrinologists and the American Thyroid Association. Endocr Pract. 2012;11:1–207.
4. Surks MI, Ortiz E, Daniels GH, Sawin CT, Col NF, Cobin RH, et al. Subclinical thyroid disease: scientific review and guidelines for diagnosis and management. JAMA. 2004;291(2): 228–38.
5. Barbesino G. Drugs affecting thyroid function. Thyroid. 2010;20(7):763–70.

# Chapter 10
# Central Hypothyroidism

Luca Persani

## Objectives

To discuss the difficulties encountered in the diagnosis and management of patients with central hypothyroidism.

## Case Presentation

In 1999, a 33-year-old woman obtains a consultation with an endocrinologist because of menstrual irregularity since 4 months (delays of 10–15 days) accompanied by an increased frequency of headache, sleep disorder, morning fatigue and dizziness. The woman was a semi-professional basketball player that recently decided to stop this sport because she was unable to follow the training program. Her gynecologist did not find any abnormality but prescribed some blood tests showing mild hyperprolactinemia on a single determination (31 ng/ml), a slight LDL-cholesterol elevation (always normal on previous determinations) and normal serum TSH (Table 10.1). Her physical examination revealed a normal blood pressure (110/70 mmHg) and heart rate (66 beats/min), the body mass index was 25 kg/m$^2$, and the thyroid appeared normal for volume and soft at palpation. The consultant diagnosed a mild hypercholesterolemia, stress-dependent hyperprolactinemia and normal thyroid function, and gave dietary recommendations, rest and a short course of an anti-anxiety drug. Two years later, the woman asked a new consultation due

L. Persani, M.D., Ph.D. (✉)
Department of Clinical Sciences and Community Health, University of Milan, Milan, Italy

Division of Endocrine and Metabolic Diseases, Ospedale San Luca, Istituto Auxologico Italiano IRCCS, Piazza Brescia 20, 20149 Milan, Italy
e-mail: luca.persani@unimi.it

© Springer Science+Business Media New York 2015
T.F. Davies (ed.), *A Case-Based Guide to Clinical Endocrinology*,
DOI 10.1007/978-1-4939-2059-4_10

**Table 10.1** Biochemical values on the different blood tests

| | June 2008 | April 2010 | June 2010 | August 2010, LT4 1.0 µg/ kg bw/day | December 2010, LT4 1.4 µg/kg bw/day |
|---|---|---|---|---|---|
| PRL, ng/ml (n.v. 3–20) | 31 | Basal: 41 +60': 34 | PRL recovery after IgG precipitation: 98 % | – | – |
| TSH, mU/l (n.v.: 0.4–4.0) | 2.4 | 1.8 | 1.5 | 0.9 | 0.1 |
| Free T4, pM (n.v.: 9–20) | – | 9.0 | 8.6 | 11.4 | 16.3 |
| Free T3, pM (n.v.: 4–8) | – | 5.7 | – | 6.4 | 6.6 |
| Anti-TPO Ab, kU/l (<20) | – | – | 12 | – | – |
| LDL-Cho, mg/dl (<150) | 188 | 178 | – | 189 | 134 |
| Hemochrome | Normal | – | Normal | Normal | – |

to the persistence of the manifestations. The blood test then confirmed a normal TSH but with a FT4 value at the lower limit of normal, her PRL was above the normal range even after 1 h of rest (Table 10.1). The Endocrinologist then asked for a confirmatory test, a thyroid ultrasound, and a magnetic resonance study of the brain. The new blood test (Table 10.1) confirmed low FT4 and normal TSH, absence of macro-prolactin and normal results of the other tests for pituitary function, including ACTH/cortisol, IGF1 and urinary values; ultrasound revealed a thyroid of normal volume (9.6 ml) and structure, magnetic resonance of the pituitary sella region was normal. Central hypothyroidism accompanied by mild hyperprolactinemia of idiopathic origin was diagnosed. Subsequently, a more careful collection of the personal history revealed a traumatic head injury during a basketball match 5 years before that did not however require hospitalization.

The consultant started LT4 treatment for central hypothyroidism up to 1.0 µg/kg bw/day. On July 2010, the patient reported poor subjective improvement and mood depression. The TSH and free thyroid hormone values were in the normal range, the LDL-cholesterol levels were still elevated despite the dietary restrictions. The consultant confirmed the LT4 regimen explaining that other factors accounted for the persistence of the manifestations. After another 3 months without any improvement, the woman asked the advice of another consultant, who augmented the daily dose of LT4 up to 1.4 µg/kg on the basis of the symptoms and biochemical testing. Few weeks later, the patient observed the normalization of menses and the recovery of mood and physical performance, and she expressed the intention to restart the basketball training. The biochemical tests of December 2010 revealed a TSH value below but the FT4/FT3 levels at the mid of their normal range, the LDL-cholesterol was normal. The new consultant confirmed the current LT4 replacement.

# Review of the Management of This Case

## *Diagnosis*

This case describes a young woman with a central hypothyroidism and mild hyperprolactinemia. In this condition, the serum TSH screening alone cannot reveal the dysfunction of the hypothalamic–pituitary–thyroid axis, as TSH levels are most frequently normal [1–3]. Central hypothyroidism is presently known to account for about 1:1,000 hypothyroid patients, but is still probably underestimated and the Endocrinologists should always consider this possibility when hypothyroid manifestations coexist with biochemical alterations or clinical manifestations pointing to a pituitary origin. In this case, the first consultant initially gave little attention to the mild hyperprolactinemia and considered to check more appropriately and extensively thyroid function tests and PRL levels only 2 years after the start of symptoms. Indeed, the correct diagnosis could be suggested by the presence of a pituitary mass or history of pituitary disease, but a more careful recording of the personal history of this woman reporting the head trauma could have helped to anticipate the diagnosis. Indeed traumatic head injury or vascular accidents even of minor entity can account for several cases of central hypothyroidism previously classified as idiopathic. Most frequently, central hypothyroidism is combined with other pituitary hormone deficiencies that may mask the manifestations of a mild hypothyroid state, but their presence would support the central origin of thyroid dysfunction. In this case, the mild hypercholesterolemia was a finding supporting the recent onset of hypothyroidism, while the hyperprolactinemia, the absence of antithyroid autoantibodies and the normal findings at thyroid ultrasound were indeed pointing to the central origin.

## *Treatment*

LT4 replacement therapy was correctly started. The initial daily dose was mistakenly judged sufficient by the consultant based on normal values of all thyroid function tests. Indeed, TSH determination is not a reliable marker of thyroid hormone action at the hypothalamic–pituitary level in patients with central hypothyroidism but the finding of unsuppressed TSH levels during thyroxine therapy is strongly suggestive of an insufficient regimen [1, 4–6]. Accordingly, LDL-cholesterol was still abnormal despite the dietary restriction. Due to the persistence of hypothyroid manifestations, the patients went to another consultant that correctly interpreted the biochemical results and augmented the daily dose of thyroxine. The regimen of 1.4 µg/kg bw was effective in restoring the wellbeing, normal menstrual activity, and physical performance in this sportswoman. The finding of suppressed TSH accompanied by thyroid hormone levels in the central part of normal range and the normalization of LDL-cholesterol were supporting the correct replacement.

# Lessons Learned

Isolated central hypothyroidism can occur in a young sportswoman as a likely consequence of a mild head trauma. The diagnosis of central hypothyroidism should always be considered when hypothyroid-like manifestations coexist with low/normal TSH concentrations in the serum, but it should not completely discarded also in the presence of slightly elevated TSH, as in the cases with prevalent hypothalamic defect [1, 3]. Hyperprolactinemia, combined pituitary hormone deficiencies, or nonhormonal manifestations of a pituitary or hypothalamic mass should raise the suspect of a defective TSH secretion. However, nontumoral causes of pituitary dysfunction, including traumatic injuries, ictus, lymphocytic hypophysitis, other inflammatory diseases or genetic forms, should be kept in mind [1–3]. The finding of FT4 values below or at the lower limit of normal should then be correctly interpreted, particularly when these data are accompanied by an unexplained and persistent rise of cholesterol levels. The normal findings at thyroid ultrasound and the absence thyroid autoimmunity are also supporting the central origin of the disease.

As in primary hypothyroidism, treatment of central hypothyroidism should restore appropriate serum concentrations of thyroid hormones. Thyroxine treatment should be given to the same doses used in primary hypothyroidism, but this is frequently not the case mainly because this corresponds in most of central hypothyroid patients to the suppression of their circulating TSH levels [1, 4–6]. This phenomenon is most likely due to the reduced pituitary TSH reserve [7, 8]. Therefore, the finding of normal TSH concentrations should raise the suspect that the thyroxine regimen is not sufficient for that particular central hypothyroid patient. Other conditions that can cause the need to adjust the daily thyroxine doses are illustrated in Table 10.2 and include the treatment of combined pituitary hormone deficiencies,

**Table 10.2** Conditions associated with the risk of a revision of L-T4 regimen

| |
|---|
| *Possible undertreatment* |
| • Serum TSH above 0.5 mU/l, in particular if associated with serum FT4 values below the lower tertile of normal range |
| • Decrease of serum FT4 values below the lower tertile of normal range |
| • Start of oral contraceptives or estrogen replacement therapy |
| • Start of GH replacement therapy in patients with combined pituitary hormone deficiencies |
| • Start of treatments affecting LT4 absorption or thyroid hormone metabolism |
| • Unexplained increases of serum cholesterol |
| • Manifestations suggestive of hypothyroidism, in particular when associated with one of the above conditions |
| *Possible overtreatment* |
| • Values of FT4 and/or FT3 above the upper tertile of normal range |
| • Stop of oral contraceptives |
| • Stop of GH or estrogen replacement therapy |
| • Stop of treatments affecting LT4 absorption or thyroid hormone metabolism |
| • Unexplained increases of sex hormone binding globulin in the hyperthyroid range |
| • Clinical manifestations suggestive of thyrotoxicosis, in particular when associated with one of the above conditions |

such as GH or estradiol replacement [1, 3, 9]. Several studies (reviewed in [1, 3]) compared the levels of FT4 in primary and central hypothyroid subjects with those found in controls matched for age and sex; these data indicate that central hypothyroids are frequently underreplaced [6]. Thyroxine treatment should therefore aim to bring the FT4 values in the central part of the normal range, underreplacement should be suspected when FT4 is in the lowest tertile and overreplacement when the free thyroid hormone is in the highest tertile. The suspect may be confirmed by the contemporary determination of clinical and/or biochemical parameters of thyroid hormone action, such as heart rate, cholesterol levels, and sex hormone-binding globulin.

## Questions

1. Which of the following thyroid function tests pattern is most suggestive of central hypothyroidism?

   (a) Low TSH, normal FT4, low T3
   (b) Normal TSH, low FT4, low T3
   (c) Normal TSH, low FT4, normal T3
   (d) High TSH with normal FT4, normal T3

2. A 27 y/o woman with hypercholesterolemia, fatigue, hair loss, and amenorrhea, who has undergone external beam radiation to the head 10 years earlier, has the following test results: Low FSH, low estradiol, normal TSH, normal prolactin, low IGF-1, and normal ACTH stimulation test. Besides starting hormone replacement therapy with estradiol and progesterone, you:

   (a) Reassure the patient that only yearly adrenal and thyroid function tests will be needed
   (b) Order a TRH stimulation test
   (c) Order a FT4
   (d) Order glycoprotein hormone alpha-subunit levels

3. A 35 y/o man who has undergone a hypophysectomy 6 years ago because of craniopharyngioma is evaluated. He is currently on transdermal testosterone, oral hydrocortisone, and oral levothyroxine. His tests show low testosterone and prolactin and suppressed TSH. Besides increasing the testosterone dose, you:

   (a) Decrease the levothyroxine dose.
   (b) Order FT4
   (c) Ask him to repeat the TSH 3 months after the increase in testosterone dose
   (d) Decrease the hydrocortisone dose

## Answers to Questions

1. (b) In central hypothyroidism, TSH is often normal, while FT4 is low. Central hypothyroidism results from direct damage to the pituitary thyrotrophs, as the theory is that the few remaining exhausted thyrotrophs, while maximally stimulated by TRH and lack of thyroxine, produce a TSH molecule that is quantitavely adequate, but not as bioactive in stimulating thyroid hormone production as normal TSH. As a result, TSH levels are "inappropriately normal" in relation to the low thyroxine level. As a compensatory mechanism, peripheral conversion of T4 to T3 is enhanced, maintaining low normal T3 level in all but the most extreme forms of the condition.
2. (c) While in most situations a normal TSH level predicts normal thyroid function, when there is significant clinical suspicion of central hypothyroidism, measuring FT4 levels is necessary to rule out the condition.
3. (b) In central hypothyroidism, adequate replacement with levothyroxine in physiologic doses rapidly and thoroughly suppresses TSH levels. Therefore, overtreatment with levothyroxine can only be ruled out or ruled in with FT4 levels.

## References

1. Persani L. Central hypothyroidism: pathogenic, diagnostic, and therapeutic challenges. J Clin Endocrinol Metab. 2012;97:3068–78.
2. Yamada M, Mori M. Mechanisms related to the pathophysiology and management of central hypothyroidism. Nat Clin Pract Endocrinol Metab. 2008;4:683–94.
3. Persani L, Beck-Peccoz P. Central hypothyroidism. In: Braverman LE, Cooper D, editors. Werner and Ingbar's the thyroid: a fundamental and clinical text, Chap. 38. 10th ed. Philadelphia, PA: Lippincott, Williams, Wilkins/Wolters Kluwer Health; 2012. p. 560–8.
4. Ferretti E, Persani L, Jaffrain-Rea ML, Giambona S, Tamburrano G, Beck-Peccoz P. Evaluation of the adequacy of L-T4 replacement therapy in patients with central hypothyroidism. J Clin Endocrinol Metab. 1999;84:924–9.
5. Shimon I, Cohen O, Lubetsky A, Olchovsky D. Thyrotropin suppression by thyroid hormone replacement is correlated with thyroxine level normalization in central hypothyroidism. Thyroid. 2002;12:823–7.
6. Koulouri O, Auldin MA, Agarwal R, Kieffer V, Robertson C, Falconer Smith J, Levy MJ, Howlett TA. Diagnosis and treatment of hypothyroidism in TSH deficiency compared to primary thyroid disease: pituitary patients are at risk of underreplacement with levothyroxine. Clin Endocrinol (Oxf). 2011;74:744–9.
7. Horimoto M, Nishikawa M, Ishihara T, Yoshikawa N, Yoshimura M, Inada M. Bioactivity of thyrotropin (TSH) in patients with central hypothyroidism: comparison between in vivo 3,5,3-triiodothyronine response to TSHand in vitro bioactivity of TSH. J Clin Endocrinol Metab. 1995;80:1124–8.
8. Persani L, Ferretti E, Borgato S, Faglia G, Beck-Peccoz P. Circulating TSH bioactivity in sporadic central hypothyroidism. J Clin Endocrinol Metab. 2000;85:3631–5.
9. Alexopoulou O, Beguin C, DeNayer P, Maiter D. Clinical and hormonal characteristics of central hypothyroidism at diagnosis and during follow-up in adult patients. Eur J Endocrinol. 2004;150:1–8.

# Chapter 11
# Treatment of Hypothyroidism: Utility of Adding T3 (Liothyronine)

**Joy Tsai and Nikolaos Stathatos**

## Objectives

- To understand the utility of liothyronine replacement treatment in patients already on levothyroxine for the treatment of hypothyroidism

## Case Presentation

A 41-year-old man presented initially for the evaluation and management of a thyroid nodule, which was noted incidentally on imaging. Further evaluation revealed the presence of a papillary thyroid carcinoma. A total thyroidectomy was performed and he immediately started taking levothyroxine as the standard replacement therapy. Based on his stage of cancer, TSH suppression was not required and therefore the TSH goal was to remain within the normal reference range. The initial dose was calculated based on his weight, and he started taking 150 µg of levothyroxine daily.

Two months after starting levothyroxine, his TSH was normal at 0.89 µIU/mL (reference range 0.40–5.00). At that time, he complained of some fatigue, particularly at the end of the day, which he characterized as unusual for him in comparison to his baseline prior to surgery. No change was made in his regimen as the serum TSH concentration was in the lower end of normal range.

Four months after starting levothyroxine, his symptoms progressed. He described his fatigue as "extreme" and he reported weight gain. He was unable to complete his

J. Tsai, M.D. • N. Stathatos, M.D. (✉)
Thyroid Unit, Massachusetts General Hospital, Harvard Medical School,
15 Parkman Street, WAC 7-730S, Boston, MA 02114, USA
e-mail: nstathatos@partners.org

© Springer Science+Business Media New York 2015
T.F. Davies (ed.), *A Case-Based Guide to Clinical Endocrinology*,
DOI 10.1007/978-1-4939-2059-4_11

usual workout at the gym. His TSH remained in the normal range at 3.11 μIU/mL. At that time, the possible management options included watchful waiting with the same therapy or the addition of liothyronine to his replacement regimen. After discussion with the patient, he chose to wait and monitor his symptoms without further intervention.

However, 6 months after starting levothyroxine, his symptoms persisted without any improvement. Based on a repeat discussion with the patient, 5 μg of liothyronine once daily in the morning was added to the levothyroxine 125 μg daily. A TSH level was not checked at this time as the TSH level had been consistently within normal reference range on the stable levothyroxine dose and the liothyronine trial was for symptomatic improvement. After 4 weeks, he reported no improvement. The liothyronine dose was increased to 5 μg twice a day and the levothyroxine was decreased by 75 μg/week. After this change, he started noticing improvement. His fatigue improved and he was able to go to gym again.

As he was not yet back to baseline, 3 months after adding liothyronine to his regimen, the liothyronine dose was increased to 10 μg in the morning and 5 mcg in the early afternoon. He then reported feeling "almost back to my old self again." His subsequent TSH was 0.1 μIU/mL. Given his excellent overall physical status and the significant clinical improvement on the current regimen, no further changes were immediately planned. The option of slightly lowering the levothyroxine dose further in order to allow the TSH to return within reference range could be discussed at future visits. His case illustrates the utility of adding liothyronine to patients already on levothyroxine for the treatment of hypothyroidism.

## Review of How the Diagnosis Was Made

Under normal circumstances, the main hormone product of the thyroid gland is thyroxine (T4). About 90 % of the total daily hormone product of the thyroid gland is thyroxine and 10 % is liothyronine (T3). T3 is the biologically active hormone. Thyoxine is converted into liothyronine in the periphery, the liver being a major site. After documentation of this peripheral conversion of T4 to T3, levothyroxine has become the mainstay of thyroid hormone replacement. However, as some patients report hypothyroid symptoms despite T4 replacement and a serum TSH concentration within normal reference range, as in this patient's case, the use of combination T4 and T3 therapy could be considered. In this case, as the liothyronine was increased, the levothyroxine dose was decreased. The liothyronine was dosed as a twice a day dose given its short half-life and rapid gastrointestinal absorption in comparison. Peak levels of liothyronine are 2–4 h after administration and steady-state cannot be achieved with once daily dosing. The dose changes of liothyronine were in small increments and increased gradually, similar to the standard practice with levothyroxine. As this was a trial to determine symptomatic improvement with only small dose changes, the dose of liothyronine was titrated mainly to symptoms only. As he reported improvement with the combination therapy, he proved to be a patient who benefited with combination therapy. As discussed in detail below, there are no other current clinically available options to distinguish responders prior to initiation of combination therapy. A trial of adding liothyronine with gradual dose changes is the only available way to determine who will respond positively to combination therapy of T3 and T4.

## Lessons Learned

### *Combination Therapy Trials*

As in the case described, practitioners have patients who report persistent symptoms despite a serum TSH concentration within normal limits on levothyroxine therapy alone. Several randomized trials have been conducted to answer the question of whether T3 and T4 combination therapy is beneficial. A review of nine controlled trials showed only one study with beneficial effects of combination therapy on mood, quality of life, and psychometric performance when compared with T4 therapy alone [1]. Also, a meta-analysis of eleven studies in which 1,216 patients were randomized showed no difference in the effectiveness of combination therapy versus T4 therapy alone [2].

Specifically, in a large, double-blind, randomized controlled trial of 697 hypothyroid patients, a group assigned to partial substitution of 50 μg of T4 by 10 μg of T3 was compared to a group on the original T4 dose [3]. At baseline, the serum TSH concentrations were within normal limits and similar between groups. At 3 months, there was significant improvement in the General Health Questionnaire (GHQ) in both groups, demonstrating a large placebo effect. This improvement was sustained at 12 months in both groups. This study did not demonstrate conclusive evidence of a beneficial effect of combining T3 and T4 therapy. However, a limitation of this study is the result of rise in TSH and a fall in serum T4 in the intervention group, indicating under replacement with T4 in this group for the duration of the study.

### *Effect of Polymorphisms in Type-2 Deiodinase*

Despite the lack of available consistent evidence showing benefit of combination T3 and T4 therapy, anecdotally, some patients prefer combination therapy. More recently, an analysis of the effect of variants of type-2 deiodinase, which converts T4 to T3, on psychological well-being and response to combined therapy, may explain these anecdotal observations. In the study described above, the relationship between common variants in three deiodinase genes and the baseline psychological well-being and improvement on combined T4–T3 therapy was examined [4]. The CC genotype of the rs225014 polymorphism in the deiodinase 2 gene (DIO2) was present in 16 % of the study population and was associated with worse baseline

General Health Questionnaire (GHQ) scores in patients on T4. Interestingly, this genotype showed greater improvement on combination therapy compared to patients on T4 alone. This variant in type-2 deiodinase could explain why some patients prefer combination therapy. It is not yet known if genotyping patients with hypothyroidism who are clinically and biochemically euthyroid will identify which patients are most likely to benefit from combination therapy.

## Treatment

Adding T3 to a regimen can be done by using preparations of T3 alone, combination preparations, or desiccated thyroid. Adding T3 alone to patients already on levothyroxine allows for adjustment of the T3 to T4 ratio tailored to each individual patient. The optimal ratio of T3 to T4 is not yet determined and may range from approximately 1:3 to 1:5. Caution should be taken against oversuppression of the serum TSH concentration in order to avoid both short-term and long-term adverse effects. In this patient described, he was of a relatively young age and could therefore be expected to tolerate some TSH suppression in comparison to an elderly patient with the same serum TSH concentration level. If he developed adverse effects or had further TSH suppression to undetectable levels, decreasing the levothyroxine dose could be considered as the next change in management.

In summary, current guidelines recommend levothyroxine as the mainstay of treatment for hypothyroid patients [5]. However, treatment decisions should be individualized and combination therapy can be considered in hypothyroid patients who are biochemically euthyroid but symptomatic. Although reviews of combination therapy studies generally show no benefit, more recent studies on the polymorphisms of the DIO2 gene offer a direction for future management for therapy tailored to patients. Currently, a trial of combination of liothyronine and levothyroxine is reasonable after careful discussion with the patient. The optimal ratio of T3:T4 is not yet certain and usually ranges from 1:3 to 1:5. The dose should be titrated to symptoms and excessive over suppression of serum TSH concentration should be avoided.

## Questions

1. A 64 y/o woman with hypothyroidism complains of ongoing fatigue and "brain fog." She asks you for advice on T4/T3 combination therapy. You explain that:

   (a) This therapy is restricted to patients with documented type 2 deiodinase deficiency.
   (b) It is associated with significant weight loss, but no effect on energy level and well-being.

(c) It has been shown not to be superior to thyroxine alone in several studies, but because of anecdotic reports of benefit it can be tried on an individual basis.

(d) It is contraindicated in patients requiring complete TSH suppression.

2. In comparison with levothyroxine, lyothyronine (T3) has the following characteristics:

(a) It is less potent and longer lasting.

(b) Its effects are most prominent on the heart and bone primarily, while T4 is more active in the CNS.

(c) It is the active hormone on all thyroid hormone-sensitive tissues, while T4 in itself does not bind the thyroid hormone receptor in any organ.

(d) It requires activation in the nucleus of sensitive cells to exert its effects.

3. A 65 y/o man has had a total thyroidectomy 8 months ago for a benign multinodular goiter. Four months ago, he reported fatigue and weight gain of 4 lbs since the operation. You added liothyronine, 5 mcg bid, to his replacement regimen of levothyroxine 112 mcg daily. He now reports feeling well. His TFTs show normal FT4 and low TSH at 0.1 mcU/mL. You take the following measure:

(a) Stop the liothyronine.

(b) Decrease the levothyroxine.

(c) Make no changes to his regimen stating that minimal TSH suppression is not harmful.

(d) Add a beta-blocker.

## Answers to Questions

1. (c) Several studies have addressed the addition of T3 to T4 in the treatment of hypothyroid patients. Most placebo-controlled studies have failed to show a statistically significant benefit. However, most experts agree that those studies may not be powered enough to identify subpopulations of patients benefiting from this regimen. Therefore, recent guidelines indicate that a trial of combination T4/T3 might be tried in selected cases.

2. (c) Thyroid hormone action is entirely mediated by T3, which is the only natural hormone able to bind the thyroid hormone receptor. T4, the main product of the thyroid gland, acts as a prohormone. T4 is transformed into T3 by activating deiodinases. While thyroid secretes a small amount of T3, most T3 in the body derives from deiodination in the target tissues and in the liver. The differential regulation of this process remains only partially understood.

3. (b) When T4/T3 combination therapy is instituted and found to be beneficial, caution needs to avoid excessive TSH suppressions in categories at risk. The goal of thyroid hormone replacement in a patient older than 60 with benign thyroid disease is normalization of TSH. A suppressed TSH carries an increased

risk of atrial fibrillation in this category and should be avoided. While stopping the liothyronine is an option, the same can be achieved by decreasing the thyroxine dose. This would at least in theory allow to maintain the benefits achieved without exposing the patient to the consequences of overtreatment.

# References

1. Escobar-Morreale HF, Botella-Carretero JI, Escobar del Rey F, Morreale de Escobar G. REVIEW: treatment of hypothyroidism with combinations of levothyroxine plus liothyronine. JCEM. 2005;90(8):4946–54.
2. Grozinsky-Glasberg S, Fraser A, Nahshoni E, Weizman A, Leibovici L. Thyroxine-triiodothyronine combination therapy versus thyroxinemonotherapy for clinical hypothyroidism: meta-analysis of randomized controlled trials. JCEM. 2006;91(7):2592–9.
3. Saravanan P, Simmons D, Greenwood R, Peters TJ, Dayan CM. Partial substitution of thyroxine (T4) with tri-iodothyronine in patients on T4 replacement therapy: results of a large community-based randomized controlled trial. JCEM. 2005;90(2):805–12.
4. Panicker V, Saravana P, Vaidya B, Evans J, Hattersley AT, Frayling TM, Dayan CM. Common variation in the DIO2 gene predicts baseline psychological well-being and response to combination thyroxine plus triiodothyronine therapy in hypothyroid patients. JCEM. 2009;94(5): 1623–9.
5. Garber JR, Cobin RH, Gharib H, Hennessey JV, Klein I, Mechanick JI, Pessah-Pollack R, Singer PA, Woeber KA, American Association of Clinical Endocrinologists and American Thyroid Association Taskforce on Hypothyroidism in Adults. Clinical practice guidelines for hypothyroidism in adults: cosponsored by the American Association of Clinical Endocrinologists and the American Thyroid Association. Endocr Pract. 2012;18(6):988–1028.

# Chapter 12
# Hypothyroidism in Pregnancy

**Raffaella M. Colzani**

## Objectives

This case history aims to illustrate the treatment of hypothyroidism in pregnancy, in particular the recommendation for levothyroxine rather than triiodothyronine (T3) containing thyroid hormone replacement. It will then address the recommendation for iodine supplementation in pregnancy.

## Case Presentation

The patient is a 33-year-old woman with past medical history of depression and herniated discs who was diagnosed with subclinical hypothyroidism 2 years ago at her yearly physical (Table 12.1). At the time of diagnosis, she had no symptoms except for several years of cold intolerance, occasional palpitations, and insomnia. The recommendation was made to start thyroid hormone replacement but she refused treatment.

At the 3 months follow-up, she complained of cold intolerance, constipation, dry skin, and feeling fatigued to the point of requiring a nap in the afternoon. The laboratory tests confirmed overt hypothyroidism (Table 12.1). Again, the recommendation was made to start levothyroxine. She opted not to be treated conventionally with levothyroxine. Rather, after consulting with an alternative medicine physician, she started Nature-Throid (N-T) 16.25 mg BID. Nature-Throid® (Thyroid USP) tablets of desiccated thyroid for oral use is a preparation derived from porcine thyroid glands. The preparation provides 38 mcg levothyroxine (T4) and 9 mcg liothyronine

R.M. Colzani, M.D. (✉)
Mount Auburn Endocrinology, 355 Waverley Oaks Road, Suite 250, Waltham, MA, USA
e-mail: rcolzani@mah.harvard.edu

© Springer Science+Business Media New York 2015
T.F. Davies (ed.), *A Case-Based Guide to Clinical Endocrinology*,
DOI 10.1007/978-1-4939-2059-4_12

**Table 12.1** Thyroid hormone levels before and during treatment with Nature-Throid. Thyroid hormone levels in pregnancy during treatment with N-T and during treatment with levothyroxine. Anti-thyroid antibodies levels

| | TSH (0.3–4.7 mIU/mL) | FT4 (0.8–1.8 ng/dL) | TT3 (60–180 ng/dL) | FT3 (2.3–4.2 pg/mL) | TgAb (<60 U/mL) | TPOAb (<60 U/mL) |
|---|---|---|---|---|---|---|
| At diagnosis | 8.2 | 0.9 | | | | |
| 3 months follow-up | 10.1 | 0.9 | | | | |
| 6 months follow-up On N-T 16.25 mcg BID | 8.1 | | | | | |
| 1 year follow-up On N-T 32.5 mcg BID | 0.8 | 0.8 | 164 | | | |
| 18 month follow-up 7 weeks 5 days pregnant On N-T 32. mcg BID | 2.18 | | | | | |
| 8 weeks pregnant On N-T 32.5 mcg BID | 3.32 | 0.6 | 216 | 4.1 | 143 | 38 |
| 12 weeks pregnant On levothyroxine 137 mcg/day | 1.5 | 1 | | | | |

(T3) for each 65 mg (1 Grain) tablet. T3 is approximately four times as potent as T4 on a microgram for microgram basis.

Subsequently, TSH was monitored approximately every 3–6 months. N-T was adjusted accordingly once after 3 months of treatment when it was increased to 32.5 mg BID, as at that point TSH was still elevated (Table 12.1).

At the 1 year follow up, after 6 months on desiccated thyroid 32.5 mg BID: TSH, FT4, TT3 were obtained and were normal (Table 12.1).

At the 18th month mark, 6 months after the last TSH was obtained, the patient became pregnant. She established care with a nurse midwife at the local natural birth center. At the initial pregnancy visit, 7 weeks, 5 days of gestation, the TSH was normal for the first trimester of pregnancy at 2.18 mIU/mL. The patient was referred for endocrinology consultation for treatment of hypothyroidism in pregnancy, as the nurse midwife was unfamiliar with adjusting desiccated thyroid.

Two days later, the patient was seen in endocrinology consultation. She was 8 weeks pregnant. She complained of feeling stressed and fatigued; she continued to complain of cold intolerance, palpitations, and insomnia, all of which were present long before the diagnosis of hypothyroidism. She reported a new complaint of nausea without vomiting in the morning, which she attributes to her pregnancy.

She was taking Nature-Throid 32.5 mg BID and prenatal vitamins at bedtime containing iodine derived from kelp.

Her family history and social history were unremarkable.

On exam, she was well appearing with a nontender palpable thyroid without nodules. No neck lymphadenopathy. She had a fine tremor of the outstretched fingers. The remainder of the physical exam was unremarkable.

Laboratory tests done when the patient was 8 weeks pregnant are reported in Table 12.1.

After reviewing the laboratory tests, the patient was informed that her hypothyroidism was due to Hashimoto's thyroiditis and that one of her thyroid hormone, T4 was low. She was advised that her current treatment with desiccated thyroid did not provide sufficient thyroid hormone to the fetus. I explained that the total T3 was still within normal range for pregnancy (upper range for pregnancy 1.5× upper normal range).

Desiccated thyroid was discontinued and brand name levothyroxine was recommended instead.

Her N-T 65 mg daily was converted to levothyroxine 100 mcg/day using a conversion chart. In addition, a 30–40 % increase in her pre-pregnancy thyroid hormone replacement dose was calculated. As a result, she was prescribed brand name levothyroxine, 137 mcg/day.

In addition, after noticing that her prenatal vitamin contained iodine derived from kelp, recommendation was made to switch to a multivitamin containing iodine in the form of potassium iodide 150 mcg/day.

One week later, at the ninth week of pregnancy, she called to discuss her worries. After viewing her laboratory tests on the patient portal, she searched online the effects of low maternal thyroid hormone in pregnancy. She was seeking advice on termination of her pregnancy. I explained to her that it is still debated whether hypothyroxinemia alone causes adverse effects on the developing fetus. I advise her against termination of pregnancy.

At her 12th weeks of pregnancy laboratory tests were obtained and both TSH and free T4 were in normal range for pregnancy (Table 12.1).

Recommendation was made to continue brand name levothyroxine 137 mcg/day.

## Review on How the Diagnosis Was Made

The fetal thyroid begins concentrating iodine at 10–12 weeks of gestation and is controlled by pituitary TSH by approximately 20 weeks of gestation. Fetal serum levels of TSH, TBG, FT4, and FT3 increase throughout gestation, reaching mean adult levels at approximately 36 weeks of gestation.

Maternal thyroid stimulating hormone does not cross the placenta, and only small amounts of maternal thyroxine (T4) and minimal amount of triiodothyronine (T3) cross the placenta. T4 crosses the placenta much more than T3 does [1]. Maternal T4 is therefore the only significant source of thyroid hormone before the development of the fetal thyroid at 13–15 weeks gestation.

When assessing a pregnant woman with hypothyroidism, appropriate maternal TSH levels in patients treated with T3 or T4/T3 combinations may be accompanied by insufficient fetal thyroid hormone levels. In the case presented, the diagnosis was made by obtaining not only the TSH but also FT4 by immunoassay. In spite of a normal TSH, FT4 was low. The results were confirmed by equilibrium dialysis. The normal TSH measured at week 8 of pregnancy was misleading. The maternal TSH was disproportionately affected by the orally administered T3 which exerts a negative feedback on the maternal TSH while only minimally reaching the fetus. In other words, a normal TSH was achieved in this woman with lower than usual daily T4 dose. Indeed her FT4 was low reflecting the abnormal T4/T3 ratio contained in desiccated porcine thyroid.

Women with hypothyroidism are at increased risk for both complications of pregnancy and adverse neonatal outcomes. If the hypothyroidism is not treated, there is increased risk of a miscarriage, gestational hypertension, placental abruption, and postpartum hemorrhage. Overt untreated maternal hypothyroidism is associated with premature birth, low birth weight, and neonatal respiratory distress. Just as importantly, a study showed that children born from untreated women with hypothyroidism had an IQ a few points below the IQ of children born from healthy women and the IQ of children born from adequately treated women with hypothyroidism [1]. Other studies observed an IQ reduction in the offspring of mothers with hypothyroidism and with isolated hypothyroxinemia in the first trimester [2–4].

Regarding our patient's iodine status, one may be tempted to assume that since she has always lived in the USA, her iodine intake is probably sufficient. A study done in the Boston area, however, surprisingly found that approximately 40 % of the women sampled may have mild iodine deficiency [5].

## Lessons Learned

### *Thyroid Hormone Preparations for Treatment of Hypothyroidism in Pregnancy*

The appropriate treatment and follow up of hypothyroidism in pregnancy is extremely important in order to avoid the consequences of lack of thyroid hormone on the mother, on the pregnancy, on the neonate, and on the fetal brain development. One should not assume that normal TSH in pregnant women treated with T3 or T4/ T3 combination reflects fetal exposure to normal maternal thyroid hormone. In this case the developing fetus was likely exposed to insufficient levels of maternal T4.

For the reasons listed above, the American Thyroid Association (ATA) guidelines strongly recommend against the use of thyroid preparations other than levothyroxine in pregnancy. In women who are well-maintained on levothyroxine, T4 can cross the placenta, as it would do in normal, euthyroid, pregnant women.

Although this is a case of maternal pre-existing hypothyroidism, indeed treatment with dessicated thyroid resulted in isolated hypothyroxinemia in our patient, when she was 8 weeks pregnant. In patients without known thyroid disease, there is controversy on whether isolated hypothyroxinemia in pregnancy should be treated. The ATA guidelines do not recommend treatment for women with hypothyroxinemia [6], while the Endocrine Society 2012 Updated guidelines state that "in the opinion of the committee, partial replacement therapy may be initiated at the discretion of the caregiver, with continued monitoring" [7].

### *Adjusting Levothyroxine Treatment in Pregnancy in Women with Preexisting Hypothyroidism*

In preexisting maternal hypothyroidism, a study aimed at calculating and timing the increase in thyroid hormone in pregnancy concluded that levothyroxine should be increased by 30–50 % once pregnancy is confirmed in order to timely meet the increased requirement of thyroid hormone in pregnancy [8].

The goal of treatment with levothyroxine is to normalize maternal serum TSH values within the trimester specific pregnancy reference range (first trimester 0.1– 2.5 mIU/L, second trimester 0.2–3 mIU/L, third trimester 0.3–3 mIU/L) [6, 7, 9]. Frequency of follow-ups in pregnancy should be every 4–6 weeks with measurement of TSH and FT4. Levothyroxine dose should be adjusted accordingly.

In our patient, the pre-pregnancy thyroid hormone dose could have been calculated based on the patient weight or by converting her current Nature-Throid dose to levothyroxine with the help of a "desiccated thyroid to levothyroxine conversion guide" or simply by multiplying by 4 the T3 content and adding it to the T4 content. Once calculated, the pre-pregnancy levothyroxine dose (approximately 100 mcg) was immediately increased by 30–40 % (137 mcg/day). After 4 weeks on this dose of levothyroxine, at week 12 of gestation, TSH and FT4 were both within pregnancy normal levels (Table 12.1).

As patients who take generic levothyroxine may, with each prescription refill, receive product from any one of the various manufacturers of generic levothyroxine, brand name levothyroxine was recommended to this patient to maintain the narrow therapeutic range required in pregnancy.

## Iodine Supplementation in Pregnancy

In iodine-sufficient areas, maternal iodine intake must be increased during pregnancy in order to compensate for the 20–40 % increase in thyroid hormone need and to provide for the fetal thyroid hormone synthesis. Therefore, iodine stores should be replete at conception with an iodine intake of more than 150 µg/day [10]. In pregnant women, the Institute of Medicine recommends daily iodine intake of 220 µg, the World Health Organization recommends daily iodine intake of 250 µg, while the ATA recommends a multivitamin with iodine level of 150 µg/day [11]. The patient presented was taking a prenatal vitamin with iodine derived from kelp. An analysis of various over-the-counter and prescription prenatal vitamins concluded that kelp did not deliver reliable iodine levels and varied by as much as 50 % from the stated levels. Ten brands had iodine values that delivered less than half the stated iodine level [10]. Hence the recommendation to discontinue the current prenatal vitamin and to start one with 150 µg iodine not derived from kelp in this patient.

## Termination of Pregnancy Not Recommended for Maternal Hypothyroidism

There is no available data to support termination of pregnancy in maternal hypothyroidism. The ATA, the Endocrine Society, and the American College of Obstetrics and Gynecologists (ACOG) all agree that aggressive thyroid hormone replacement should be given as soon as possible but early termination is not warranted [6, 7, 12]. When counseling pregnant women who have been exposed to hypothyroidism early during the pregnancy, it is important to observe that the study published in the NEJM by Haddow et al. included women with a wide range of TSH elevations, and that the IQ of their offspring, while slightly lower than the control group, was still in the normal range [13]. Another recent study does not exclude subtle changes in intellectual function but agrees that children born from women with maternal hypothyroidism likely have a normal cognitive outcome [14].

In summary, this is a case of a woman diagnosed with hypothyroidism and treated with desiccated porcine thyroid (T4/T3) during her reproductive years, then later found to be pregnant. Complication of treatment and the possibility of congenital hypothyroidism with T4/T3 and T3 during pregnancy were discussed. The recommendation of treatment with levothyroxine in pregnancy, and perhaps in all women of reproductive age, and optimization of iodine intake during pregnancy are also discussed.

## Questions

1. A 26 y/o woman with a history of hypothyroidism presents on consultation at the 28th week of her first pregnancy. She is currently taking levothyroxine 175 mcg daily and a multivitamin containing iodine. She shows you results of thyroid function tests obtained earlier during pregnancy by another physician. Her TSH has been consistently in the 0.8–1.5 mU/L range. She is extremely worried, as she has just received her latest TSH results, which came back at 2.85 mU/L. You:

    (a) Increase the levothyroxine dose to 200 mcg daily, as the TSH goal in pregnancy is < 2.5 mU/L.
    (b) Reassure her that in the last trimester of pregnancy a TSH <3 is adequate.
    (c) You stop the multivitamin, as it is most likely decreasing the absorption of levothyroxine.
    (d) Order a fetal ultrasound to assess the fetus for intrauterine growth restriction.

2. You examine a 28 y/o woman who seeks prenatal counseling regarding management of her hypothyroidism during pregnancy. Since her surgery for Graves' disease 3 years ago, she has been on levothyroxine and liothyronine. Besides recommending measurement of TSH receptor antibodies, you advise her that:

    (a) Any thyroid hormone replacement regimen keeping her TSH in the normal range is acceptable.
    (b) An increase in the relative T3 content of the regimen will be necessary as soon as she becomes pregnant.
    (c) She should switch to a thyroxine-only regimen, and adjust to a normal TSH level, before she becomes pregnant.
    (d) She should switch to a thyroxine-only regimen, and adjust to a normal TSH level, after the first trimester.

3. With regard to iodine supplementation in pregnancy:

    (a) Only women with hypothyroidism should supplement their diet with iodine.
    (b) Women who are taking thyroid hormone do not need iodine supplementation, as their thyroid function is being replaced already.
    (c) The W.H.O. recommends daily supplementations with up to 250 mcg iodine in all women to prevent untoward fetal effects of severe or moderate iodine deficiency.
    (d) A kelp-derivate iodine supplement provides an ideal form of iodine supplementation.

# Answers

1. (b) Normal TSH range and TSH goals for thyroid hormone replacement therapy vary with the pregnancy trimester. In the first trimester, TSH levels tend to be lower in normal pregnancy, due to high HCG levels stimulating the thyroid gland and therefore slightly increasing thyroid hormone production. More importantly, the fetal thyroid starts secreting thyroid hormone only around the 14th week, while the fetal neurological development requires small amounts of thyroid hormone early on. Therefore, in the first trimester, the fetus entirely relies on the maternal thyroid hormone and all efforts should be made to maintain TSH levels in the normal range for that trimester, 0.1–2.5 mU/L. In the third trimester, declining HCG levels are associated with a wider TSH normal range. In addition, the fetal thyroid is now fully functional, making the maternal thyroid hormone contribution negligible and therefore irrelevant. For this reason, strict adherence to a narrow TSH goal is not necessary in the third trimester.
2. (c) T4/T3 combination replacement is contraindicated during pregnancy. Women on combination therapy will require a relatively lower T4 dose to achieve euthyroidism. Since only T4 crosses the placenta in significant amounts, T4/T3 combination therapy carries the risk of exposing the fetus to suboptimal T4 levels. This is thought to be particularly critical during the first trimester, when the fetal thyroid has not started producing thyroid hormone yet.
3. (c) Pregnancy is a state of increased iodine need, as the maternal thyroidal function increases early on. In addition, the developing fetal thyroid uses a quota of the total maternal dietary iodine. This puts women at risk for marginal iodine deficiency in pregnancy, even in geographic areas considered to be iodine sufficient. Even mild iodine deficiency is associated with an increased maternal and neonatal thyroidal volume, and with defective neurological development of the fetus. Therefore, the W.H.O. recommends that all pregnant women receive iodine supplementation, up to 250 mcg daily. Iodine-sufficient regions like the United States may require lower doses.

# References

1. de Escobar GM, Obregon MJ, del Rey FE. Maternal thyroid hormones early in pregnancy and fetal brain development. Best Pract Res Clin Endocrinol Metab. 2004;18(2):225–48.
2. Pop VJ, Brouwers EP, Vader HL, Vulsma T, van Baar AL, de Vijlder JJ. Maternal hypothyroxinaemia during early pregnancy and subsequent child development: a 3-year follow-up study. Clin Endocrinol (Oxf). 2003;59(3):282–8.
3. Li Y, Shan Z, Teng W, Yu X, Fan C, Teng X, et al. Abnormalities of maternal thyroid function during pregnancy affect neuropsychological development of their children at 25-30 months. Clin Endocrinol (Oxf). 2010;72(6):825–9.
4. Henrichs J, Bongers-Schokking JJ, Schenk JJ, Ghassabian A, Schmidt HG, Visser TJ, et al. Maternal thyroid function during early pregnancy and cognitive functioning in early childhood: the generation R study. J Clin Endocrinol Metab. 2010;95(9):4227–34.

5. Pearce EN, Leung AM, Blount BC, Bazrafshan HR, He X, Pino S, et al. Breast milk iodine and perchlorate concentrations in lactating Boston-area women. J Clin Endocrinol Metab. 2007;92(5):1673–7.

6. Stagnaro-Green A, Abalovich M, Alexander E, Azizi F, Mestman J, Negro R, et al. Guidelines of the American Thyroid Association for the diagnosis and management of thyroid disease during pregnancy and postpartum. Thyroid. 2011;21(10):1081–125.

7. Endocrine Society, American Association of Clinical Endocrinologists, Asia & Oceania Thyroid Association, American Thyroid Association, European Thyroid Association, Latin American Thyroid Association. Management of thyroid dysfunction during pregnancy and postpartum: an Endocrine Society Clinical Practice Guideline. Thyroid. 2007;17(11):1159–67.

8. Alexander EK, Marqusee E, Lawrence J, Jarolim P, Fischer GA, Larsen PR. Timing and magnitude of increases in levothyroxine requirements during pregnancy in women with hypothyroidism. N Engl J Med. 2004;351(3):241–9.

9. Panesar NS, Li CY, Rogers MS. Reference intervals for thyroid hormones in pregnant Chinese women. Ann Clin Biochem. 2001;38(Pt 4):329–32.

10. Leung AM, Pearce EN, Braverman LE. Iodine content of prenatal multivitamins in the United States. N Engl J Med. 2009;360(9):939–40.

11. Becker DV, Braverman LE, Delange F, Dunn JT, Franklyn JA, Hollowell JG, et al. Iodine supplementation for pregnancy and lactation-United States and Canada: recommendations of the American Thyroid Association. Thyroid. 2006;16(10):949–51.

12. American College of Obstetrics and Gynecology. ACOG practice bulletin. Thyroid disease in pregnancy. Number 37, August 2002. American College of Obstetrics and Gynecology. Int J Gynaecol Obstet. 2002;79(2):171–80.

13. Haddow JE, Palomaki GE, Allan WC, Williams JR, Knight GJ, Gagnon J, et al. Maternal thyroid deficiency during pregnancy and subsequent neuropsychological development of the child. N Engl J Med. 1999;341(8):549–55.

14. Downing S, Halpern L, Carswell J, Brown RS. Severe maternal hypothyroidism corrected prior to the third trimester is associated with normal cognitive outcome in the offspring. Thyroid. 2012;22(6):625–30.

# Chapter 13
# Hypothyroid Myopathy and Thelogen Effluvium

**Giuseppe Barbesino**

## Objectives

Describing common and uncommon manifestations of hypothyroidism and rapid changes in thyroid function.

## Case

A 20-year-old woman received 8 mCi I-131 for Graves' disease. She had received methimazole for the 2 months preceding the treatment and was euthyroid at the time of her treatment. However she had developed a rash while on methimazole and this prompted the I-131 treatment. Four weeks after I-131 treatment she presented for a scheduled follow-up appointment. She felt well and her TFTs demonstrated euthyroidism, albeit with a suppressed TSH (Table 13.1). One month later, she presented with severe muscle pains, rated at 8/10. Pains were most prominent in the left calf, which appeared slightly larger in diameter than the right, and in the right thigh, which appeared normal. Her laboratory tests (see Table 13.1) showed markedly elevated TSH, undetectable FT4 and extremely low T3 and Vitamin D. Her CPK was markedly elevated and her creatinine was in the normal range. Thyroxine, 100 mcg orally daily was prescribed. In addition, she was treated with lyothyronine 25 mcg twice a day orally for 10 days, with the purpose or restoring euthyroidism rapidly. High dose Vitamin D supplementation was also administered. Her symptoms improved rapidly and resolved completely in 1 week. Two months later blood

G. Barbesino, M.D. (✉)
Thyroid Unit, Massachusetts General Hospital, ACC730S, 15 Parkman St., Boston, MA 02114, USA
e-mail: gbarbesino@partners.org

© Springer Science+Business Media New York 2015
T.F. Davies (ed.), *A Case-Based Guide to Clinical Endocrinology*,
DOI 10.1007/978-1-4939-2059-4_13

**Table 13.1** Thyroid function test and CPK course. Levothyroxine replacement treatment was started on day 60

| Days after I-131 | TSH (mcU/L), 0.4–5.0 | FT4 (ng/mL), 0.9–1.8 | T3 (ng/dL), 60–181 | CK (IU/L), 40–150 |
|---|---|---|---|---|
| 0 | 0.01 | 1.2 | 192 | |
| 28 | <0.01 | 1.2 | 145 | |
| 60 | 170.88 | <0.4 | 13 | |
| 61 | | | | 4,878 |
| 64 | 119.30 | 0.7 | 49 | 3,405 |
| 94 | 0.15 | | | |
| 175 | 0.04 | 1.7 | | 83 |

tests showed normal thyroid function and her CPK was in the normal range. She felt very well. One month later, she presented with complaint of severe hair loss. She described clumps of hair falling with each shower and was worried that she "would go bald." On exam there were no patches of baldness or male pattern alopecia. The hair was slightly thinner all over. Her thyroid function tests remained normal. She was reassured that this was a transient phenomenon. Three more months later, the hair loss had stopped and 6 months later she reported a complete restoration of her previous hair quality.

## Review of How the Diagnosis Was Made

This patient presented with severe muscle aches and objective findings of muscle swelling. Her muscle enzymes demonstrated severe hypothyroid myopathy, in association with rapid onset post-I-131 hypothyroidism. Her subsequent course was characterized by hair loss. The exam of her scalp revealed only mild hair thinning and no focal areas of alopecia, leading to a diagnosis of telogen effluvium.

## Lessons Learned

Statistically, the symptoms of hypothyroidism are correlated to the severity of the hormonal deficiency [1]. However there is significant variability [2]. Some patients may report prominent fatigue with modest TSH elevations, while others may be surprisingly free of symptoms, even when profoundly hypothyroid. Unrecognized individual factors may play a role in this variability. The rate of thyroid hormone loss may also be important, with patients in whom hypothyroidism develops rapidly being more symptomatic. Patients with thyroid cancer and surgical hypothyroidism whose thyroxine replacement dose is suddenly held in preparation of radioiodine scanning become typically very symptomatic in a short period of time. Of course these patients are also profoundly hypothyroid, more so than the average patient with Hashimoto's thyroiditis, whose milder hypothyroidism develops over a long period of time.

Mild muscle and joint aches are common in hypothyroidism. In a study from Canaris [1] muscle aches were among the most specific symptoms in identifying patients with hypothyroidism. Moderately to markedly elevated creatine phosphokinase (CPK) levels are observed in up to 60 % of patients with overt hypothyroidism [3]. These manifestations have been loosely referred to as "hypothyroid myopathy." The etiology of hypothyroid myopathy remains unclear. A few pathology studies have shown selective loss of type-II fibers, increased nuclear counts and diffuse glycogen inclusions [4]. The range of clinical manifestations is wide, ranging from patients being completely asymptomatic with minimal CPK elevation, some others with significant but nonprogressive myalgias and a small minority developing severe myopathy, rhabdomyolisis, compartment syndrome, and renal failure [5]. The concurrent use of statins may be a risk factor for the development of hypothyroid myopathy. This is demonstrated in several case reports of patients who developed the condition after many years of statin treatment when the hypothyroidism occurred [6]. Thus so far one can draw the following clinical suggestions:

1. Hypothyroidism should always be considered in the evaluation of a myopathy, whether in the setting of clinically silent CPK elevation, or in the presence of symptomatic muscle damage.
2. Patients who develop hypothyroidism while taking statins should be monitored carefully for evidence of muscle damage. Special caution should be used in thyroid cancer patients in whom rapid and profound hypothyroidism is purposely precipitated for radioiodine scanning and treatment.
3. Patients who develop significant muscle aches with severe hypothyroidism should be carefully monitored for the development of compartment syndrome and renal failure. Euthyroidism should be restored as quickly as possible. Lyothyronine in addition to thyroxine may prove beneficial although caution should be used in the elderly or cardiac patient.

After restoration of euthyroidism, the patient reported concerning hair loss. Hair changes are common in hypothyroidism. In the era of sensitive TSH testing and frequent screening, most patients with hypothyroidism are diagnosed with early and mild forms. The classical finding of coarse, brittle, and sparse hair, which is typically seen only in profound and prolonged hypothyroidism, is nowadays rarely observed. Alopecia areata can be observed with increased frequency in patients with Hashimoto's thyroiditis [7]. The association is independent of thyroid function status and reflects the common autoimmune background of the two conditions. Alopecia areata is characterized by patchy hair loss developing over a period of weeks or months. The condition is self-limited and remitting in a majority of cases, but it may result in partial or total permanent scalp hair loss (alopecia totalis) [8]. In our patient, the absence of patchy hair loss made alopecia areata unlikely. The history of sudden hair loss, without focal or regional baldness, in coincidence with recent rapid changes suggests the diagnosis of telogen effluvium. Human adult hair cycle is asynchronous, in that at any given moment there is a fraction of hair in the anagen, catagen, or telogen phase, respectively. As a consequence a small constant number of hairs is shed every day, as they end the telogen phase. In telogen effluvium, hair becomes synchronized and the majority of hair rapidly enters the telogen phase at the same time and is subsequently shed. This phenomenon is observed after pregnancy. During pregnancy hair is held in prolonged anagen as a consequence of the hormonal changes associated with pregnancy. This larger-than-normal proportion of hair in anagen then progresses to telogen synchronously after delivery. When the telogen phase is completed, some 3–4 months later, this hair is shed simultaneously, resulting in the distressing observation of large clumps of hair in the shower. However the intact follicles start producing new hair right away and over the next few months the hair is restored to its original thickness and quality. A similar phenomenon occurs after acute illnesses, except that the pathophysiology is sudden and synchronous exit from anagen [9]. This variety of telogen effluvium is particularly common after rapid changes in thyroid hormone levels. It is seen both after correction of hyperthyroidism or hypothyroidism, and after patients become suddenly hypothyroid, for example in preparation of whole body scanning. It is quite common to receive the distressed phone call from a patient who has noticed "clumps and clumps of hair coming off my scalp every day." In spite of the frequency of this observation, the literature on this topic is surprisingly limited. A few months after stable normal levels of thyroid hormone are achieved, hair regrowth and restoration of previous hair quality are observed. Since there is no known treatment or prevention for this self-limited condition, patients need only be counseled on its reversible nature. Rare forms of chronic telogen effluvium occur, but can be only diagnosed when failure of remission is observed. Understanding of this phenomenon by the endocrinologist will spare unnecessary dermatological consultations.

## Questions

1. A 68 y/o woman is referred for evaluation of hyperlipidemia. Her only medical problem is hypertension, controlled with hydrochlothiazide and a beta-blocker. Her total cholesterol is elevated at 312 mg/dL, her HDL is normal at 46 mg/dL, and her triglycerides are slightly elevated at 202 mg/dL. Her TSH is markedly elevated at 79 mU/L. As a next step, you:

   (a) Start levothyroxine, adjust the dose at 6 weeks intervals until her TSH is normalized, and then recheck her lipid profile
   (b) Start levothyroxine and a statin; recheck her TSH at 6 weeks intervals until her TSH is normalized.
   (c) Measure her FT4, then start a statin only if her FT4 is in the normal range, and start levothyroxine.
   (d) Measure thyroid-peroxydase antibody.

2. In hypothyroidism, multiple symptoms and signs can be present. In general:

   (a) Symptoms and manifestations are directly correlated to the thyroid hormone level.
   (b) Symptoms and manifestations occur in a ordinated fashion, with cardiovascular symptoms appearing with minimal thyroid dysfunction, metabolic symptoms with moderate thyroid dysfunction, and muscular-skeletal symptoms only present with profound thyroid dysfunction.
   (c) Symptoms and manifestations are highly variable from patient to patient and are not correlated to the thyroid hormone level.
   (d) Male-pattern baldness occurs in most females with hypothyroidism.

3. Which of the following is not a typical manifestation of hypothyroidism:

   (a) Myalgias
   (b) Arthralgias
   (c) Hair thinning
   (d) Bradycardia

## Answers

1. (a) Marked hypothyroidism is a possible cause of hyperlipidemia. The hyperlipidemia associated with hypothyroidism is reversible with restoration of euthyroidism. Therefore, in patients with hypothyroidism, treatment of hyperlipidemia should be instituted only if the hypercholesterolemia persists after euthyroidism is restored. Starting a statin in a hypothyroid patient increases the risk of myopathy.
2. (c) Classical symptoms of hypothyroidism are for the most part nonspecific and are present with surprising variability in different patients.
3. (c) Hair thinning is not typically seen in hypothyroidism. The classical description includes "sparse coarse hair."

## References

1. Canaris GJ, Steiner JF, Ridgway EC. Do traditional symptoms of hypothyroidism correlate with biochemical disease? J Gen Intern Med. 1997;12(9):544–50.
2. Tachman ML, Guthrie Jr GP. Hypothyroidism: diversity of presentation. Endocr Rev. 1984;5(3):456–65.
3. Hekimsoy Z, Oktem IK. Serum creatine kinase levels in overt and subclinical hypothyroidism. Endocr Res. 2005;31(3):171–5.
4. McKeran RO, Slavin G, Ward P, Paul E, Mair WG. Hypothyroid myopathy. A clinical and pathological study. J Pathol. 1980;132(1):35–54.
5. Croxson MS, Muir P, Choe MS. Rapid development of anterotibial compartment syndrome and rhabdomyolysis in a patient with primary hypothyroidism and adrenal insufficiency. Thyroid. 2012;22(6):651–3.

6. Lando HM, Burman KD. Two cases of statin-induced myopathy caused by induced hypothy-roidism. Endocr Pract. 2008;14(6):726–31.
7. Kurtev A, Iliev E. Thyroid autoimmunity in children and adolescents with alopecia areata. Int J Dermatol. 2005;44(6):457–61.
8. Finner AM. Alopecia areata: clinical presentation, diagnosis, and unusual cases. Dermatol Ther. 2011;24(3):348–54.
9. Harrison S, Sinclair R. Telogen effluvium. Clin Exp Dermatol. 2002;27(5):389–95.

# Part IV
# Thyroid Cancer

# Chapter 14
# Introduction

Kenneth D. Burman

In this Thyroid Section, we have presented several cases and clinical scenarios that are commonly encountered by clinicians. Drs. Chindris and Bernet describe a patient with a recently discovered thyroid nodule. Thyroid nodules are frequent and by autopsy study occur in about 12–37 % of individuals with 2.1 % having thyroid cancer [1]. The important issue is how to discriminate a thyroid nodule that is likely to be benign that can be monitored from a nodule more likely to harbor malignancy and should be more aggressively treated with thyroid surgery. Clinical history and features play an important role in this discrimination with, for example, a history of neck radiation, a family history of thyroid cancer, and local compression symptoms being worrisome for the presence of thyroid cancer [2]. Thyroid ultrasound characteristics are also important with shape (taller than wide), hazy borders, hypoechogenicity, increased internal vascularity, and microcalcifications suggesting (but not proving) the presence of thyroid cancer [3]. Serum TSH in the upper portion of the normal range is statistically correlated with the presence of thyroid cancer [4]. Of course, the cornerstone of the diagnostic approach is the performance of a thyroid Fine Needle Aspiration (FNA) [2]. Drs. Chindris and Bernet discuss the interpretation of an FNA in detail, but, in general, a thyroid FNA will be interpreted as benign, indeterminate, or consistent with malignancy (usually papillary thyroid cancer). Benign nodules generally can be monitored (with some exceptions) and malignant nodules (e.g., papillary thyroid cancer) require a thyroidectomy. The approach to an indeterminate cytology has improved recently due to the ability to perform molecular diagnostics. The likelihood of an indeterminate nodule harboring cancer is about 5–15 % for Atypia of Undetermined Significance (AUS), 15–30 % for follicular lesion, and 60–75 % for suspicious for papillary thyroid cancer [5]. There are two available molecular diagnostic tests or approaches presently available that can

K.D. Burman, M.D. (✉)
Endocrine Section, Medstar Washington Hospital Center, Washington, DC, USA

Department of Medicine, Georgetown University, Washington, DC, USA
e-mail: kenneth.d.burman@medstar.net

© Springer Science+Business Media New York 2015
T.F. Davies (ed.), *A Case-Based Guide to Clinical Endocrinology*,
DOI 10.1007/978-1-4939-2059-4_14

assist in helping to determine if an indeterminate nodule contains cancer [5, 6]. Drs. Chindris and Bernet discuss the molecular analysis and its clinical applicability in detail. They also discuss the appropriate management and monitoring for each type of thyroid nodule.

Drs. Goyal and Burman then discuss a patient with about a 3 cm nodule that on thyroid FNA was suspicious for papillary thyroid cancer. Thyroid cancer is increasing at an alarming rate with about 60,220 new cases projected to occur in 2013 [7]. The stages of thyroid cancer are reviewed. The TNM staging system is commonly utilized. Interestingly, patients under age 45 can only have Stage 1 (disease localized to the neck) or Stage 2 disease (disease outside of the neck). However, patients; 45 years and above are classified as having Stage 1 through 4 disease, where Stage 1 is localized to the thyroid and Stage 4 represents metastatic disease outside the neck area [2]. This TNM Staging System has been useful in predicting mortality, but it may not accurately represent recurrence rates. The TNM Staging System (as noted above), however, has been noted to have discrepancies in predicting mortality, especially in some (but not all) patients with metastatic thyroid cancer who are under age 45. In an effort to improve prognostication, it has now become commonplace to reassess patients approximately a year after treatment [8]. This risk adapted strategy seems to aid in the long term assessment of patients. That is, a patient, for example, may have metastatic disease to the lungs and bones at presentation, but then responds to the initial treatment (e.g., surgery and radioactive iodine and perhaps external radiation therapy to selected sites). If re-evaluation at 1 year reveals resolution of the metastatic lesions, these patients are considered to have a good long-term prognosis as compared to their original evaluation. Drs. Goyal and Burman review the common somatic molecular mutations that occur in thyroid cancer, with approximately 40–70 % of patients with papillary thyroid cancer having a BRAF mutation (BRAF V600E) and a lesser percentage having a RAS or Ret/PTC or a PAX8/PPAR gamma translocation (that occurs more frequently in follicular thyroid cancer) [5]. There is active debate whether a somatic BRAF mutation is associated with a worse prognosis as compared to patients who do not possess this mutation. Indications, benefits, and possible side effects of treatment modalities, surgery, and radioactive iodine are discussed [9–11].

Dr. Burch discusses a patient who presents with osseous metastasis from papillary thyroid cancer. This situation is serious and appropriate diagnosis and therapy are discussed. When analyzing tissue from a patient with metastatic disease and when it is relevant to consider thyroid cancer, tissue staining with thyroglobulin may be very useful. Patients who present with a distant metastatic lesion from thyroid cancer, after the diagnosis of thyroid cancer is confirmed, a total thyroidectomy is recommended following by radioactive iodine [2]. Dr. Burch discusses the importance of assessing such a patient for exposure to recent previous radiocontrast dye (e.g., CT with IV contrast). Such a dye load will preclude radioactive iodine scanning and treatment for perhaps 4–8 weeks and such patients should have serial spot urine iodine measurements to help determine when it would be appropriate to proceed with radioiodine scans and treatment. Preparation for radioactive iodine therapy may be either levothyroxine withdrawal or maintenance of levothyroxine therapy and the use of rhTSH stimulation [12]. Use of rhTSH stimulation for metastatic disease is not presently approved by the FDA but it is increasingly frequently being used clinically in this circumstance. Levothyroxine withdrawal may be associated with symptoms of fatigue, electrolyte abnormalities (e.g., hyponatremia) and decreased ability to perform routine daily activities including work. Two recent articles suggest that the use of rhTSH preparation for radioactive iodine therapy is associated with comparable beneficial effects as levothyroxine withdrawal [12, 13]. Further treatment of patients with distant metastatic lesion depends on the site, location, size, and clinical associations. External radiation may be effective as it is usually performed in patient with large osseous lesions, especially if they are impinging on vital structures (e.g., spinal cord) and/or are painful. Newer treatment techniques include radiofrequency ablation, laser ablation and/or tumor embolization [14]. Patients with osseous thyroid cancer metastases are also treated with bisphosphonates (usually IV) or denosumab (SQ) [14]. The frequency of these treatments is controversial in thyroid cancer.

Dr. Jonklaas reviews a patient with medullary thyroid cancer. Medullary thyroid cancer is distinct from differentiated thyroid cancer (papillary and follicular) in that is may occur sporadically or may be part of a familial genetic syndrome in which a germline RET oncogene mutation is present [15]. The pathologic and clinical manifestations and treatment modalities may be different than differentiated thyroid cancer. For example, medullary thyroid cancer does not respond to and is not treated with radioactive iodine therapy. Further, a normal serum TSH is maintained, rather than TSH suppression which is the goal in many patients with differentiated thyroid cancer. Depending on the series and the referral patterns, perhaps 20–30 % of patients with medullary thyroid cancer will have a germline RET mutation. RET mutations are most commonly part of the Multiple Endocrine Neoplasia (MEN) 2 syndrome, but also may be part of familial medullary thyroid cancer [15]. All patients with medullary thyroid cancer should be screened for a germline RET oncogene mutation. Frequently it is clear a patient has a family history of medullary thyroid cancer or a relevant genetic syndrome, but even some patients with apparently sporadic medullary thyroid cancer may actually have a RET mutation. Patients with a RET mutation must be screened initially and periodically for an associated pheochromocytome and hyperparathyroidism with hypercalcemia. It is recommended that a detected pheochromocytoma be removed prior to a thyroidectomy [15]. Moreover, all first degree relatives of a patient with a RET mutation must similarly be screened. A prophylactic thyroidectomy is considered in a screened RET oncogene positive first degree relative of a patient with known RET positive medullary thyroid cancer. Specific RET mutations are classified as low, medium and high risk disease and the timing of the thyroidectomy in the screened RET oncogene positive relative depends on clinical factors and the genetic site of the mutation [15]. The most important aspect of care of a medullary thyroid cancer patient is an expeditious total thyroidectomy with removal of lateral and central compartment lymph nodes as appropriate [15]. The prognosis of medullary thyroid cancer depends on the initial clinical and pathological findings. Patient with medullary thyroid cancer are monitored closely with serial calcitonin and CEA levels, neck ultrasounds, and neck examinations. Serum calcitonin is an excellent marker for the presence and extent of persistent or recurrent disease. The doubling time of serum calcitonin helps predict the progression and course of disease [16]. If the serum calcitonin is higher than approximately 250–400 pg/ml CT scans of neck and chest as well as MRI of the spine and liver (or a liver protocol CT) are indicated as medullary thyroid cancer typically metastasizes to these locations [15]. Appropriate therapy may include external radiation, chemo-or bland embolization of hepatic lesions, and/or directed therapy at a specific lesion (e.g., cryotherapy, laser therapy). Recently, two multikinase inhibitors, Vandetanib and Cabozantanib, have been approved by the FDA for systemic therapy for metastatic, progressive medullary thyroid cancer [17, 18]. These agents have multiple potential adverse effects, including fatigue, neutropenia, proteinuria, hypertension, and hand–foot syndrome. Prolongation of the QT interval may occur and there are specific physician requirements to administer Vandetanib and for EKG and cardiac monitoring of both of these agents. Further, they generally cause temporary stabilization of disease and experience with their long term use is limited [19–21].

In summary, these related thyroid nodule and cancer articles bring us up to date on how to diagnose, evaluate, treat, and monitor common presentations of thyroid cancer. This effort to manage aggressive thyroid cancer is optimally integrated into a multidisciplinary team. Entry into an appropriate clinical trial should also be considered when appropriate. Future studies will no doubt focus on improved molecular analysis of thyroid FNAs and histologically obtained thyroid tissue, and on better treatment modalities, for example, the development of better more targeted TKIs and, also, on combination TKI therapy in an attempt to decrease the development of thyroid cancer resistance to single TKI therapy.

# References

1. Mortensen JD, Woolner LB, Bennett WA. Gross and microscopic findings in clinically normal thyroid glands. J Clin Endocrinol Metab. 1955;15:1270–80.
2. Cooper DS, Doherty GM, Haugen BR, et al. Revised American Thyroid Association management guidelines for patients with thyroid nodules and differentiated thyroid cancer. Thyroid. 2009;19:1167–214.
3. Kim GR, Kim MH, Moon HJ, Chung WY, Kwak JY, Kim EK. Sonographic characteristics suggesting papillary thyroid carcinoma according to nodule size. Ann Surg Oncol. 2013;20: 906–13.
4. Jonklaas J, Nsouli-Maktabi H, Soldin SJ. Endogenous thyrotropin and triiodothyronine concentrations in individuals with thyroid cancer. Thyroid. 2008;18:943–52.
5. Nikiforov YE, Steward DL, Robinson-Smith TM, et al. Molecular testing for mutations in improving the fine-needle aspiration diagnosis of thyroid nodules. J Clin Endocrinol Metab. 2009;94:2092–8.
6. Alexander EK, Kennedy GC, Baloch ZW, et al. Preoperative diagnosis of benign thyroid nodules with indeterminate cytology. N Engl J Med. 2012;367:705–15.
7. Davies L, Welch HG. Increasing incidence of thyroid cancer in the United States, 1973–2002. JAMA. 2006;295:2164–7.

8. Tuttle RM, Tala H, Shah J, et al. Estimating risk of recurrence in differentiated thyroid cancer after total thyroidectomy and radioactive iodine remnant ablation: using response to therapy variables to modify the initial risk estimates predicted by the new American Thyroid Association staging system. Thyroid. 2010;20:1341–9.

9. Xing M, Alzahrani AS, Carson KA, et al. Association between BRAF V600E mutation and mortality in patients with papillary thyroid cancer. JAMA. 2013;309:1493–501.

10. Guerra A, Sapio MR, Marotta V, et al. The primary occurrence of BRAF(V600E) is a rare clonal event in papillary thyroid carcinoma. J Clin Endocrinol Metab. 2012;97:517–24.

11. Sarne DH. A piece of the puzzle: what does BRAF status mean in the management of patients with papillary thyroid carcinoma? J Clin Endocrinol Metab. 2012;97:3094–6.

12. Klubo-Gwiezdzinska J, Burman KD, Van Nostrand D, Mete M, Jonklaas J, Wartofsky L. Radioiodine treatment of metastatic thyroid cancer: relative efficacy and side effect profile of preparation by thyroid hormone withdrawal versus recombinant human thyrotropin. Thyroid. 2012;22(3):310–7.

13. Tala H, Robbins R, Fagin JA, Larson SM, Tuttle RM. Five-year survival is similar in thyroid cancer patients with distant metastases prepared for radioactive iodine therapy with either thyroid hormone withdrawal or recombinant human TSH. J Clin Endocrinol Metab. 2011; 96:2105–11.

14. Wexler JA. Approach to the thyroid cancer patient with bone metastases. J Clin Endocrinol Metab. 2011;96:2296–307.

15. Kloos RT, Eng C, Evans DB, et al. Medullary thyroid cancer: management guidelines of the American Thyroid Association. Thyroid. 2009;19:565–612.

16. Gawlik T, d'Amico A, Szpak-Ulczok S, et al. The prognostic value of tumor markers doubling times in medullary thyroid carcinoma – preliminary report. Thyroid Res. 2010;3:10.

17. Durante C, Paciaroni A, Plasmati K, Trulli F, Filetti S. Vandetanib: opening a new treatment practice in advanced medullary thyroid carcinoma. Endocrine. 2013;44(2):334–42.

18. Viola D, Cappagli V, Elisei R. Cabozantinib (XL184) for the treatment of locally advanced or metastatic progressive medullary thyroid cancer. Future Oncol. 2013;9:1083–92.

19. Wells Jr SA, Robinson BG, Gagel RF, et al. Vandetanib in patients with locally advanced or metastatic medullary thyroid cancer: a randomized, double-blind phase III trial. J Clin Oncol. 2012;30:134–41.

20. Haddad RI. New developments in thyroid cancer. J Natl Compr Canc Netw. 2013;11:705–7.

21. Nixon IJ, Shaha AR, Tuttle MR. Targeted therapy in thyroid cancer. Curr Opin Otolaryngol Head Neck Surg. 2013;21:130–4.

# Chapter 15
# Approach to the Patient with an Incidentally Discovered Thyroid Nodule

**Ana Maria Chindris and Victor Bernet**

## Objectives

To review steps in evaluation of a newly discovered thyroid nodule, ultrasound characteristics and indications for fine needle aspiration, to understand cytology results and role of molecular analysis and to discuss management options and long-term follow-up based on nodule characteristics and cytology.

## Case Presentation

A 71-year-old Caucasian male is referred to the endocrine department for a newly diagnosed right thyroid nodule found at palpation during a routine physical examination. He had no associated symptoms such as voice changes, hoarseness, and neck swelling. No systemic type symptoms were reported. The patient was without any history of radiation exposure or family history of thyroid cancer. At physical examination, thyroid was normal in size, with irregular surface and a 2 cm discrete nodule palpable in the right lower lobe. No cervical lymphadenopathy was noted. The remaining of the physical examination was unremarkable.

TSH was 1.6 µIU/mL [0.3–5.0 µIU/mL]. An ultrasound of the neck revealed two heterogeneous solid nodules in the mid and lower pole of the right lobe. The largest, located in the lower pole measured $3.0 \times 2.1 \times 2.3$ cm and had coarse internal calcifications, the second, located in the mid pole measured $1.3 \times 1.1 \times 1.1$ cm and had peripheral calcifications. A third nodule, hypoechoic and less than 1 cm in size, was located in the right upper pole. Left lobe contained a single solid nodule measuring $1.2 \times 0.9 \times 0.9$ cm without worrisome features.

A.M. Chindris (✉) • V. Bernet
Mayo Clinic, Jacksonville, FL, USA

© Springer Science+Business Media New York 2015
T.F. Davies (ed.), *A Case-Based Guide to Clinical Endocrinology*,
DOI 10.1007/978-1-4939-2059-4_15

Based on ultrasound features it was decided to perform FNA on the two larger right lobe nodules. The cytology was assessed as being indeterminate (atypia) and molecular analysis using a gene expression classifier was requested. The molecular results were assessed as being suspicious for malignancy in the case of the 3 cm nodule, while in the case of the 1.3 cm nodule no result was obtained secondary to inadequate RNA in the sample.

The patient was referred for thyroid surgery, and the final pathology indicated a 0.5 cm papillary thyroid cancer in the right lobe and also three subcentimeter foci of PTC in the left lobe with findings consistent with Stage 1 differentiated thyroid cancer. After discussion it was decided to forego treatment with radioactive iodine and patient was started on suppressive doses of thyroxine.

## How the Diagnosis Was Made

Thyroid nodules are very common, with 40 % of patients in their 50s having a thyroid nodule detected by ultrasound [1] and with autopsy studies reporting a prevalence ranging between 13 and 57 % [2]. As in our case, they are typically found during routine physical examination, noted by the patient or family, or incidentally diagnosed on radiological studies performed for unrelated reasons [carotid Doppler, neck/chest computed tomography (CT)]. Advances in imaging techniques and increased use of radiologic studies led to a further increase in rate of detection of thyroid incidentalomas, from about 5 % by palpation to ten times more frequently with the use of high resolution ultrasound [1, 2].

Ultrasound examination is the preferred imaging modality to evaluate newly discovered thyroid abnormalities. In one study, one in six thyroid abnormalities noted on palpation did not correspond to a defined thyroid nodule on the ultrasound. Conversely US uncovered additional non-palpable nodules over 1 cm in 27 % of patients [3]. Incidence in thyroid nodules appears to increase with age, female sex, history of iodine deficiency, and exposure to head and neck radiation [2]. Solitary nodules are about four times more common in women than in men [1].

Assessing for presence of malignancy followed by presence of autonomous overactivity are the main objectives in evaluating a thyroid nodule. The incidence of thyroid cancer has been rising over the past three decades, only partly due to increase in use and performance of imaging [4]. Estimates indicate that about 5–13 % of all thyroid nodules harbor malignancy [5]. Fine needle aspiration remains the gold standard in assessing thyroid nodules for presence of cancer, however, up to 20 % of cytology results fall into the "indeterminate" category where the presence of cancer remains in doubt. A growing number of investigations over the last 10–15 years have focused on the potential use of molecular markers to confirm or exclude the presence of cancer in thyroid nodules. Several molecular tests are now available for the evaluation of thyroid nodules.

# Lessons Learned

## *Clinical Evaluation of a Newly Discovered Thyroid Nodule*

When evaluating a newly diagnosed thyroid nodule, the physician should start by obtaining a careful history with emphasis on risk factors for malignancy (exposure to radiation, family history of thyroid cancer, MEN 2a or 2b syndromes or, familial adenomatous polyposis) along with a description of nodule growth and of abnormal cervical lymph nodes if present. A review of systems should address symptoms consistent with hypo- and hyperthyroidism along with any compression related symptoms such as: dysphagia, positional dyspnea, voice changes/hoarseness, and/or cervical lymphadenopathy.

Physical examination should focus on location, size, mobility, and firmness of the nodule, presence of cervical lymphadenopathy, as well as signs of hypo- or hyperthyroidism.

## *Biochemical Tests*

A serum thyroid-stimulating hormone (TSH) should be obtained. A TSH in the upper half of normal range or above has been correlated with increased risk of thyroid malignancy [6]. If suppressed, an elevated free thyroxine would confirm hyperthyroidism, and radioactive iodine uptake and scan are indicated as to determine the presence of a toxic/hyperfunctioning nodule or nodules [6]. In the case of hyperfunctioning nodules, fine needle aspiration (FNA) is not typically recommended as the risk of malignancy is extremely rare, although in the face of concerning ultrasound characteristics FNA may be appropriate in select cases. Measurement of serum thyroglobulin levels is not recommended as it is not specific for thyroid cancer in the presence of an intact thyroid and can be elevated secondary to benign conditions such as thyroiditis. A consensus does not exist with respect to routine measurements of unstimulated serum calcitonin levels for the evaluation of thyroid nodules. Selective use in case of family history of thyroid cancer or family history of MEN syndromes is indicated. Although the two-site, two step chemiluminiscent immunometric assays used currently are much less susceptible to interferences, they still display significant inter assay variability, and heterophilic antibodies have been described to cause falsely elevated, and occasionally low, calcitonin levels. However, it is generally accepted that values above 100 pg/mL are suggestive of medullary thyroid cancer, in which case surgery is indicated [6].

## *Ultrasound Characteristics and Malignancy Risk*

All newly diagnosed or suspected thyroid nodules should be evaluated by ultrasound, as it provides the most accurate imaging technique in evaluating the structure of the thyroid gland. In the case of substernal extension, additional CT evaluation is appropriate.

A thyroid nodule typically represents thyroid tissue that has become distinct from surrounding parenchyma. Nonthyroidal entities can also appear as thyroid nodules such as: metastases from other primary malignancies, sarcoma, lymphoma, and intrathyroidal parathyroid. Likewise, chronic lymphocytic thyroiditis can appear on ultrasound as hyper- or hypoechoic areas separated by fibrotic strands, which may be mistakenly diagnosed as nodules. These areas also called pseudonodules do not have a halo or a sharp border and are not visualized in both longitudinal and transverse views.

Thyroid ultrasound should document the appearance and size of the thyroid lobes and any nodules or cysts and abnormal cervical lymph nodes, if noted. Sonographic features of thyroid nodules include: size (AP, transverse, and longitudinal diameter), shape (round, taller than wide), margins (borders/halo), echogenicity (hypo-, iso-, or hyperechoic), echostructure (homogenous vs. mixed solid/cystic vs. spongiform), presence of calcifications and internal vascularity. Several studies focused on identifying associations between certain US characteristics and malignancy, as summarized in Table 15.1. As seen, certain ultrasound features can be suggestive, but not definitively characterize a thyroid nodule as malignant or benign, for this purpose the gold standard remains FNA.

The size of the nodule does not predict risk of malignancy in a linear fashion. In a recent study including over 7,300 thyroid nodules the incidence of malignancy was 10.5 % in those measuring 1–1.9 cm and 15 % in thyroid nodules over 2 cm, incidence that remained relatively stable for sizes above 2 cm. Histopathology however, did change significantly, with follicular and Hurthle cell cancers being notably more frequent as the nodules got larger [9]. Micronodules (less than 1 cm) have a reported malignancy rate ranging between 2.1 and 7 % [10]. The American Thyroid

**Table 15.1** Thyroid nodule ultrasound features

| Ultrasound feature of the thyroid nodule | Sensitivity (%) | Specificity (%) | PPV (%) | NPV (%) |
|---|---|---|---|---|
| Microcalcifications | 26–59 | 85–95 | 24–77 | 42–94 |
| Irregular borders | 17–78 | 39–85 | 9–60 | 39–98 |
| Increased intranodular vascularity | 54–74 | 79–81 | 24–42 | 86–97 |
| Solid | 69–75 | 52–56 | 16–27 | 88–92 |
| Hypoechogenicity | 26–87 | 43–94 | 11–79 | 68–94 |
| Taller than wide (transverse view) | 33–40 | 91–93 | 68–77 | 67–75 |

Adapted from Frates [7], Moon [8]
*PPV* positive predictive value, *NPV* negative predictive value

Association (ATA) generally recommends biopsy of the nodules 1 cm and larger in size, with FNA of micronodules reserved for cases with high risk history, suspicious ultrasound findings or abnormal cervical lymph nodes [6].

Shape of the nodule was also assessed as predictor of malignancy; a taller than wide shape being found significantly specific for malignancy however with a low sensitivity.

Thyroid nodules may have either smooth or irregular margins. Most benign nodules will appear as well defined sonographically, while a blurred contour may indicate malignancy. The halo represents compressed perinodular blood vessels and appears as a thin iso- or hypoechoic rim surrounding usually a benign nodule. Absence of halo or a thick irregular halo (>2 mm) is, however, suggestive of follicular neoplasm [11, 12].

Echogenicity of a nodule describes its brightness compared to normal thyroid parenchyma. Solid nodules can therefore be hypo-, iso-, or hyperechoic. Hypoechogenicity has been associated with an increased risk of malignancy, although this feature is not specific [5]. Cystic fluid is anechoic. It may contain bright echogenic spots with reverberation artifact ("comet tail") which represent colloid crystal aggregates and signify a benign character. Pure thyroid cysts are rare; most thyroid nodules are complex, having both solid and cystic components. A particular mention should be made of "spongiform" or "honeycomb" nodules, which consist of multiple cystic areas, separated by septae, and are considered to be benign.

Calcifications can be divided in microcalcifications and macro (coarse) calcifications. Microcalcifications are echogenic foci without acoustic shadowing, considered to be the equivalent of psammoma bodies on histology and highly suggestive of papillary thyroid cancer. Coarse (eggshell) calcifications are associated mainly with benign disease; however, disruption of rim calcification may be seen in cases of malignancy [13].

Thyroid nodule vascularity is most commonly evaluated by Color Flow Doppler (CFD). In case of nodules with slow intranodular flow, Power Doppler, which is independent of velocity, can be used to better characterize internal vascularity. Several studies indicate that increased internal flow increases the probability that a thyroid nodule is malignant [11, 14, 15]. One suggested classification describes the pattern of nodular flow, as absent (grade I), perinodular (grade II), and peri and intranodular (grade III) [11]. In a study on over 200 thyroid nodules, Frates et al. [15] reports the nodule vascularity as absent (0), minimal internal flow without peripheral ring (1), peripheral ring of flow (defined as >25 % of the nodule's circumference) but minimal or no internal flow (2), peripheral ring of flow and small to moderate amount of internal flow, (3) and extensive internal flow with or without a peripheral ring (4).

Thyroid nodules that are hard to palpation have been recognized to have a higher malignant potential. Ultrasound elastography assesses tissue stiffness, by measuring the degree of distortion when a tissue is subjected to external pressure. It has been initially developed to evaluate other tissues including breast and prostate nodules, liver fibrosis and lymph nodes for malignancy. In recent years elastography has been used in evaluation of thyroid nodules and emerging data suggest that, it could represent an independent predictor for thyroid nodule malignancy, to be used in conjunction with conventional ultrasound techniques [16].

## Indications for FNA Sampling: Interpretation of the FNA Results—Role of Molecular Analysis

ATA 2009 guidelines summarize indications for biopsy of thyroid nodules based on various levels of evidence. Indications for FNA are based on a combination of patient's clinical history (e.g., exposure to radiation or personal or family history of thyroid cancer) and nodule size and appearance [6]. For example, a 1.5 cm nodule with increased intravascular flow and irregular margins would be favored for biopsy over a 2.5 cm spongiform nodule. Similarly, a 1.8 cm solid hypoechoic nodule with microcalcifications would take priority over a spongiform nodule (honeycomb appearance) 2 cm in size. Current guidelines recommend against FNA of completely cystic nodules.

Nonpalpable nodules have the same risk of malignancy as the palpable ones of similar size [17]. Similarly, solitary thyroid nodules carry the same risk of malignancy as individual nodules from a multinodular goiter [3]. Deciding which of the nodules to choose for FNA can represent a challenge. In the setting of multiple nodules without worrisome characteristics, it is generally accepted that the largest nodule should be biopsied. Radioactive iodine scan can be used in case of multinodular goiters in the setting of low or low–normal TSH. In this case, hypofunctioning nodules are identified for FNA.

FNA is a simple and safe procedure essential for thyroid nodule evaluation, with an overall accuracy exceeding 95 %. There are several techniques currently employed [parallel vs. perpendicular approach, free hand or with a needle guide, closed suction aspiration vs. "needle only"], all regarded as equally effective. It can be performed by palpation or under US guidance. Two to six passes with 27 or 25G needles are usually done, dictated by technique and operator's preference. Specimen adequacy can be assessed on site. Complications are rare, and consist of local pain and hemorrhage/hematoma. Isolated case reports in the literature note infection, acute thyroid inflammation, tumor seeding (needle tract), and recurrent laryngeal nerve injury with vocal cord paralysis. Anticoagulants should be preferentially discontinued 4–7 days prior to the procedure if possible, although cases of massive hematomas with airway obstruction are exceedingly rare, and hemostasis can be usually obtained by compression against the trachea.

Cytology results are currently reported using Bethesda system for reporting thyroid cytopathology [18]. At least 6 groups of benign follicular cells, with at least 10 follicular cells per group are required in order for the pathologist to make a benign diagnosis. In our institution, 10 follicular groups with ~10 cells per group are required for an adequate specimen with cells being present on two slides being preferred. The following diagnostic categories are reported [18] (Table 15.2):

**Table 15.2** Bethesda diagnostic categories

| Bethesda 2007 diagnostic category | Risk of malignancy (%) | Management previously recommended | Management currently recommended |
|---|---|---|---|
| Nondiagnostic | 1–4 | Repeat FNA with US | Repeat FNA with US |
| Benign | 0–3 | Clinical follow-up | Clinical follow-up |
| Atypia of undetermined significance (AUS) or follicular lesion of undetermined significance (FLUS) | 5–15 | Repeat FNA | GEC/mutation analysis |
| Follicular neoplasm (FN) or suspicious for a follicular neoplasm (SFN) | 15–30 | Surgical lobectomy | GEC/mutation analysis |
| Suspicious for malignancy (SMC) | 60–75 | Near total thyroidectomy or surgical lobectomy | Mutation analysis |
| Malignant | 97–99 | Near total thyroidectomy | Near total thyroidectomy |

Although most biopsies are adequate for a cytologic diagnosis, 5–20 % will be nondiagnostic or unsatisfactory [19]. Reported causes include large cystic component [19]; colloid nodules that are acellular or hypocellular or artifacts. In case of a nondiagnostic FNA performed by palpation; the ATA recommends use of ultrasound guidance for the repeated procedure. In case of mixed nodules with large cystic component, sampling the solid portion of the nodule will yield a better specimen. Likewise, in case of large nodules with cystic degeneration, sampling the periphery of the nodule may avoid obtaining a nondiagnostic sample. In a series of 189 nodules with indeterminate cytology at first biopsy, Alexander et al. reports a success rate of 48 % (cystic nodules) to 76 % (solid nodules) with the second attempt [19]. Some advocate ultrasound guided core needle biopsy in cases where repeat FNA remains nondiagnostic, with one study on 21 nodules showing 86 % diagnostic yield by core biopsy following two or more nondiagnostic FNAs [20]. If repeat cytology remains nondiagnostic, surgical excision should be taken into consideration, as the risk of malignancy can be as high as 10 % [18].

Although small (about 5 %), false-negative rates are not negligible therefore clinical and sonographic follow-up in 6–18 months is essential [6]. The causes are sampling error, which occurs mainly with very small (<1 cm) or very large (>4 cm) nodules [1] and interpretation error. Significant growth (50 % in volume or at least 2 mm in two diameters) should prompt repeat FNA [6].

FNA has substantially reduced the number of required thyroid surgeries for thyroid nodules with an expected increase in the number of malignancies diagnosed at surgery from 3.1 % to 34 % [21]. Still a significant number of thyroid surgeries are performed to obtain a definitive histopathology diagnosis. Research over the past years focused on identifying molecular markers that will identify all benign from malignant thyroid nodules and make distinction between adenoma and carcinoma, therefore offering prognostic information and guiding management. There are three methods currently available:

Mutation detection (miRinform, Asuragen), "rules in" malignancy by using a panel of somatic mutations that collectively occur in about 70 % of thyroid cancers. They include point mutations (BRAF V600E, NRAS codon 61, HRAS codon 61, and KRAS codons 12/13) and rearrangements (RET/PTC1, RET/PTC3 and PAX8/PPARgamma). In a study of 1,056 FNA samples with indeterminate cytology, this method yielded a specificity ranging from 99 % (AUS/FLUS) to 96 % (SMC), with a corresponding PPV of 88–95 %, thus having the potential to correctly identify malignant nodules that would need total thyroidectomy. The authors propose a clinical algorithm for managing thyroid nodules with indeterminate cytology based on the results of this mutational analysis [22]. The main drawback of this method is the limited sensitivity of only 60 %, with as many as 40 % of thyroid cancers being missed at diagnosis, possibly due to lacking in the somatic mutations included in this panel [23].

Multigene expression classifier (Afirma, Veracyte)- is a "rule-out" test that measures expression levels of 167 genes using a thyroid gene microarray analyzed with a classification algorithm. The test reports the result as benign or suspicious and is designed to identify benign nodules within the "indeterminate cytology" category, therefore reducing the number of unnecessary surgeries. A validation trial on over 4,800 FNA samples from supracentimeter thyroid nodules, of which 265 were indeterminate, reported a sensitivity of 90–94 %, with a NPV ranging from 95 % (AUS/FLUS) to 85 % (SMC), respectively. The study reported false negative results in six cases of papillary carcinoma, and suggested that sampling method, especially in small nodules may be the culprit [24].

Thyrotropin Receptor mRNA (TSHR-mRNA) was developed at Cleveland Clinic as a molecular marker of thyroid cancer that is measured in the peripheral blood. In case of follicular neoplasm and suspicious for follicular neoplasm cytology, TSHmRNA in association with high quality neck ultrasound improved sensitivity to 97 %, with 84 % specificity. The data on using TSHR-mRNA for assessment of thyroid nodule cancer risk would benefit from confirmation as it is presently limited to a single institution.

## Management Considerations: Intervention Versus Observation—Role of LT4 Suppressive Therapy

Management of a thyroid nodule is dictated by clinical presentation and cytology assessment.

(a) **Suspicious** cytology or molecular analysis results represent indications for surgery. In case of indeterminate cytology with suspicious mutation detection result (miRinform), proceeding with total thyroidectomy as opposed to standard diagnostic lobectomy may be considered.

(b) **Asymptomatic** thyroid nodules with benign cytology should be followed up for stability, with repeat ultrasound in intervals between 6 and 12 months (because of low but not negligible risk of a false-negative FNA result). Repeat biopsy is indicated in case of a volume increase ≥50 % or if the nodule increases by 2 mm in at least two dimensions. For large benign nodules >4 cm and nodules with associated compression symptoms, surgical removal with hemithyroidectomy is recommended. Newer methods of treatment of thyroid nodules include laser and radiofrequency ablation (RFA) and high-intensity focused ultrasound (HIFU) ablation however, at present they are mainly used in Europe and have not gained wide acceptance in the USA [5].

(c) **Management of thyroid cysts** management poses particular problems. As already mentioned, pure cysts do not require FNA, however drained fluid should be sent for cytology. Small asymptomatic cyst can be followed with periodic ultrasound. Large cysts that were drained should be followed for fluid reaccumulation. In such case, especially if associated with symptoms, a more definitive treatment is needed. Options include hemithyroidectomy and percutaneous ethanol ablation; in the latter case, more than one treatment may be required for successful nodule shrinkage.

(d) **Management of micro nodules (<1–1.5 cm)** continues to represent a particular challenge. The frequency of thyroid microcarcinoma is reported to be as high as 35 %. Although most cases are asymptomatic and diagnosed by chance, up to 43 % may have associated cervical lymphadenopathy, and up to 2.8 % are noted to have distant metastases [25]. Cytological malignancy rate reported in the literature for nodules <1.5 cm ranges between 7 and 13 %. Currently, ATA recommends FNA of nodules as small as 0.5 cm in the case of high risk history, concerning ultrasound characteristics in the presence of abnormal lymph nodes. Nodules <1.5 cm that are solid and hypoechoic or contain microcalcifications should also be biopsied.

(e) **Suppressive treatment with thyroid hormone to induce shrinkage or halt growth of benign thyroid nodules in euthyroid patients is no longer advocated.** Widely used in the past, it is now out of favor as risks associated with excess thyroid hormone (e.g., osteoporosis and atrial fibrillation) outweigh the potential benefits. Use of LT4 is justified in hypothyroid patients in whom TSH normalization can be also associated with reduction in thyroid nodule size. In addition, LT4 suppressive therapy can shrink cancerous nodules offering a false sense of comfort and delay in diagnosis.

(f) **Autonomously functioning thyroid nodules** should be evaluated for the presence of clinical or subclinical hyperthyroidism and managed accordingly.

# Questions

1. Which of the following thyroid nodules is more likely to be malignant on cytology? (nodule size reported as transverse × antero-posterior × longitudinal)

    (a) A 3×2×2 cm round nodule with honeycomb appearance in a multinodular goiter
    (b) A 2.5×2.8×2.8 cm solid hypoechoic nodule with irregular margins and punctate internal calcifications
    (c) A 1×1.5×1.5 cm mixed nodule with bright internal echogenic foci
    (d) A 1.5×1.5×1.2 cm nodule with eggshell calcification

2. A 43-year-old patient with a recently discovered TN during routine physical examination, has a TSH of 0.06 mIU/L, FT4 = 1.5 (0.6–1.6) FT3 = 3.9 (2.6–7.5). He is otherwise asymptomatic. What test would you order next? OK

    (a) Antithyroid peroxidase (TPO) antibody titers
    (b) Serum thyroglobulin
    (c) Radioactive iodine uptake and scan
    (d) Palpation-guided FNA

3. A 52-year-old patient with a palpable TN undergoes a neck ultrasound. This notes a heterogenous thyroid gland with a hypoechoic nodular area located in mid left lobe and measuring 2×1.5 cm on transverse view. Rotating the probe longitudinally fails to identify the nodule. Her TSH is 3.8 mIU/L, and she is otherwise asymptomatic. What would you recommend to the patient?

    (a) Repeat neck ultrasound in 3 months
    (b) Thyroglobulin level
    (c) Antithyroid peroxidase and thyroglobulin antibody levels
    (d) Radioactive iodine uptake and scan

4. A 44-year-old patient presents with an incidentally found thyroid nodule. Her TSH is 1.2 mIU/L and she is asymptomatic. Neck ultrasound reveals a 2.5×3.0×2.5 cm right lower lobe hypoechoic nodule with irregular margins and increased internal vascularity that pushes against the thyroid capsule. Ultrasound guided FNA yields indeterminate result and gene expression classifier returns as benign. What would you advise the patient?

    (a) Repeat FNA in 6 months
    (b) Start LT4 suppressive therapy
    (c) Reassure the patient and recommend repeat ultrasound and TSH in 1 year.
    (d) Perform thyroid lobectomy for histological diagnosis.

## Answers to Questions

1. b: Explanation: Amongst ultrasound features associated with increased risk of malignancy, microcalcifications in a hypoechoic, taller-than-wide nodule, have been associated with a higher specificity for cancer. Spongiform nodules are almost always benign, continuous eggshell calcifications are also associated with benign nodules as well as the echogenic foci (comet tail artifact)
2. c: Explanation: In the setting of a suppressed TSH, the next step in evaluating a thyroid nodule is a radioactive iodine uptake and scan to assess whether the nodule is hyperfunctioning. In such case, FNA is not indicated. An ultrasound should, however be performed in every newly diagnosed thyroid nodule.
3. c: Explanation: Pseudonodules appear as nodular structures in one ultrasound view, but not on the other, and do not need FNA. They can be seen in Hashimoto thyroiditis, therefore it is reasonable to test for markers of autoimmunity, even if TSH is within normal range, as they may indicate if patient is a risk of developing hypothyroidism.
4. d: Explanation: The reported sensitivity of the gene expression classifier is 90–94 %. This nodule displays several ultrasound characteristics suggestive for malignancy therefore surgery for histological diagnosis, as opposed to follow-up in 1 year, is indicated. Repeat FNA would be indicated if the FNA was nondiagnostic/unsatisfactory. Suppressive therapy with thyroxine would not be beneficial in case the nodule is malignant.

## References

1. Mazzaferri EL. Management of a solitary thyroid nodule. N Engl J Med. 1993;328(8):553–9.
2. Dean DS, Gharib H. Epidemiology of thyroid nodules. Best Pract Res Clin Endocrinol Metab. 2008;22(6):901–11.
3. Marqusee E, et al. Usefulness of ultrasonography in the management of nodular thyroid disease. Ann Intern Med. 2000;133(9):696–700.
4. Chen AY, Jemal A, Ward EM. Increasing incidence of differentiated thyroid cancer in the United States, 1988–2005. Cancer. 2009;115(16):3801–7.
5. Sipos JA. Advances in ultrasound for the diagnosis and management of thyroid cancer. Thyroid. 2009;19(12):1363–72.
6. Cooper DS, et al. Revised American Thyroid Association management guidelines for patients with thyroid nodules and differentiated thyroid cancer. Thyroid. 2009;19(11):1167–214.
7. Frates MC, et al. Management of thyroid nodules detected at US: Society of Radiologists in Ultrasound consensus conference statement. Ultrasound Q. 2006;22(4):231–8. discussion 239–40.
8. Moon WJ, et al. Benign and malignant thyroid nodules: US differentiation–multicenter retrospective study. Radiology. 2008;247(3):762–70.
9. Kamran SC, et al. Thyroid nodule size and prediction of cancer. J Clin Endocrinol Metab. 2013;98(2):564–70.
10. Butros R, et al. Management of infracentimetric thyroid nodules with respect to ultrasonographic features. Eur Radiol. 2007;17(5):1358–64.

11. Cerbone G, et al. Power Doppler improves the diagnostic accuracy of color Doppler ultrasonography in cold thyroid nodules: follow-up results. Horm Res. 1999;52(1):19–24.
12. Bonavita JA, et al. Pattern recognition of benign nodules at ultrasound of the thyroid: which nodules can be left alone? AJR Am J Roentgenol. 2009;193(1):207–13.
13. Kim BM, et al. Sonographic differentiation of thyroid nodules with eggshell calcifications. J Ultrasound Med. 2008;27(10):1425–30.
14. Papini E, et al. Risk of malignancy in nonpalpable thyroid nodules: predictive value of ultrasound and color-Doppler features. J Clin Endocrinol Metab. 2002;87(5):1941–6.
15. Frates MC, et al. Can color Doppler sonography aid in the prediction of malignancy of thyroid nodules? J Ultrasound Med. 2003;22(2):127–31. quiz 132–4.
16. Azizi G, et al. Performance of elastography for the evaluation of thyroid nodules: a prospective study. Thyroid. 2013;23(6):734–40.
17. Hagag P, Strauss S, Weiss M. Role of ultrasound-guided fine-needle aspiration biopsy in evaluation of nonpalpable thyroid nodules. Thyroid. 1998;8(11):989–95.
18. Cibas ES, Ali SZ. The Bethesda system for reporting thyroid cytopathology. Am J Clin Pathol. 2009;132(5):658–65.
19. Alexander EK, et al. Assessment of nondiagnostic ultrasound-guided fine needle aspirations of thyroid nodules. J Clin Endocrinol Metab. 2002;87(11):4924–7.
20. Samir AE, et al. Ultrasound-guided percutaneous thyroid nodule core biopsy: clinical utility in patients with prior nondiagnostic fine-needle aspirate. Thyroid. 2012;22(5):461–7.
21. Carpi A, et al. Aspiration needle biopsy refines preoperative diagnosis of thyroid nodules defined at fine needle aspiration as microfollicular nodule. Biomed Pharmacother. 1996;50(8):325–8.
22. Nikiforov YE, et al. Impact of mutational testing on the diagnosis and management of patients with cytologically indeterminate thyroid nodules: a prospective analysis of 1056 FNA samples. J Clin Endocrinol Metab. 2011;96(11):3390–7.
23. Hodak SP, Rosenthal DS, For The American Thyroid Association Clinical Affairs Committee. Information for clinicians: commercially available molecular diagnosis testing in the evaluation of thyroid nodule fine-needle aspiration specimens. Thyroid. 2013;23(2):131–4.
24. Alexander EK, et al. Preoperative diagnosis of benign thyroid nodules with indeterminate cytology. N Engl J Med. 2012;367(8):705–15.
25. Bernet V. Approach to the patient with incidental papillary microcarcinoma. J Clin Endocrinol Metab. 2010;95(8):3586–92.

# Chapter 16
# Papillary Thyroid Cancer

**Rachna M. Goyal and Kenneth D. Burman**

## Objectives

1. To understand the presentation of papillary thyroid cancer (PTC)
2. To examine the high-risk features of PTC
3. To discuss the molecular genetics of PTC
4. To understand the surgical indications for PTC
5. To discuss the utility of radioactive iodine remnant ablation
6. To review the appropriate long-term follow-up for patients with PTC

## Case Presentation

A 41-year-old male with a history of hypertension and multinodular goiter was found to have concerning features on a follow-up thyroid ultrasound. His thyroid ultrasound showed bilateral enlarging nodules with calcifications. The nodule in the right upper pole was $2.8 \times 2.0 \times 2.0$ cm and in the left lower pole was $3.0 \times 1.7 \times 1.1$ cm. He subsequently underwent ultrasound guided fine-needle aspiration of these nodules, revealing cellular adenomatoid nodule in the right nodule and findings highly suspicious for papillary carcinoma in the left nodule (i.e., areas of moderate cellularity, enlarged cells with focal nuclear pleomorphism, and single cells with dense

R.M. Goyal, M.D. (✉)
Division of Endocrinology, Washington Hospital Center,
110 Irving Street, NW, Washington, DC 20010, USA
e-mail: Rachnamgoyal@gmail.com

K.D. Burman, M.D.
Department of Endocrinology, Medstar Washington Hospital Center, Washington, DC, USA

Georgetown University, Washington, DC, USA

© Springer Science+Business Media New York 2015
T.F. Davies (ed.), *A Case-Based Guide to Clinical Endocrinology*,
DOI 10.1007/978-1-4939-2059-4_16

cytoplasm, intranuclear inclusions, multinucleated giant cells, and psammoma bodies). Physical exam was notable for palpable bilateral thyroid nodules. He had no known family history of thyroid disease or malignancy and no personal history of radiation exposure. He also denied neck compressive symptoms or symptoms of hyper-or hypothyroidism. CBC-d and CMP were normal. Thyroid-stimulating hormone was 1.6 mU/L and free thyroxine ($FT_4$) was 1.5 ng/dL, both within the normal range.

A total thyroidectomy was recommended. Pathology from the total thyroidectomy showed the right side contained an adenomatoid nodule and the left side contained a 2.8 cm papillary thyroid cancer (PTC) with extrathyroidal extension, inked surgical margin, and skeletal muscle negative for malignancy; and 3 cm PTC on the left side, 10/28 lymph nodes positive (4 of 14 positive right level 3; 6/14 positive left level 3). Patient has Stage I PTC (T3N1). He proceeded to receive 150 mCi radioactive iodine ablation therapy under rhTSH stimulation. He was administered suppressive doses of levothyroxine to maintain a TSH of <0.01 mIU/L. His post-therapy whole body 131-I scan noted two foci of radioiodine uptake in the thyroid bed which were unchanged from his pretherapy scan. His stimulated thyroglobulin was 2.0 ng/mL and thyroglobulin antibody was <20 IU/mL.

One year after his initial surgery, his laboratory studies revealed TSH of <0.01 mU/L (at goal) and FT4 1.8 ng/dL with unstimulated serum thyroglobulin level of 0.4 ng/mL and the absence of thyroglobulin antibodies. He then underwent a rhTSH stimulated whole body scan, which showed no evidence of local recurrence or distant metastases. Neck ultrasound was also unremarkable. However, his stimulated thyroglobulin increased to 5.0 ng/mL, which will be followed closely.

## Fundamentals of Well-Differentiated Thyroid Cancer

Thyroid cancer is the most common endocrine malignancy, and its incidence and prevalence are on the rise. According to the American Cancer Society, the projected incidence of thyroid cancer for 2013 is 60,220 new cases (45,310 in women, and 14,910 in men) with 1,850 deaths from thyroid cancer (1,040 women and 810 men) [1]. Differentiated thyroid cancer includes both papillary and follicular thyroid cancer, which accounts for more than 90 % of all thyroid cancers, with papillary thyroid cancer prevailing (about 80–90 % of differentiated thyroid cancer are PTC). The higher incidence of papillary thyroid cancer, in part, is attributed to increased detection of small papillary thyroid carcinomas and more frequent use of neck and chest imaging leading to incidentally found thyroid nodules [2]. In the Unites States, there is no significant difference in the risk of thyroid cancer between solitary nodules and multinodular goiter [3]. Therefore, patients with multinodular goiter should be monitored closely as well, as in the case described above. However, the increasing frequency is not thought to be related to enhanced detection alone. If detection alone was the predominant factor, it is expected that most of the detected thyroid cancers would be Stage 1 disease. Yet, the mortality rate of older men with differentiated thyroid cancer is increasing at an alarming rate. Further, a recent molecular analysis of the frequency of BRAF mutations in PTC tissues samples has increased over the last 10–15 years [4].

There are several risk factors associated with PTC. These include female gender (three times more common in women), previous exposure to ionizing radiation, and rare hereditary conditions (e.g., Cowden's syndrome). Approximately 5 % of patients with PTC will have familial PTC; the exact genetic cause has not yet been determined. Although mortality from thyroid cancer is low, the recurrence rate is 25–35 %, making risk stratification a priority. Prognostic factors such as age <15 or ≥45 years, male gender, tumor size >4 cm, follicular histology or tall and columnar cell variants, multifocality, initial local tumor invasion, and regional lymph node metastasis are associated with increased risk of recurrence [5]. Staging is an extremely important tool in management of patients with malignancy. Currently, the TMN (tumor, node, and metastasis) staging system is used which was proposed by the American Joint Committee on Cancer (AJCC) and the International Union against Cancer Committee (UICC). Patients under the age of 45 are subdivided into stage I or II, with the only difference being the presence of distant metastasis (stage II).

In patients 45 years and older: Stage I: Cancer is located only within the thyroid gland and is 2 cm or less. Stage II: intrathyroidal cancer larger than 2 cm and less than 4 cm. Stage III: Either the tumor is larger than 4 cm and only in the thyroid or the tumor is any size and cancer has spread to tissues just outside the thyroid, but not to lymph nodes; or the tumor is any size and cancer may have spread to tissues just outside the thyroid and has spread to lymph nodes near the trachea or the larynx. Stage IVA: Either the tumor is any size and cancer has spread outside the thyroid to tissues under the skin, the trachea, the esophagus, the larynx, and/or the recurrent laryngeal nerve; cancer may have spread to nearby lymph nodes; or the tumor is any size and cancer may have spread to tissues just outside the thyroid. Cancer has spread to lymph nodes on one or both sides of the neck or between the lungs. Stage IVB: cancer has spread to tissue anterior to the spinal column or has surrounded the carotid artery or the blood vessels in the area between the lungs; cancer may have spread to lymph node. Stage IVC: the tumor is any size and cancer has spread to distant sites, such as the lungs and bones, and may have spread to lymph nodes.

The American Thyroid Association (ATA) has developed a risk stratification system into low, intermediate, and high-risk patients. Low-risk patients have no metastases, all their macroscopic tumor has been resected, there is no tumor invasion of locoregional tissues or structures, the tumor lacks aggressive histology, and if I-131 remnant ablation is performed, there is no uptake outside the thyroid bed on the first post-treatment whole-body scan. The characteristics for intermediate-risk patients include either microscopic tumor invasion into the perithyroidal soft tissue, cervical lymph node metastases, I-131 uptake outside the thyroid bed on the first post-treatment whole-body scan, or tumor with aggressive histology or vascular invasion. High-risk patients have macroscopic tumor invasion, incomplete tumor resection, distant metastases, and elevated thyroglobulin levels out of proportion to what is seen on the post-treatment scan [6]. Patients can also be restratified based on their response to initial therapy following thyroidectomy and radioactive iodine remnant ablation and potentially be downstaged. This allows a more individualized risk assessment strategy. Based on clinical outcomes during the first 2 years of follow-up including suppressed Tg, stimulated Tg, and imaging studies patients are further re-staged according to their initial response into three groups: excellent response, acceptable response, or incomplete response. This has been proven to be especially useful in intermediate and high-risk patients since those who have an initial excellent response have a very low likelihood of disease recurrence [7].

## Molecular Genetics of Papillary Thyroid Cancer

Recently, advances have been made in identifying molecular markers from FNA samples that carry both diagnostic and prognostic value in the management of PTC. BRAF gene mutations occur in PTC, and in several other carcinomas as well, such as pulmonary carcinoma, although the exact BRAF mutations may vary. BRAF is a B-type Raf kinase, which is located in chromosome 7 and plays a role in regulating the mitogen-activated protein kinase/extracellular-signal-regulated kinase (MEK–ERK) pathway, which affects cell division, differentiation, and secretion [8]. The incidence of BRAF gene mutations in patients with sporadic PTC ranges from about 40 % to 70 %. The most common BRAF mutation is a change in valine to glutamic acid at codon 600, designated BRAF$^{V600E}$, and accounts for more than 90 % of occurrences. BRAF mutations often insinuate a poorer prognosis and are associated with older age, tall cell variant, extrathyroidal extension, and later disease stage presentation (stage III and IV) [9]. In a recent retrospective, multicenter study by Xing, et al., 1,849 patients with PTC were studied and the presence of BRAF$^{V600E}$ mutation was significantly associated with increased cancer-related mortality (5.3 % in the mutation-positive group vs. 1.1 % in the mutation-negative patients) [10]. Additionally, nearly 40 % of patients with micropapillary carcinoma (<10 mm) have the BRAF$^{V600E}$ mutation, suggesting that it could be a useful tool for staging in the future [11]. However, some studies suggest that BRAF mutation is a rare clonal event, indicating that using BRAF separately as a prognostic factor remains controversial [12]. BRAF is not the only genetic variation found in PTC, as many as 70 % of patients with non-familial PTC have some type of gene mutation (ex. RET, Ras genes, NTRK1, Ret/PTC).

Several commercial molecular genetic tests are now available that purport to have improved diagnostic sensitivity and specificity for indeterminate thyroid FNAs. There are presently two commercially available tests currently on the market that may be used in conjunction with fine-needle aspiration: Veracyte *Afirma®* gene classifier and Asuragen *miRInform™* thyroid panel. Veracyte uses a multigene expression classifier that compares gene expression from mRNA isolated from needle washings during a standard FNA to 167 genes that have been identified by Veracyte as characteristic of the genetic signatures of both benign and malignant thyroid nodules. These specific genes analyzed in this assay are not identified in their publications. In one study, the sensitivity is 92 % and specificity is 52 %, making this a useful rule-out test that can effectively identify benign nodules [13]. However, the clinical applicability of this test needs further confirmation. For example, does this high sensitivity to detect benign nodules apply in select groups of patients (e.g., older patients with a 5 cm nodule). The Asuragen panel, on the other hand, detects several of the key mutations involved with PTC, including BRAF, Ras, RET, and PAX8/PPar gamma. It is primarily used as a rule-in test with a high predictive specificity (98 %), meaning a positive test is likely malignant [14]. However, perhaps 50–70 % of PTC does not harbor one of these mutations. Therefore, a test that identifies a mutation is helpful whereas a negative test does not exclude the presence of thyroid cancer. These tests have promising roles in the management of PTC, but experience with molecular genetics remains limited, and should be interpreted on a case by case basis. At present, most clinicians may use one of these molecular tests and there are limited studies assessing the utility of using both tests in the same patient. There are, of course, additional cost considerations.

## Surgical Considerations in Papillary Thyroid Cancer

According to the American Thyroid Association (ATA) revised guidelines on the management and treatment of differentiated thyroid cancer from 2009, the initial surgical option for those with a tumor size of >1 cm, is a near-total or total thyroidectomy, as was done in the case of this patient. Thyroid lobectomy should be reserved for those with low risk disease, micropapillary carcinoma, unifocality, absence of lymph nodes, and no personal history of head and neck irradiation. All patients with FNA-proven differentiated thyroid cancer should be staged preoperatively and undergo a neck ultrasound with node mapping evaluating the contralateral lobe and lymph nodes for the presence of disease [6]. Performing lymph node dissection at the time of thyroidectomy is controversial, and surgical expertise is warranted. Postoperatively, serum thyroglobulin and thyroglobulin antibodies should be monitored serially on all patients.

## Utility of Radioactive Iodine Ablation

The initial dose of radioactive iodine 131 ($^{131}$I) after total thyroidectomy is primarily utilized for one of three reasons: (1) remnant ablation, (2) adjuvant therapy, or (3) RAI therapy. Remnant thyroid ablation after total thyroidectomy is the mainstay of treatment for patients with high-risk disease (evidence of distant metastasis, extrathyroidal extension, tumor size >4 cm). For low-risk patients (unifocal or multifocal tumor burden <1 cm without high-risk features), the use of remnant ablation is usually not necessary [6]. Its utility is more controversial for those patients with intermediate-risk disease. In one retrospective study, select patients with PTC and intermediate risk of disease according to GAMES staging criteria, who also had an undetectable serum thyroglobulin after total thyroidectomy, were managed safely without adjuvant treatment with RAI [15]. The GAMES (Grade, Age, Metastases, Extent, Size) staging system stratified patients into low-, intermediate-, or high-risk categories and age of 45 and size of 4 cm were the cutoff points for continuous variables [16].

Remnant ablation requires TSH stimulation via recombinant human TSH (rhTSH) or withdrawal of thyroid hormone. Both methods are thought to be equally successful for remnant ablation and rhTSH may be associated with fewer clinical side effects related to hypothyroidism [17]. rhTSH stimulation is approved by the FDA for remnant ablation but not for use in metastatic thyroid cancer. However, two recent studies have suggested rhTSH and levothyroxine withdrawal are equivalent as adjunct to 131-I therapy relating to progression free survival and disease related mortality in patients with metastatic disease [18]. During levothyroxine withdrawal, serum TSH >30 mU/L is required and is associated with an increased RAI uptake in tumors, although this precise cut off value has not been studied rigorously. Additionally, regardless of the method of preparation for RAI ablation, a low iodine diet should be consumed 7–10 days before ablation and 1–2 days after I-131 administration [6]. Checking urine iodine levels is important, since excessive urinary iodine excretion often results in ablation failure, and this is particularly important in regions with high iodine consumption [19]. Indeed, there may be considerable iodine in many foods, such as bread and pastry, milk, and seafood. IV radiocontrast agents contain very high levels of iodine that persist at least for several weeks, and would preclude the use of radioiodine. Since the dietary habits of a patient, as well as previous recent exposure, may be not always be apparent, we recommend routinely measuring a spot urine iodine before administering RAI. Although the exact cutoff value has not been determined rigorously, we recommend that a urine iodine value of less than about 150–200 μg/L be used to decide whether to proceed with RAI scans and treatment.

Determining the dose of RAI is controversial and is clinically relevant given the dose-dependent increased risk of secondary primary malignancies. However, the absolute risk of secondary malignancies is very low although statistically significant. Among patients with differentiated thyroid cancer who have received RAI ablation therapy, the standardized incidence ratio is of a secondary primary malignancy is 1.18, compared to those who did not receive RAI. The most common secondary malignancies include cancer of the salivary glands, melanoma, kidney cancer, leukemia, and lymphoma [20]. The 2009 ATA revised guidelines suggest using low dose (30–100 mCi) I-131 for low-risk patients and higher doses (100–200 mCi) for those with residual microscopic disease or aggressive tumor histology (e.g., tall cell, columnar cell carcinoma, insular). Two to ten days following RAI ablation, a post-therapy scan is recommended [6]. With adjunctive rhTSH stimulation, recent evidence even suggests that 30 mCi is as effective as 100 mCi for 131-I ablation in low-risk patients and is associated with fewer adverse outcomes [21, 22]. In regard to the above case, the patient has metastatic disease to the lymph nodes and therefore received RAI remnant ablation therapy with 150 mCi.

## Hormone Suppressive Therapy and Long-Term Follow-Up

Typically, after initial therapy for PTC, patients are started on exogenous oral levo-thyroxine ($LT_4$) with a goal to suppress serum thyrotropin (TSH). Suppressing TSH with supraphysiologic doses of $LT_4$ has been shown to decrease the risk of recurrence and helps decrease the likelihood of major adverse events relating to progression of the cancer. The ATA recommends an initial TSH of <0.1 mU/L for intermediate-risk and high-risk patients; and an initial TSH of 0.1–0.5 mU/L for low-risk patients [6]. Of course, clinical judgment should be used particularly in the case of elderly patients and those with multiple comorbidities. In one cross-sectional study, the rate of atrial fibrillation in PTC patients over the age 60 on TSH suppressive therapy was 17.5 % [23]. In a longitudinal study of the Framingham cohort, the risk of developing atrial fibrillation was increased approximately threefold (in patients taking exogenous thyroid hormone or who had endogenous hyperthyroidism) if serum TSH was less than 0.1 mU/L as compared to a population that had normal serum TSH values [24]. Additionally, women >50 years of age with PTC on TSH suppression can have a significant decrease in their bone mineral density (BMD) 1 year post-thyroidectomy [25]. Thus, the risk of thyroid cancer recurrence should be balanced against the dangers of atrial fibrillation, bone loss and fractures. The long-term benefit of TSH suppressive therapy needs to be further delineated. However the ATA suggests that in the absence of contraindications, those patients with persistent disease should maintain a TSH below 0.1 mU/L. Patients who initially presented with high-risk disease should aim to keep their TSH between 0.1–0.5 mU/L for at least 5–10 years, and those free of disease who are low risk can have a TSH in the low normal range (0.3–2 mU/L) [6]. Two to three months after definitive treatment, thyroid function tests (TFTs) should be checked to determine the adequacy of TSH suppressive therapy. These general comments regarding suppressive therapy may vary in select patients groups (e.g., elderly, children and adolescents, pregnancy).

Follow-up at 6 months should ascertain disease status of the patient by undergoing a physical exam, neck ultrasound, basal (and in some cases TSH-stimulated) thyroglobulin (Tg) and thyroglobulin antibody (Tg Ab) measurement. Tg is only produced within the thyroid gland and is recognized as an excellent biomarker for the presence of residual disease in patients who do not have Tg antibodies. A diagnostic whole body RAI scan (WBS) is not necessary in all patients, especially those with negative neck ultrasounds and undetectable basal Tg with absence of Tg Ab. It should, however, generally be performed in high and intermediate-risk patients, usually at 1 year post 131-I treatment. The requirement of a second TSH-stimulated Tg in patients free of disease is still debated, but yearly TFT's, Tg, and neck ultrasounds should be performed. In the subset of patients with detectable Tg, if this value increases then imaging techniques for localization of disease should be pursued [6]. It is controversial whether performing serial rhTSH stimulated Tg levels that increase over time helps to detect progressive, recurrent disease. In a recent study, the chance of a detectable stimulated serum Tg level after having an undetectable stimulated Tg was about 3 % [26].

One of the major pitfalls in using serum Tg as a biomarker is that measuring Tg in the presence of Tg Ab using an enzyme linked immunoabsorbent method has been shown to be unreliable. Newer assays are becoming available that diminish this concern. One particular method is a novel liquid chromatography-tandem mass spectrometry-based assay that allows a more accurate determination of Tg levels in patients with Tg Ab [27]. This assay requires further evaluation in clinical studies. Further clinical studies using this assay are required to confirm its validity. A Tg radioimmunoassay was developed at the University of Southern California that has shown to give useful results in Tg Ab-positive patients as well [28].

The patient outlined in the case above has had an increase in his stimulated Tg at 1 year. He will, therefore, need to remain on TSH suppression with goal TSH less than 0.01 mU/L and have a physical exam, repeat TFTs, a neck ultrasound, perhaps TSH-stimulated Tg, and another WBS the following year to screen him for local recurrence. Given these findings, the likelihood that he will have detectable neck recurrences requiring surgery or repeat 131-I can be quite high. Therefore, it is imperative that this patient receives close surveillance moving forward.

## Questions

1. A 40-year-old female was recently diagnosed with PTC. She was found to have a 2.5 cm focus of PTC in the left lobe of her thyroid with metastasis to her level VI lymph nodes, but no evidence of distant metastases.

   What stage is she?

   (A) Stage I
   (B) Stage II
   (C) Stage III
   (D) Stage IV

2. What is the goal TSH for the patient described in the case above?

   (A) <0.1 mU/L
   (B) 0.1–2.0 mU/L
   (C) 1.0–2.0 mU/L

3. The presence of antithyroglobulin antibodies increases the accuracy for thyroglobulin antibodies. True or False?

   (A) True
   (B) False

4. Which of the following characteristics seen in a nodule on neck ultrasound is NOT suspicious for malignancy?

   (A) Microcalfications
   (B) Irregular margins
   (C) Spongioform appearance
   (D) Central vascularity

5. What is the most common molecular marker found in PTC?

   (A) RET
   (B) Ras genes
   (C) NTRK1
   (D) BRAF

## Answers to Questions

1. A
2. B
3. B
4. C
5. D

## References

1. American Cancer Society. Thyroid cancer overview. 2013. Available at: http://www.cancer.org/cancer/thyroidcancer/overviewguide/thyroid-cancer-overview-key-statistics. Accessed 31 Mar 2013
2. Davies L, Welch HG. Increasing incidence of thyroid cancer in the United States, 1973–2002. JAMA. 2006;295(18):2164–7.
3. Brito JP, Yarur AJ, Prokop LJ, McIver B, Murad MH, Montori VM. Prevalence of thyroid cancer in multinodular goiter versus single nodule: a systematic review and meta-analysis. Thyroid. 2013;23(4):449–55. doi:10.1089/thy.2012.0156.
4. Romei C, Fugazzola L, Puxeddu E, Frasca F, Viola D, Muzza M, et al. Modifications in the papillary thyroid cancer gene profile over the last 15 years. J Clin Endocrinol Metab. 2012; 97(9):E1758–65.
5. Pacini F, Castagna MG. Approach to and treatment of differentiated thyroid carcinoma. Med Clin North Am. 2012;96(2):369–83.
6. American Thyroid Association (ATA) Guidelines Taskforce on Thyroid Nodules and Differentiated Thyroid Cancer, Cooper DS, Doherty GM, Haugen BR, Kloos RT, Lee SL, Mandel SJ, Mazzaferri EL, McIver B, Pacini F, Schlumberger M, Sherman SI, Steward DL, Tuttle RM. Revised American Thyroid Association management guidelines for patients with thyroid nodules and differentiated thyroid cancer. Thyroid. 2009;19(11):1167–214.
7. Tuttle RM, Tala H, Shah J, Leboeuf R, Ghossein R, Gonen M, et al. Estimating risk of recurrence in differentiated thyroid cancer after total thyroidectomy and radioactive iodine remnant ablation: using response to therapy variables to modify the initial risk estimates predicted by the new American Thyroid Association staging system. Thyroid. 2010;20(12):1341–9.

8. Davies H, Bignell GR, Cox C, Stephens P, Edkins S, Clegg S, et al. Mutations of the BRAF gene in human cancer. Nature. 2002;417(6892):949–54.
9. Nikiforova MN, Kimura ET, Gandhi M, Biddinger PW, Knauf JA, Basolo F, et al. BRAF mutations in thyroid tumors are restricted to papillary carcinomas and anaplastic or poorly differentiated carcinomas arising from papillary carcinomas. J Clin Endocrinol Metab. 2003;88(11): 5399–404.
10. Xing M, Alzahrani AS, Carson KA, Viola D, Elisei R, Bendlova B, et al. Association between BRAF V600E mutation and mortality in patients with papillary thyroid cancer. JAMA. 2013;309(14):1493–501.
11. Basolo F, Torregrossa L, Giannini R, Miccoli M, Lupi C, Sensi E, et al. Correlation between the BRAF V600E mutation and tumor invasiveness in papillary thyroid carcinomas smaller than 20 millimeters: analysis of 1060 cases. J Clin Endocrinol Metab. 2010;95(9):4197–205.
12. Guerra A, Sapio MR, Marotta V, Campanile E, Rossi S, Forno I, et al. The primary occurrence of BRAF(V600E) is a rare clonal event in papillary thyroid carcinoma. J Clin Endocrinol Metab. 2012;97(2):517–24.
13. Alexander EK, Kennedy GC, Baloch ZW, Cibas ES, Chudova D, Diggans J, et al. Preoperative diagnosis of benign thyroid nodules with indeterminate cytology. N Engl J Med. 2012;367(8):705–15.
14. Nikiforov YE, Ohori NP, Hodak SP, Carty SE, LeBeau SO, Ferris RL, et al. Impact of mutational testing on the diagnosis and management of patients with cytologically indeterminate thyroid nodules: a prospective analysis of 1056 FNA samples. J Clin Endocrinol Metab. 2011;96(11):3390–7.
15. Ibrahimpasic T, Nixon IJ, Palmer FL, Whitcher MM, Tuttle RM, Shaha A, et al. Undetectable thyroglobulin after total thyroidectomy in patients with low- and intermediate-risk papillary thyroid cancer–is there a need for radioactive iodine therapy? Surgery. 2012;152(6): 1096–105.
16. Shaha AR, Loree TR, Shah JP. Intermediate-risk group for differentiated carcinoma of thyroid. Surgery. 1994;116(6):1036–40. discussion 1040–1.
17. Sabra MM, Tuttle RM. Recombinant human thyroid-stimulating hormone to stimulate 131-I uptake for remnant ablation and adjuvant therapy. Endocr Pract. 2013;19(1):149–56. doi:10.4158/EP12278.RA.
18. Klubo-Gwiezdzinska J, Burman KD, Van Nostrand D, Mete M, Jonklaas J, Wartofsky L. Radioiodine treatment of metastatic thyroid cancer: relative efficacy and side effect profile of preparation by thyroid hormone withdrawal versus recombinant human thyrotropin. Thyroid. 2012;22(3):310–7.
19. Sohn SY, Choi JY, Jang HW, Kim HJ, Jin SM, Kim SW, et al. Association between excessive urinary iodine excretion and failure of radioiodine thyroid ablation in patients with papillary thyroid cancer. Thyroid. 2013;23(6):741–7.
20. Iyer NG, Morris LG, Tuttle RM, Shaha AR, Ganly I. Rising incidence of second cancers in patients with low-risk (T1N0) thyroid cancer who receive radioactive iodine therapy. Cancer. 2011;117(19):4439–46.
21. Schlumberger M, Catargi B, Borget I, Deandreis D, Zerdoud S, Bridji B, et al. Strategies of radioiodine ablation in patients with low-risk thyroid cancer. N Engl J Med. 2012;366(18): 1663–73.
22. Mallick U, Harmer C, Yap B, Wadsley J, Clarke S, Moss L, et al. Ablation with low-dose radioiodine and thyrotropin alfa in thyroid cancer. N Engl J Med. 2012;366(18):1674–85.
23. Abonowara A, Quraishi A, Sapp JL, Alqambar MH, Saric A, O'Connell CM, et al. Prevalence of atrial fibrillation in patients taking TSH suppression therapy for management of thyroid cancer. Clinical & Investigative Medicine – Medecine Clinique et Experimentale. 2012; 35(3):E152–6.
24. Sawin CT, Geller A, Wolf PA, Belanger AJ, Baker E, Bacharach P, et al. Low serum thyrotropin concentrations as a risk factor for atrial fibrillation in older persons. N Engl J Med. 1994;331(19):1249–52.

25. Sugitani I, Fujimoto Y. Effect of postoperative thyrotropin suppressive therapy on bone mineral density in patients with papillary thyroid carcinoma: a prospective controlled study. Surgery. 2011;150(6):1250–7.
26. Klubo-Gwiezdzinska J, Burman KD, Van Nostrand D, Wartofsky L. Does an undetectable rhTSH-stimulated Tg level 12 months after initial treatment of thyroid cancer indicate remission? Clin Endocrinol (Oxf). 2011;74(1):111–7.
27. Clarke NJ, Zhang Y, Reitz RE. A novel mass spectrometry-based assay for the accurate measurement of thyroglobulin from patient samples containing antithyroglobulin autoantibodies. J Investig Med. 2012;60(8):1157–63. doi:10.231/JIM.0b013e318276deb4.
28. Spencer CA, Takeuchi M, Kazarosyan M, Wang CC, Guttler RB, Singer PA, et al. Serum thyroglobulin autoantibodies: prevalence, influence on serum thyroglobulin measurement, and prognostic significance in patients with differentiated thyroid carcinoma. J Clin Endocrinol Metab. 1998;83(4):1121–7.

# Chapter 17
# Metastatic Papillary Thyroid Cancer

Henry B. Burch

## Objectives

1. To become familiar with unusual presentations of papillary thyroid cancer
2. To recognize challenges associated with the management of thyroid cancer with spinal metastases
3. To review the indications and methodology of thyrogen-stimulated radioiodine remnant ablation and therapy
4. To review the management of iodine excess in a patient awaiting radioiodine therapy

## Case Presentation

A 59-year-old male with a history of toxic multinodular goiter presents to his primary care physician with progressive low back pain. An MRI of the spine reveals a 4.0 cm left paraspinal mass with nearly complete obliteration of the L3 vertebral body (Fig. 17.1). CT-guided biopsy shows the lesion metastatic papillary thyroid cancer and serum thyroglobulin levels are greater than 2,100 ng/mL. The patient's past medical history is significant for type-1 diabetes mellitus complicated by advanced retinopathy and peripheral vascular disease as well as chronic renal failure. Five years earlier he underwent combined kidney and pancreatic transplantation and has remained insulin-free and off dialysis ever since. His toxic multinodular

H.B. Burch, M.D. (✉)
Medical Corps, U.S. Army, Bethesda, MD, USA

Endocrinology Division, Uniformed Services University of the Health Sciences,
Bethesda, MD, USA
e-mail: hankburch@gmail.com; henry.burch@us.army.mil

© Springer Science+Business Media New York 2015     151
T.F. Davies (ed.), *A Case-Based Guide to Clinical Endocrinology*,
DOI 10.1007/978-1-4939-2059-4_17

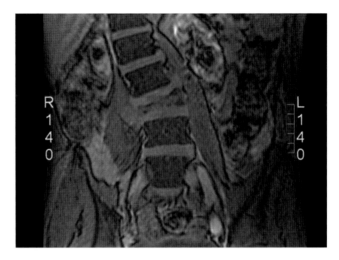

**Fig. 17.1** An unsuspected paraspinal mass in a patient with a history of toxic multinodular goiter and progressive low back pain. A paraspinal mass is shown at L3, with complete obliteration of the L3 vertebral body by tumor

goiter was treated 6 years earlier with radioiodine therapy, resulting in hypothyroidism. He also has a history of severe scoliosis of the lower thoracic and lumbar spine. Neck exam reveals a nodular thyroid bilaterally and no cervical adenopathy. Thyroid ultrasound shows a large calcified right thyroid nodule and smaller nodules bilaterally. Additional staging studies show multiple subcentimeter pulmonary nodules as well as metastatic foci in the boney pelvis. MRI of the head is negative for metastatic disease. The patient undergoes tumor embolization followed by complete extirpation of the L3 vertebral body and paraspinal mass, with basket insertion in the L2–L4 spinal region and spinal fusion from T-12 to S1. After a prolonged hospital course with several transfers to the surgical intensive care unit for congestive heart failure and volume overload, suspected superior vena cava syndrome, wound dehiscence, and upper extremity venous thrombosis, the patient recovered and was released to home. During the course of his hospital stay he was exposed to iodinated contrast on three occasions. He was subsequently readmitted for total thyroidectomy with findings of a 1.2 cm papillary thyroid cancer. Postoperatively the patient recovered and was released to home. Urinary iodine excretion measured prior to discharge was markedly elevated at 7,810 µg/24 h. He was placed on a low iodine diet, furosemide therapy at 40 mg daily, and after 4 months, when the urinary iodine level fell to less than 100 µg daily (Fig. 17.2), he underwent thyrogen-assisted dosimetry followed by thyrogen-stimulated therapy with 192 mCi $^{131}$I. Post-therapy scan shows uptake in the neck and physiological uptake in the bowel. Six months later the patient rhTSH-stimulated thyroglobulin testing and is noted to have a peak thyroglobulin at 180 ng/mL; whole body scan shows thyroid

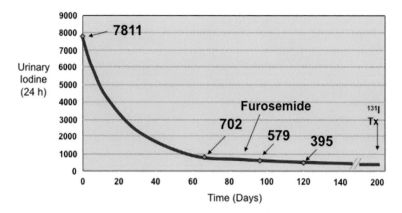

**Fig. 17.2** Prolonged clearance of iodine in a patient awaiting therapy with radioiodine following multiple exposures to iodinated contrast

bed uptake only. He again underwent thyrogen-assisted dosimetry followed by thyrogen-stimulated therapy, this time with 187 mCi $^{131}$I. Post-treatment scan showed uptake in the neck, mediastinum. Six months later a PET-CT showed recurrent nonradioiodine-avid disease in the pararaspinal region at the site of the original tumor resection and he received 10 Gy external beam radiotherapy to this region for palliation.

## Review of How the Diagnosis Was Made

The diagnosis of papillary thyroid cancer is generally straightforward. Thyroid FNA is both sensitive and specific for the detection of papillary thyroid cancer within a thyroid nodule. However, occasionally the first presentation for thyroid cancer is with either locoregional or distant metastases. This patient's paraspinal mass led to the discovery of an otherwise unsuspected thyroid cancer. CT-guided biopsy revealed a follicular lesion and was subjected to special immunohistochemical staining (Fig. 17.3) to pinpoint the primary source. Specifically, TTF-1 staining was positive, indicating either pulmonary or thyroid etiologies, and thyroglobulin staining was strongly positive, confirming metastatic thyroid cancer. Ultimately, thyroidectomy confirmed the presence of a small innocuous appearing primary papillary thyroid cancer.

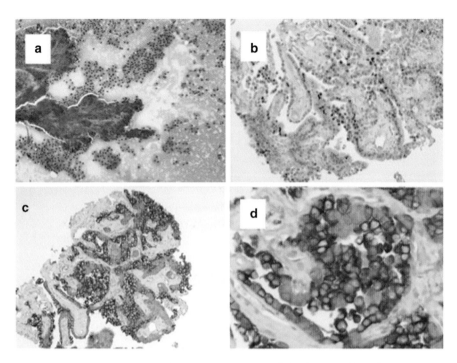

**Fig. 17.3** Histology and special staining of tumor obtained following CT-guided biopsy of a 4 cm paraspinal mass. (**a**) Typical appearance of papillary thyroid cancer; (**b**) TTF1 immunostaining; (**c**) thyroglobulin immunostaining, low magnification; (**d**) thyroglobulin immunostaining, high magnification

## Lessons Learned

1. Papillary thyroid cancer may have unusual presentations. When metastatic to bone, thyroid cancer may present with a large paraspinal mass, as occurred in the present case. Failure to perform special staining might have resulted in a misdiagnosis of adenocarcinoma of unknown primary and the patient would not have received therapy with radioiodine. Likewise, had the patient presented with colon or lung cancer metastatic to spine, he may not have been considered for the extensive tumor extirpation and spine stabilization performed in this case, which were only undertaken after consideration of the comparatively favorable prognosis and efficacy of treatment for thyroid cancer.
2. Exposure to iodinated contrast results in a delay of the delivery of effective radioiodine therapy. This patient's protracted and complicated hospital course necessitated exposure to iodinated contrast during the performance of diagnostic studies deemed critical to the patient's acute management. The resultant iodine overload required a prolonged period of iodine restriction and introduction of furosemide therapy, which has been shown to augment urinary excretion of iodine in animal studies, to facilitate attainment of a low iodine state in preparation for radioiodine therapy.

3. Spinal metastases from thyroid cancer present unique therapeutic challenges. Bone tissue provides a rich environment for metastatic disease, with high blood flow and elaboration of local growth factors in response to tumor damage to bone. Approximately 2 % of papillary thyroid cancer patients experience bone metastases compared to 7–20 % of patients with follicular thyroid cancer. The spine and pelvis are the most frequently involved sites, followed by the rib cage. Approximately half of these patients present with bone pain, 23 % are asymptomatic, and the remainder present with local edema, fracture, or cord compression. Patients with spinal metastases from thyroid cancer tend to present with radicular pain and less commonly, paresis or paraplegia. Paraspinal masses due to thyroid cancer metastases may be quite large and hypervascular. A 2012 series of 22 patients with spinal cord compression due to metastatic thyroid cancer showed clinical improvement in all patients following surgical intervention [1]. Patients with bone metastases from differentiated thyroid cancer tend to have higher serum thyroglobulin levels and 40–80 % have visible uptake on radioiodine imaging. Treatment modalities considered for bone metastases from thyroid cancer include surgery to remove the focus (extirpation), tumor embolization, radioiodine, external beam radiotherapy, and bisphosphonate therapy. Complete tumor extirpation has been shown to positively affect overall survival. In the present case, extensive spine stabilization was required to prevent acute cord compression in the course of surgical extirpation and radioiodine therapy. In general, patients with radioiodine uptake within bone metastases tend to be younger and have improved survival, although radioiodine therapy per se has not always been shown to improve survival in these patients. It has been argued that radioiodine may not be able to deliver a tumoricidal dose to boney metastases. In one example in the literature, dosimetric evaluation showed that a dose of 400 mCi $^{131}$I would deliver a radiation dose of 3,500 cGy to a thoracic spine metastasis, yet a 10,000 cGy would be needed for a tumoricidal effect. Tumor embolization provides prompt relief of pain and improvement in neurological symptoms in many patients without affecting long-term survival. Likewise, external beam radiation therapy can deliver high doses of radiation to a metastatic deposit in bone, resulting in pain relief but no demonstrable effect on survival. Bisphosphonate therapy for the treatment of bone metastases is discussed in another case in this section.

4. rhTSH-stimulated radioiodine remnant ablation is increasingly being used to avoid morbidity associated with conventional therapy under conditions of thyroid hormone withdrawal [2]. Two randomized controlled trials published in 2012, comparing rhTSH-assisted thyroid remnant ablation to thyroid hormone withdrawal therapy using either 30 or 100 mCi, found similar rates of successful remnant ablation at 1 year of follow-up, and no differences between the two doses used [3, 4]. Conversely, rhTSH-stimulated radioiodine therapy for persistent local or metastatic disease has traditionally been reserved for patients unable to tolerate thyroid hormone withdrawal, as in our patient, or those unable to achieve sufficient endogenous TSH elevation due to pituitary or hypothalamic dysfunction. A large 2012 retrospective study compared outcomes of remnant ablation using rhTSH-stimulated $^{131}$I therapy or withdrawal in thyroid cancer patients

with AJCC stages I-IV and found no differences in recurrence rates at a median follow-up period of 9 years [5]. An earlier review of radioiodine therapy of metastatic disease using of rhTSH found that 75 % of 138 patients with post-treatment scan results showed uptake in the metastatic deposits, and 65 % of 115 patients had either improved disease (tumor shrinkage or decreased serum thyroglobulin levels) or disease stability [6]. Currently, rhTSH-stimulated radioiodine remnant ablation is being increasingly used in patients with more advanced tumors, but generally not in patients known to have distant metastatic disease prior to administration of radioiodine therapy.

## Questions

1. A 69-year-old woman with papillary thyroid cancer experiences progressive right hemiparesis while undergoing rhTSH-stimulated whole body scanning. Which one of the following is the most likely explanation for her acute presentation?

   A. Hypertensive urgency due to rhTSH administration
   B. A thromboembolic event due to hypercoagulability
   C. An unsuspected brain metastasis has expanded under the influence of serum TSH
   D. Cerebral ischemia due to vascular effects of hypothyroidism
   E. Thyroid storm due to rhTSH stimulation of functional metastases

2. A 58-year-old male with hypopituitarism due to a craniopharyngioma is found to have papillary thyroid cancer with lung metastases. He undergoes total thyroidectomy and central lymph node resection.

   Which one of the following is the best means of preparing this patient for radioiodine therapy?

   A. Withdrawal therapy using 200 mCi $^{131}I$
   B. rhTSH therapy using 200 mCi $^{131}I$
   C. rhTSH therapy using 350 mCi $^{131}I$
   D. Change modalities to external beam radiotherapy
   E. Use rhTSH to perform both dosimetry and subsequent radioiodine therapy

3. A 42-year-old woman undergoes surgery for a suspicious thyroid nodule and is found to have a T3, N1b, Nx papillary thyroid cancer. While awaiting radioiodine remnant ablation with rhTSH, the patient presents to the emergency department experiencing acute shortness of breath, and undergoes a CT-scan with contrast to exclude pulmonary embolism. Which one of the following is the best approach to this patient's radioiodine remnant ablation?

   A. Proceed with rhTSH-stimulated remnant ablation
   B. Change to thyroid hormone withdrawal proceed with remnant ablation
   C. Give furosemide for 5 days and proceed with remnant ablation

    D. Institute plasma exchange to remove excess iodine

    E. Continue thyroid hormone therapy and delay preparation for remnant abla-
       tion until urine iodine excretion is sufficiently low

## Answers to Questions

1. C: One of the risks associated with rhTSH scanning is stimulation of known or
   unsuspected CNS metastases resulting in tumor growth and edema. Patients with
   known CNS metastases should receive concomitant corticosteroid therapy to prevent acute tumor expansion, although this is not always successful.
2. E: This represents an example of an inability to deliver effective radioiodine therapy using withdrawal conditions, due to central hypothyroidism. The patient still
   requires radioiodine therapy, and given his pulmonary metastases should have
   dosimetry to assure against excessive lung exposure to radioactivity, which can
   cause pulmonary fibrosis. If the patient is to be treated with rhTSH augmentation,
   then the dosimetry also needs to be performed using rhTSH.
3. E: Since the iodine contained in the contrast media will compete with radioiodine therapy, she needs to clear this iodine prior to remnant ablation. Since this
   may take 2–4 months, she should be maintained on thyroid hormone and receive
   remnant ablation only when her spot urine iodine is <50–100 mcg/L.

## References

1. Zhang D, Yin H, Wu Z, Yang X, Liu T, Xiao J. Surgery and survival outcomes of 22 patients
   with epidural spinal cord compression caused by thyroid tumor spinal metastases. Eur Spine
   J. 2013;22(3):569–76.
2. Schlumberger M, Catargi B, Borget I, Deandreis D, Zerdoud S, Bridji B, et al. Strategies of
   radioiodine ablation in patients with low-risk thyroid cancer. N Engl J Med. 2012;366(18):
   1663–73.
3. Schlumberger M, Catargi B, Borget I, Deandreis D, Zerdoud S, Bridji B, Bardet S, Leenhardt L,
   Bastie D, Schvartz C, Vera P, Morel O, Benisvy D, Bournaud C, Bonichon F, Dejax C, Toubert
   ME, Leboulleux S, Ricard M, Benhamou E, Tumeurs de la Thyroïde Refractaires Network for
   the Essai Stimulation Ablation Equivalence Trial. Strategies of radioiodine ablation in patients
   with low-risk thyroid cancer. N Engl J Med. 2012;366(18):1663–73. doi:10.1056/
   NEJMoa1108586. PubMed PMID: 22551127.
4. Mallick U, Harmer C, Yap B, Wadsley J, Clarke S, Moss L, Nicol A, Clark PM, Farnell K,
   McCready R, Smellie J, Franklyn JA, John R, Nutting CM, Newbold K, Lemon C, Gerrard G,
   Abdel-Hamid A, Hardman J, Macias E, Roques T, Whitaker S, Vijayan R, Alvarez P, Beare S,
   Forsyth S, Kadalayil L, Hackshaw A. Ablation with low-dose radioiodine and thyrotropin alfa
   in thyroid cancer. N Engl J Med. 2012;366(18):1674–85. doi:10.1056/NEJMoa1109589.
   PubMed PMID: 22551128.
5. Hugo J, Robenshtok E, Grewal R, Larson S, Tuttle RM. Recombinant human thyroid stimulating hormone-assisted radioactive iodine remnant ablation in thyroid cancer patients at intermediate to high risk of recurrence. Thyroid. 2012;22(10):1007–15.
6. Luster M, Lippi F, Jarzab B, Perros P, Lassmann M, Reiners C, Pacini F. rhTSH-aided radioiodine ablation and treatment of differentiated thyroid carcinoma: a comprehensive review.
   Endocr Relat Cancer. 2005;12(1):49–64.

# Chapter 18
# Management of Metastatic Medullary Thyroid Cancer

Jacqueline Jonklaas

## Objectives

1. To understanding the staging of medullary thyroid cancer.
2. To recognize the prognostic factors associated with medullary thyroid cancer.
3. To review the laboratory testing and imaging that are helpful in the monitoring of metastatic medullary thyroid cancer.
4. To understand the prognosis of medullary thyroid cancer once disease has become metastatic.
5. To understand the treatment options for metastatic medullary thyroid cancer.

## Case Presentation

A 65-year-old female was found to have a palpable lymph node in the right posterior neck during an examination by a physician who was treating her for sinusitis. A fine needle aspiration of the lymph node showed pleomorphic, spindle-shaped cells, which stained positively for synaptophysin, carcinoembryonic antigen, and calcitonin. The patient was referred to a head and neck surgeon. The patient denied any compressive symptoms related to her neck lesion. She had no diarrhea or facial flushing. An ultrasound of the neck was performed and not only showed that the index 2 cm lymph node was suspicious without a fatty hilum, but also showed several other smaller suspicious nodes within the right neck, and a hypoechoic 3 cm right thyroid nodule with intranodular vascularity. No abnormal lymph nodes were noted within the left neck. A fine needle aspiration of the thyroid nodule yielded cells with spindled nuclei and plasmacytoid appearance. Nuclear pleomorphism and

J. Jonklaas (✉)
Division of Endocrinology, Georgetown University, Washington, DC, USA
e-mail: jonklaas@georgetown.edu

© Springer Science+Business Media New York 2015
T.F. Davies (ed.), *A Case-Based Guide to Clinical Endocrinology*,
DOI 10.1007/978-1-4939-2059-4_18

focal binucleation were also noted. Again, the cells stained positive for calcitonin. A serum calcitonin level was significantly elevated at 851 pg/mL (normal <15 pg/mL). Screening for the RET proto-oncogene was negative. Thyroidectomy and neck dissection were planned. Prior to her surgery the patient underwent a CT scan of the thorax and abdomen. The chest CT showed two tiny pulmonary nodules and the abdominal CT showed a hepatic lesion that was described as "incompletely assessed." A repeat CT scan was performed which showed a 4×2 cm liver lesion that was described as filling in with time, consistent with a hemangioma. Smaller lesions were seen along the periphery of the liver that were described as consistent with "flash-filling hemangioma."

The patient was judged to have disease limited to her neck and curative surgery was planned. The patient underwent a total thyroidectomy, central compartment neck dissection, and right modified radical neck dissection. She developed postoperative hypoparathyroidism associated with hypocalcemia requiring calcium and calcitriol therapy. She also developed hoarseness affecting her job as a high school teacher. Her pathology report confirmed medullary thyroid cancer (MTC). Multiple right-sided lymph nodes were involved by the cancer, and, in addition, vascular and lymphatic invasion were noted in all sections of the thyroid gland that were examined. The tumor penetrated into perithyroidal soft tissue and surgical margins were positive. Once she was stabilized on levothyroxine and calcitriol therapy, the patient was referred for, and received external beam radiotherapy to her neck. Following this therapy the patient developed significant odynophagia resulting in weight loss. This odynophagia was protracted, was associated with laryngeal edema documented by laryngoscopy and necessitated temporary use of narcotics for pain relief. She also temporarily required a liquid diet, use of a liquid calcium preparation, and ingestion of crushed levothyroxine and calcitriol in puddings and jello.

Despite her surgery and external beam radiotherapy, the patient's serum calcitonin levels did not decline. These were 978 pg/mL and 1,439 pg/mL 2 months and 3 months after completion of radiotherapy, respectively. These increasing calcitonin levels prompted additional cross-sectional imaging of the patient's lungs and liver. An MRI of the abdomen employing a liver protocol confirmed the presence of a large lesion with imaging characteristics of a hemangioma. However, the multiple peripheral lesions in the liver were noted to have increased signal intensity on T2-weighted images and decreased signal intensity with T1-weighted images. Additionally they were observed to have early arterial enhancement with contrast, followed by washout, but with occasional areas of contrast retention. These lesions were judged to be consistent with metastatic disease and were 50 % larger than on prior imaging.

The patient consulted with several specialists, but was reluctant to initiate therapy with a tyrosine kinase inhibitor (TKI), as was suggested. During her ongoing surveillance, both pulmonary metastases and bony metastases were detected. The patient agreed to begin therapy with vandetanib and a bisphosphonate. She initially appeared to tolerate both these therapies, but then developed severe hypocalcemia, despite adherence to her calcium supplements and calcitriol regimen. Her regimen for treatment of her hypoparathyroidism was successfully adjusted to maintain a low–normal calcium without hypocalcemic symptoms. The patient's liver and pulmonary lesions initially appeared to respond to vandetanib with slight shrinkage in the size of some lesions. However, the patient developed severe diarrhea, debilitating fatigue, and anorexia. She tolerated these symptoms for about 18 months, during which time she was too fatigued to maintain her teaching job. However, then progression of her disease and a concerning degree of QT interval prolongation were observed and her therapy was discontinued. Her calcitonin at this time was 63,000 pg/mL.

The patient was then placed on sorafenib, but eventually discontinued this therapy due to the development of painful foot lesions that limited the patient's mobility. During the 12 months of sorafenib therapy her disease initially remained stable, but then began to progress. Shortly after discontinuation of sorafenib the patient was admitted to a community hospital with hemoptysis. A gastrointestinal bleed was initially suspected, but eventually a diagnosis of carotid artery rupture was made. The patient expired despite multiple blood transfusions while arrangements were being made to transfer her to a facility with vascular surgery and interventional radiology capabilities. The patient had survived for 3 years from the time of her initial diagnosis.

## Overview of MTC

MTC originates from the parafollicular C cells. Approximately 75 % of cases are sporadic, while the remaining 25 % are familial. Sporadic cases occur as a result of clonal expansion of a single focus of tumor cells, whereas heritable MTC usually presents with multifocal disease. C-cell hyperplasia is a common finding in familial disease. It is diagnosed when there are more than six C cells per thyroid follicle. C-cell hyperplasia is thought to progress through clonal expansion and eventual transformation to malignancy. Disruption of the follicular basement membrane by C cells is thought to mark the transition to malignancy. A germ line mutation of the RET proto-oncogene, which codes for a tyrosine kinase receptor, is the cause of familial disease. It is transmitted as an autosomal dominant trait with high penetrance linked to chromosome 10. Mutations in the RET proto-oncogene can occur in the extracellular or intracellular domain. Somatic mutations may be present in sporadic cases.

MTC cells almost invariably secrete calcitonin, and frequently also secrete carcinoembryonic antigen, neuron-specific enolase, chromogranin-A, and/or adrenocorticotrophic hormone. Calcitonin is a clinically useful marker for MTC and is employed both as a serum marker and immunohistochemical marker. Although serum calcitonin may be elevated in patients with large thyroid nodules harboring MTC, it may be normal in smaller tumors and in subjects with C-cell hyperplasia. Provocative tests using pentagastrin or calcium may confirm the diagnosis in these cases. However, the use of these biochemical tests has been replaced by RET proto-oncogene testing when screening for familial disease. Furthermore, pentagastrin is not commercially available in the United States.

When not detected by screening, MTC usually presents as a thyroid nodule. The nodule is typically painless and may be accompanied by cervical adenopathy. Symptoms of ectopic hormone production such as diarrhea are uncommon. The correct diagnosis is usually reached on the basis of the cytology from a fine needle aspiration or elevated serum calcitonin levels. However, the use of serum calcitonin as routine screening in patients with thyroid nodules remains controversial. Primary treatment of MTC consists of a total thyroidectomy performed by an experienced thyroid surgeon with appropriate exploration of the neck and central compartment for affected lymph nodes.

Serum calcitonin and carcinoembryonic antigen levels nadir several months after surgery and their values are helpful in guiding the types and frequency of imaging studies. Undetectable calcitonin levels at 2–6 months after surgery are associated with the best prognosis and a 5-year recurrence rate of only 5 %, whereas detectable calcitonin levels of under 150 pg/mL may indicate residual disease in the neck. Generally calcitonin levels above 150 pg/mL should trigger a search for distant metastatic disease. Clinically occult hepatic disease may account for failure to render a cure. Distant metastases often affect multiple organs and may simultaneously affect the liver, lungs, and bones. Lung metastases may be macronodular or micronodular and are generally diffuse to both lungs. Bone metastases are osteolytic or osteoblastic and are often best seen by MRI. Liver metastases are hyperechoic when imaged by ultrasound. They may be misdiagnosed as hepatic cysts in venous phase contrast CT scans. During MRI imaging they share some characteristics with hepatic hemangiomas.

Treatment options for residual or recurrent disease include additional surgery, external radiotherapy, molecularly targeted antineoplastic agents, and cytoxic chemotherapy. The molecularly targeted TKIs are being more frequently used for patients whose imaging studies show progressive structural disease. Additional treatment for residual or recurrent disease with these agents is rarely curative. Future challenges include the need to target therapy according to RET mutational status and to develop effective combinations of drugs that overcome resistance to TKIs.

Tumor stage predicts prognosis and effectiveness of treatment and 10-year survival rates are greater than 95 % for disease confined to the thyroid, approximately 75 % for regional disease, and 40 % for distant metastases. Familial disease generally has a better prognosis than sporadic disease, but this advantage is no longer seen when adjustment is made for disease stage, suggesting that sporadic disease is usually detected in a more advanced stage.

## Review of How the Diagnosis Was Made

### Diagnosis of MTC

Accurate diagnosis of MTC solely by the cytologic features of a fine needle aspiration specimen may be difficult. MTC usually appears as a cellular specimen with clusters of pleomorphic tumors cells. Cells may be oval with eccentric nuclei, similar to plasma cells, or polygonal with granular cytoplasm, similar to Hürthle cells. They may also be spindle shaped. An aspirate from a MTC lesion, therefore, can mimic other benign and malignant entities, such as Hürthle cell tumors, poorly differentiated carcinoma, and metastatic renal cell carcinoma and melanoma. In one study, fine needle aspiration detected only 75 % of MTC cases that were suspected based on serum calcitonin screening. The diagnosis, however, can be confirmed by immunohistochemical staining for calcitonin. Immunostaining of the cytology specimen for calcitonin is considered the gold standard for preoperative diagnosis of MTC. In this case, immunostaining of both the lymph node and thyroid nodule cytology were instrumental in providing a pre-operative diagnosis of MTC. Sporadic MTC is usually diagnosed by fine needle aspiration of a palpable nodule, as occurred in this patient, or it may be diagnosed at the time of surgery. In contrast, familial MTC is usually diagnosed at the time of thyroidectomy after genetic screening has identified a RET proto-oncogene mutation.

## *Diagnosis of Metastatic MTC*

Many patients with MTC have metastases at the time of diagnosis, with approximately 50 % having lymph node metastases and 5 % having distant metastases. Because of this, a thorough preoperative evaluation is essential to guide therapy. Ultrasonography of the neck to assess for local and regional disease in the neck is recommended, as was performed in this case. In addition, imaging of the chest and mediastinum is advised in patients with cervical node metastases and/or basal calcitonin levels greater than 400 pg/mL [1], as such patients are more likely to also have involvement of mediastinal lymph nodes and liver metastases. Metastatic liver lesions were visualized, but not recognized in this patient (see lessons learned). Screening for pheochromocytoma is also often necessary preoperatively, but would not be indicated in this patient who had a negative RET mutation analysis and no family history of diseases suggestive of MEN 2.

## Lessons Learned

### *Presentation of Sporadic Disease*

Although there is a trend for MTC to be detected earlier as microscopic disease or disease without cervical node involvement, sporadic disease still generally presents with a clinically detectable thyroid nodule [2]. Approximately 50 % of patients will present with cervical node metastases, as occurred in this patient, and approximately 5–10 % will initially have distant metastases.

## Sonographic Appearance of MTC Within Thyroid Nodules

The ultrasound features that are suggestive of malignancy being harbored within a thyroid nodule are well-documented for papillary thyroid cancer. However, many of these features are not equally suggestive of MTC. A recent retrospective study suggested that hypoechogenicity and intranodular vascularity, as was documented in this patient, are predictive of MTC [3]. Irregular margins were not, however, a feature of MTC. Although microcalcifications were seen with MTC, these were much less frequent than in papillary thyroid cancer.

## Imaging Characteristics of Hepatic Metastases

MTC metastatic to the liver may have a military pattern and initially be difficult to detect. The ultrasonography appearance of hepatic metastases can be similar to hemangioma when the metastases are under 3 cm in size. Their appearance on MRI is characteristic. Peripheral enhancement with progressive centripetal fill-in similar to that seen with hemangioma can also be seen with MRI imaging (see Fig. 18.1) [4]. Single-shot fast spin-echo is a useful sequence to make the distinction between such metastases and hemangioma. In this patient, the diagnosis of liver metastases was not appreciated until her calcitonin levels failed to decrease after her thyroidectomy and neck dissection. Knowledge of these metastases beforehand may have dampened enthusiasm for the aggressive surgical approach and subsequent radiotherapy she received. Although it is difficult to know the impact of her initial therapy on her overall survival, perhaps less aggressive initial therapy would have improved her quality of life.

## Staging of MTC

The staging system most commonly used for MTC is the Tumor-Node-Metastases (TNM) staging system adopted by the American Joint Committee on Cancer. This staging system is based on tumor size, invasion of the tumor, the presence of nodal metastases, and the presence of distant metastases. Overall survival in all cases of MTC is approximately 75 %, with the TNM staging system providing good discrimination as follows in one short-term study: stage I with 0 % mortality, stage II with 13 % mortality, stage III with 56 % mortality, and stage IV with 100 % mortality. An alternate staging system developed by the National Thyroid Cancer Treatment Cooperative Study Group provides similar separation of outcomes for a population affected by MTC. Survival is significantly affected by the whether disease is confined to the thyroid, affects local and regional lymph nodes only, or involves distant sites (see Fig. 18.2). A comparison of several of these staging systems found the European Organization for Research and Treatment of Cancer

**Fig. 18.1**  MRI of the
abdomen with intravenous
contrast showing hepatic
metastases indicated by *red
arrows* measuring
approximately 1.2×1 cm
(posterior lesion) and
0.8×0.9 cm (anterior lesion)

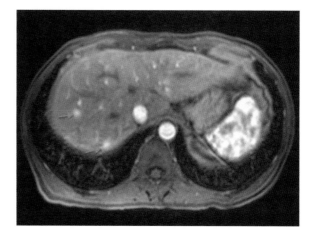

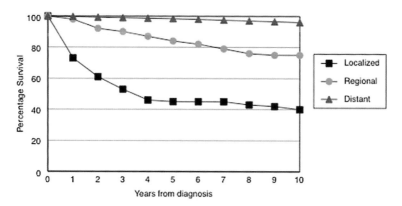

**Fig. 18.2**  Disease specific survival for patients with medullary thyroid cancer according to site of disease metastases based on Surveillance, Epidemiology, and End Results (SEER) data. From Roman et al., Cancer 107: 2134–2142, 2006, with permission

(EORTC) staging system to have the best predictive value [5]. In retrospect, our patient was stage IV by all staging systems at the time of her diagnosis. Approximately 50 % of similarly staged patients are alive at 5 years. However, such staging systems do not incorporate other important prognostic indicators such as age and calcitonin doubling time.

## Calcitonin Doubling Time

The calcitonin doubling time is a powerful prognostic indicator of survival in MTC. In one study when calcitonin doubling time was less than 6 months, as it was in our patient after her initial therapy, 25 % and 8 % of such patients survived 5 years and 10 years, respectively. In the same study, although TNM stage, EORTC score, and calcitonin doubling time were significant predictors of survival by univariate analysis, only calcitonin doubling time remained an independent predictor of survival by multivariate analysis [6]. A tool that can be used to calculate calcitonin doubling time is available on the website of the American Thyroid Association (http://www.thyroid.org/thyroid-physicians-professionals/calculators/thyroid-cancer-carcinoma/).

## Side Effects of Tyrosine Kinase Inhibitors

Molecularly targeted and orally active antineoplastic agents are increasingly used for the treatment of MTC [7]. Tyrosine kinases are involved in signaling, and thereby stimulate tumor proliferation, angiogenesis, invasion, and metastases. TKIs may have inhibitory effects at multiple levels, but inhibition of angiogenesis seems to be an important part of their action. Both vandetanib and cabozantinib are approved agents for the treatment of patients with progression of structural disease. As these agents are now available outside of clinical trials, a restricted distribution program has been put in place to monitor their use and provide oversight. Common side effects of these agents include anorexia, transaminitis, diarrhea, fatigue, weight loss, and QT interval prolongation. A comprehensive review of the experience of the University of Texas MD Anderson Cancer Center with the use of these agents for MTC and non-MTC has recently been published [8]. Our patient suffered the typical side effects of vandetanib, including anorexia, diarrhea, fatigue, and QT prolongation. The hand and foot syndrome typically affects approximately 30 % of patient taking sorafenib and sunitinib, but does not affect those taking vandetanib.

## Common and Rare Complications of External Beam Radiotherapy

Radiotherapy to the neck and mediastinum are often considered after initial surgery in those with residual disease. For example the National Comprehensive cancer Network recommends that external beam radiotherapy (EBRT) is considered for "gross extrathyroidal extension (T4a or T4b) with positive margins after resection of all gross disease and following resection of moderate- to high-volume disease in the central or lateral neck lymph nodes with extra-nodal soft tissue extension." Our patient certainly fell into that category. Slight improvements have been reported in local disease-free survival after EBRT for selected patients. In one study, high-risk patients with microscopic residual disease, extraglandular invasion, or lymph node involvement had a higher local/regional relapse free rate of 86 % at 10 years compared with a relapse free rate of 52 % in those who did not receive postoperative external beam radiation [9].

Unfortunately, there are significant toxicities associated with external beam radiotherapy. These include mucositis, radiation dermatitis, dysphagia, fatigue, taste changes, xerostomia, and hoarseness. Sometimes such side effects necessitate a break from treatment. Patients undergoing radiation therapy may require a tracheostomy or percutaneous endoscopic gastrostomy tube placement. Although this is typically due to progressive local disease, occasionally this may be due to pharyngeal or laryngeal edema associated with the therapy. Our patient suffered a catastrophic but rare complication associated with both the progression and management of head and neck cancers, namely rupture of the carotid artery [10]. This carotid "blowout" is associated with radiotherapy, nodal metastases, and neck dissection. Radiation therapy has been implicated in the pathophysiology of carotid blowout because it causes changes in the vasa vasorum and adventitia that lead to subsequent weakening of the arterial wall. In one retrospective study 14 of 17 patients with carotid artery rupture had received radiation therapy, with the rate of rupture being about eightfold higher in radiated compared with nonirradiated patients.

## Questions

1. Which of the following are true statements regarding the presentation of sporadic MTC?

    (a) 75 % of individuals with apparently sporadic MTC are generally found to have a germ line RET proto-oncogene mutation
    (b) Somatic RET proto-oncogene mutation can be documented in about 10 % of patients with sporadic MTC
    (c) The most common presentation of sporadic MTC is a solitary thyroid nodule
    (d) MTC occurs most commonly in females with a female to male ratio of 8:1
    (e) Diarrhea, facial flushing, and ectopic Cushing's syndrome are presenting manifestations in approximately 30 % of patients with sporadic MTC.

2. You are seeing a patient who underwent thyroidectomy and bilateral neck dissection for metastatic MTC 6 months ago. A serum calcitonin level was drawn this morning and is currently pending. The patient has many questions about the significance of the current calcitonin level and also about future monitoring of calcitonin levels. Which of the following statements regarding serum calcitonin measurements would present the true picture to your patient?

    (a) A nadir in serum calcitonin is reached within a few weeks of initial surgery
    (b) Increases in calcitonin levels during follow-up do not correlate with increases in carcinoembryonic antigen
    (c) A serum calcitonin level of 150 pg/mL would not trigger additional imaging at this point in time

    (d) Future imaging will not be dictated by the trajectory of the patients calcitonin and carcinoembryonic antigen levels

    (e) A high serum calcitonin level approximately 6 months after surgery is evidence of the presence of residual disease

3. A patient with MTC has been documented to have progressive disease. Which of the following would be not be considered a contraindication to use of vandetanib in this patient?

    (a) Progression documented only on the basis of increasing tumor markers

    (b) Prior history of torsades de pointes

    (c) Poor performance status measured using a reliable performance scale

    (d) Progressive structural disease demonstrated on cross-sectional imaging

    (e) Uncompensated heart failure

## Answers to Questions

1. c: The most common presentation of sporadic MTC is a solitary thyroid nodule, which occurs in about 75–80 % of patients. Typically patients present in the fifth or sixth decade of life. There may be a slight female preponderance. About 6–7 % of patients with apparently sporadic MTC are found to carry unsuspected germ line mutations in the RET proto-oncogene. Somatic (acquired) mutations in the RET proto-oncogene, on the other hand, may be found within the tumor cells in approximately 60 % of patients with sporadic MTC. Symptoms of hormonal excess such as diarrhea, flushing, and ectopic Cushing's syndrome are generally seen with progressive metastatic disease, and are not a common feature of a patient's initial presentation.

2. e: The nadir in serum calcitonin levels usually occurs several months after surgery. Undetectable calcitonin levels at 2–6 months after surgery are associated with the best prognosis and a 5-year recurrence rate of only 5 %. Detectable calcitonin levels of under 150 pg/mL may indicate residual disease in the neck, whereas levels above 150 pg/mL are suggestive of distant metastases. The postoperative calcitonin values and their rate of change can be used to guide the frequency of surveillance imaging studies. Changes in carcinoembryonic antigen levels generally correlate well with calcitonin levels.

3. d: Increasing tumor markers, in the absence of structural disease progression, are not considered an indication for treatment with vandetanib. Vandetanib carries a black box warning regarding QT interval prolongation, torsades de pointes, and sudden death. It is generally contraindicated in patients with a history of torsades de pointes, patients with a QT interval greater than 450 ms, and those with bradyarrhythmias or uncompensated congestive heart failure. Patients with a poor performance status are more likely to be unable to tolerate TKI therapy and so patient suitability for such therapy has to be carefully assessed.

# References

1. Kloos RT, Eng C, Evans DB, Francis GL, Gagel RF, Gharib H, et al. Medullary thyroid cancer: management guidelines of the American Thyroid Association. Thyroid. 2009;19(6):565–612.
2. Pacini F, Castagna MG, Cipri C, Schlumberger M. Medullary thyroid carcinoma. Clin Oncol (R Coll Radiol). 2010;22(6):475–85.
3. Trimboli P, Nasrollah N, Amendola S, Rossi F, Ramacciato G, Romanelli F, et al. Should we use ultrasound features associated with papillary thyroid cancer in diagnosing medullary thyroid cancer? Endocr J. 2012;59(6):503–8.
4. Dromain C, de Baere T, Baudin E, Galline J, Ducreux M, Boige V, et al. MR imaging of hepatic metastases caused by neuroendocrine tumors: comparing four techniques. AJR Am J Roentgenol. 2003;180(1):121–8.
5. Kebebew E, Ituarte PH, Siperstein AE, Duh QY, Clark OH. Medullary thyroid carcinoma: clinical characteristics, treatment, prognostic factors, and a comparison of staging systems. Cancer. 2000;88(5):1139–48.
6. Barbet J, Campion L, Kraeber-Bodere F, Chatal JF. Prognostic impact of serum calcitonin and carcinoembryonic antigen doubling-times in patients with medullary thyroid carcinoma. J Clin Endocrinol Metab. 2005;90(11):6077–84.
7. Tuttle RM, Ball DW, Byrd D, Daniels GH, Dilawari RA, Doherty GM, et al. Medullary carcinoma. J Natl Compr Canc Netw. 2010;8(5):512–30.
8. Carhill AA, Cabanillas ME, Jimenez C, Waguespack SG, Habra MA, Hu M, et al. The noninvestigational use of tyrosine kinase inhibitors in thyroid cancer: establishing a standard for patient safety and monitoring. J Clin Endocrinol Metab. 2013;98(1):31–42.
9. Brierley J, Tsang R, Simpson WJ, Gospodarowicz M, Sutcliffe S, Panzarella T. Medullary thyroid cancer: analyses of survival and prognostic factors and the role of radiation therapy in local control. Thyroid. 1996;6(4):305–10.
10. Powitzky R, Vasan N, Krempl G, Medina J. Carotid blowout in patients with head and neck cancer. Ann Otol Rhinol Laryngol. 2010;119(7):476–84.

# Chapter 19
# Thyroid Cancer and Bone Metastases

**Ritu Madan and Jason A. Wexler**

## Objectives

1. To discuss the incidence of bone metastases in thyroid cancer and realize their importance in prognostication of the disease
2. To discuss the role of imaging modalities and bone biopsy in establishing the diagnosis of bone metastases from thyroid cancer
3. To discuss the forms of treatment targeting eradication or palliation of the disease
4. To discuss the role of bisphosphonates, denosumab, and tyrosine kinase inhibitors in management of patients with bone metastases
5. To discuss appropriate monitoring strategies in these patients

## Case Presentation

A 47-year-old man underwent a total thyroidectomy, central and right lateral neck dissection for a 5 cm right thyroid nodule in May 2002. Pathology revealed papillary thyroid carcinoma of the right nodule with vascular invasion and positive lymph nodes in the right central compartment (10/16 lymph nodes positive) and right lateral compartment (9/19 lymph nodes positive). In September 2002, he received

R. Madan, M.D.
National Institutes of Health/National Institute of Diabetes and Digestive and Kidney Diseases, Bethesda, MD, USA

J.A. Wexler, M.D. (✉)
Section of Endocrinology, MedStar Washington Hospital Center, Washington, DC, USA

Georgetown University Medical Center, Washington, DC, USA
e-mail: Jason.A.Wexler@medstar.net

© Springer Science+Business Media New York 2015
T.F. Davies (ed.), *A Case-Based Guide to Clinical Endocrinology*,
DOI 10.1007/978-1-4939-2059-4_19

radioactive iodine ablation with 146.7 mCI of I-131 after surgery with post-therapy I-131 scan showing thyroid bed uptake as well as uptake suspicious for residual lymph node metastases in the right lateral cervical lymph node region. On 6-month follow-up in July 2003, his stimulated thyrolobulin (Tg) levels were elevated at 251 ng/ml with negative Tg antibodies. A pretherapy scan did not show any uptake. He was subsequently treated 200 mCI of I-131 in August 2003 and post-therapy scan showed two foci of uptake in right lower neck consistent with residual lymph node metastases. Subsequent to this treatment, his stimulated Tg level was elevated to 4,734 ng/ml with negative Tg antibodies. Additional tests at this time including MRI neck, CT scan of head, neck, abdomen, and pelvis and FDG-PET showed FDG-positive lymph nodes in the right lateral neck and a 3 cm mass in the left thyroid bed. A bone scan done at this time was negative. He underwent a modified radical neck dissection in which 8 out of 21 lymph nodes were positive for papillary thyroid carcinoma. After surgical debulking, he was treated with 431.5 mCI of I-131 following a radioiodine dosimetry protocol. His post-therapy scan showed abnormal tracer uptake in left lateral neck region without anatomic correlate on cross-sectional imaging. He continued to have elevated Tg levels on thyroid hormone suppression with no obvious source on various imaging studies. In June 2007, PET-CT showed a new nasopharyngeal mass and a 3 mm right apex lung nodule. A stimulated Tg at this time was 661 ng/ml. He received radiation therapy (surgical debulking was not possible) to this nasopharyngeal mass without an improvement in Tg levels. His PET/CT in 2008 showed new sclerotic lesions in the right superior pubic ramus and body of the sternum. His Tg was 80 ng/ml on levothyroxine suppression, stimulated Tg was 1,138 ng/ml and a diagnostic I-131 scan was negative. He was followed conservatively for a few months at which time suppressed Tg levels continued to rise and his lung nodule grew to more than 1 cm in size. He was started on an experimental treatment protocol with sunitinib in May 2009. He completed 11 monthly cycles of sunitinib in June 2010 at which time his Tg had risen to 1,039 ng/ml and PET/CT showed stable pelvic and sternal lesions but a new occipital bone lesion and new bilateral subpleural lung metastases had developed. He was withdrawn from the sunitinib protocol for progressive disease and started on monthly zoledronic acid infusions for his bone metastases. The occipital bone lesion was surgically resected and treated with external beam radiotherapy. A repeat PET/CT in August 2011 showed an increase in size of his pelvic and sternal lytic lesions. He received radiotherapy to these lesions and enrolled in phase-2 study with lenvatinib. Zoledronic acid was discontinued and he began therapy with monthly subcutaneous denosumab for his bone metastases. His last imaging showed stable lung and bone disease.

## Incidence of Bone Metastases in Differentiated Thyroid Cancer

Bone metastases are uncommon in thyroid cancer. While follicular thyroid cancer accounts for less than 15 % of all differentiated thyroid cancers, bone metastases occur in up to 7–20 % of these patients. Bone metastases are less common in papillary thyroid cancer, but still may be seen in up to 1–7 % of cases. In absolute terms however, the number of patients with bone metastases due to papillary thyroid cancer is higher since papillary thyroid cancer is more common. Overall, the incidence of bone metastases in well-differentiated thyroid cancer is 2–13 %. Skeletal metastases often are clinically silent but can present with pain, pathologic fracture, painful radiculopathy, bladder and bowel incontinence, and weakness of one more extremities from spinal cord compression. Spine is the most common site of bone metastases and 25 % of patients may have isolated bone metastases, with 15 % having both lung and bone metastases. It is important to be vigilant for metastatic disease since the presence of metastases lowers the 10-year survival rates for differentiated thyroid cancer from about 90 % to 40 %.

## How to Diagnose Bone Metastases

It can be difficult to detect bone metastases from thyroid cancer. Diagnostic I-131 scans are insensitive, while post-therapy scans perform better. X-rays and bone scintigraphy can be used in the evaluation of osseous metastases, but these imaging modalities are often limited by their poor specificity and their ability to detect disease only when more than half of an involved bone has been destroyed. Tc-99 bone scintigraphy can detect skeletal metastases earlier than plain radiographs when there is a predominant osteoblastic component to the lesion. But because thyroid cancer metastases are predominantly osteolytic, bone scintigraphy is of limited value in thyroid cancer with high false positive and false negative rates.

MRI of the whole body or of specific bones is an excellent modality to visualize the medullary component of bones and detailing the extra-skeletal extent of disease. Whole body MRI has higher sensitivity than PET/CT for diagnosis of osseous metastases (85–95 % vs. 62–91 %). CT alone is valuable in imaging cortical bone. In a prospective study of 80 patients comparing FDG PET/CT, I-131 SPECT/CT, and 99m Tc-MDP bone scans, FDG PET/CT and I-131 SPECT/CT were significantly superior to bone scans in detecting osseous metastases. PET scans have a role in predicting prognosis as well; a positive PET/CT increases the risk of death from thyroid cancer by fourfold.

Two future modalities for detecting bone metastases are 18F-fluoride PET/CT and Iodine-124. 18F-fluoride is a bone-seeking, positron emitting molecule with excellent sensitivity and specificity for detecting bone lesions, especially osteolytic metastases. When combined with PET/CT, 18F-fluoride can provide exquisite spatial resolution of osseous metastases with some studies suggesting better performance than PET/CT and Tc-99 bone scintigraphy. I-124 emits a positron that can be detected by PET scan. One study has demonstrated the superiority of I-124 PET/CT compared to I-131, I-124, and CT scans alone in detecting bone metastases.

We recommend that when extracervical spread is suspected, one should obtain an FDG-PET/CT. If bone metastases are discovered, then a directed MRI or CT should be employed to specifically define the lesion(s) of interest and as an aid in planning any surgical approaches or use of other modalities in the treatment of destructive osseous lesions.

## Role of Biopsy in Evaluating Bone Lesions

In most situations where the histology of primary malignancy has been established, it is usually unnecessary to biopsy new lesions that present at distant sites. However, if a bone lesion represents the first manifestation of recurrent thyroid cancer, biopsy is recommended. Bone biopsy is not necessary if the bone lesions take up radioactive iodine on diagnostic or post-therapy I-131 scans or if a patient with widespread disease has undergone bone biopsy before confirming metastases of thyroid origin.

A needle biopsy is recommended for newly detected spine and pelvis bone lesions that do not take up radioiodine. Sections of biopsy should be carefully examined for histological subtype (papillary, follicular, Hürthle cell, and poorly differentiated carcinomas). Special stains for thyroid transcription factor (TTF), Tg, cytokeratin, and calcitonin should be employed and the need for supplemental stains like prostate-specific antigen should be individualized. Another simple technique that can be used in evaluating distant metastases is detection of thyroglobulin in the washout of fine needle aspirates of nonthyroidal masses. While not specifically studied in bone metastases, the value of the technique is probably similar. Once a bone biopsy has confirmed the origin of the tumor, I do not recommend biopsies of subsequent skeletal lesions except in rare circumstances.

## Therapy with I-131 for Bone Metastases

There is no prospective study evaluating the effect of I-131 therapy on survival in patients with metastatic differentiated thyroid cancer. A retrospective study of 444 patients by Durante et al. showed that only 7 % of patients with bone metastases achieved remission with I-131 therapy and even 43 % of patients who had iodine avid lesions still did not achieve remission with radioactive iodine therapy. The factors that predicted response to I-131 therapy were age <40 years, solitary lesion and well-differentiated cancer. 10-year survival rates for complete responders, partial responders, and nonresponders were 92 %, 29 %, and 10 %, respectively.

The efficacy of I-131 treatment may be improved by using dosimetry protocols. Several studies have demonstrated that skeletal metastases treated under a dosimetry protocol achieved greater reduction in tumor volume and Tg levels than a historical control group that was treated with a fixed dose of radioiodine. Also, dosimetry may identify lesions that do not concentrate radioiodine to a degree that would allow the delivery of a therapeutic radiation dose, thus distinguishing patients who may not benefit from I-131 therapy.

But some investigators have reported more successful results with I-131 in subgroups of patients with bone metastases. A retrospective review of 107 patients with an initial skeletal metastasis demonstrated significantly higher rates of total or partial remissions in patients younger than 45 years old (62.5 %) compared to patients over 45 years of age (49.5 %). In younger patients with three or fewer bone lesions, 75 % achieved complete remission, suggesting that I-131 can be used with curative intent in specific situations.

## Role of Surgery and Other Local Treatment Modalities for Bone Metastases

Several studies have reported survival benefit if resection of metastases is undertaken. There is potential for considerable bias in this conclusion since in many cases surgical resection is never contemplated since complete resection is unachievable given the burden of the disease; these patients may have poor prognosis to begin with. Some authors have suggested that resection of basal skull metastases should not be undertaken. Nevertheless, surgery is indicated for intractable pain, neurological deficit, and cervical instability. On a case to case basis, this may include complete metastatectomy, anterior spine reconstruction and stabilization, percutaneous vertebroplasty, and balloon kyphoplasty.

Selective arterial embolization therapy is a minimally invasive procedure that is particularly useful for preparing selected patients for open surgery of targeted metastatic lesions. It decreases the blood flow to the lesion thus significantly lowering the intraoperative blood loss. Embolization has been associated with decreasing serum Tg levels. However, embolization therapy alone does not appear to confer a survival benefit though it helps achieve improvement in pain and neurological symptoms.

Percutaneous spinal tumor ablation can be accomplished by various techniques which include radiofrequency ablation (RFA), cryotherapy, and ethanol ablation.

During radiofrequency ablation, high-frequency alternating current passes from a needle electrode to the tissue, resulting in frictional heating and necrosis. In a study of 43 patients at Mayo clinic, radiofrequency ablation was able to control pain in 95 % of cases. Complications occurred in three patients and included a second-degree burn at the grounding pad site, fracture at the site of ablation, and transient bowel and bladder incontinence after treating a sacral lesion. RFA can be considered for pain palliation or as an adjunct to surgery.

Cryotherapy has also been used for palliation of symptoms from metastatic bone disease. Studies with cryotherapy specifically in thyroid cancer related bone metastases are lacking. But a prospective study of 12 patients with bone metastases who were treated with argon-based cryotherapy showed lesser incidence of fractures compared to conventional nitrogen-based therapy and no complications of infection or tissue necrosis. All treated patients experienced a significant improvement in pain. After cryotherapy treatment, cavities created by treatment may need to be filled with bone cement or other substitutes in bones that are weight bearing.

## Adjunctive Therapy with Bisphosphonates and Denosumab

Regardless of the form of definitive treatment chosen, one should consider the use of bisphosphonates or denosumab to prevent the secondary complications of bone metastases and also to reduce pain.

Bisphosphonates inhibit osteoclast activity, so it has been proposed that these agents slow or prevent the skeletal complications of bone metastases. There is a paucity of data on treatment of bone metastases from thyroid cancer with these agents but they are being used in management of bone metastases from other solid malignancies.

In a study by Vitale et al., pamidronate 90 mg was administered intravenously to 10 thyroid cancer patients with bone metastases every month for 12 months. The patients had a significant decrease in bone pain and partial radiographic response was observed in 2/10 patients while 5/10 patients had stabilization of their bone lesions. In a retrospective study by Orita et al. in thyroid cancer patients with metastatic bone disease, zoledronic acid 4 mg intravenously every month for average of 16 months significantly delayed the onset of skeletal-related events (SRE) compared to patients who did not get zoledronic acid. The SREs included pathological fracture, need for orthopedic surgery or radiation, and spinal cord compression. The SRE free 3-year survival rate was 86 % in the treated group compared to 50 % in the untreated group. Intravenous and oral ibandronate have also been studied in other cancers and have demonstrated effectiveness in reducing bone pain and time to SRE.

Side effects associated with intravenous bisphosphonates are fever, myalgias, nausea, and bone pain. They are usually mild and can be managed with antipyretics and they tend to become uncommon on subsequent infusions. Renal toxicity is the main concern with intravenous bisphosphonates and is directly related to dose and infusion time. It is advisable to monitor renal function and creatinine clearance with every cycle of IV bisphosphonate. Adequate supplementation with calcium and vitamin D can prevent most cases of hypocalcemia. For those who measure 25-hydroxyvitamin D levels, the target range should be approximately >30 ng/ml to reduce the risk of hypocalcemia.

Denosumab is a fully human monoclonal antibody of IgG2 subtype. It acts by neutralizing RANKL, preventing its binding to RANK on osteoclasts and their precursor cells, thereby inhibiting osteoclast proliferation and function and reducing bone resorption.

In a phase-3 trial comparing subcutaneous denosumab 120 mg every 4 weeks to intravenous zoledronic acid 4 mg every 4 weeks for 1 year in patients with bone metastases from solid tumors, denosumab delayed the onset of a SRE event by 27.66 months and this was significantly higher than zoledronic acid which delayed the onset of a skeletal related event by 19.45 months. There were no differences between denosumab and zoledronic acid groups in terms of overall disease progression.

The common side effects associated with administration of denosumab are fever, fatigue, nausea, and anorexia. Hypocalcemia is more common with denosumab than with zoledronic acid with an incidence as high as 9.6 %. As with bisphosphonates, adequate supplementation with calcium and vitamin D can prevent most cases of hypocalcemia.

Osteonecrosis of the jaw (ONJ) has been associated with IV bisphosphonates and subcutaneous denosumab. ONJ is defined as the presence of exposed bone in the maxillofacial region that does not heal within 2 months after identification. The risk of ONJ in cancer patients treated with monthly doses of these agents may be as high as 1–10/100 patients. Risk factors for ONJ include head and neck radiotherapy, periodontal disease, dental procedures involving bone surgery, edentulous regions, and trauma from poorly fitting dentures. Malignancy, chemotherapy, corticosteroids, and systemic infections are additional risk factors.

Atypical fractures of the femoral diaphysis have been reported in patients on long-term (3–8 years) bisphosphonates and those on denosumab. Atypical femoral fractures are rare, low energy fractures of either the subtrochanteric region of the hip or the femoral shaft. Although these fractures have been reported mostly in patients who have been treated with bisphosphonates (especially those on glucocorticoids), atypical femoral fractures have occurred in patients with no history of bisphosphonate use.

Given the lack of comprehensive clinical trial data on the efficacy of bisphosphonates and denosumab for patients with bone metastases from thyroid cancer, the optimal treatment regimen and duration of therapy is unknown. For those who suffer an acute pathologic fracture or have extensive, symptomatic bone metastases, or short life expectancy, we think it is reasonable to follow the prescribing information for both agents and give full doses (zoledronic acid 4 mg intravenously or denosumab 120 mg subcutaneously) every 4 weeks. Based on trial data for other malignancies, we are prepared to treat severely affected patients with metastatic disease to bone monthly for 2–4 years.

For patients who have a solitary bone metastasis or stable bone metastases, particularly if asymptomatic, and with a life expectancy more than 5 years, we think a prudent course would be to administer zoledronic acid 4 mg twice yearly and denosumab 120 mg twice yearly. For those who develop new bone metastases or progression of older metastases, we recommend treating with zoledronic acid 4 mg every 1–3 months or denosumab 120 mg every 1–3 months. If patients go on to develop stable disease, then it seems reasonable to reduce the dosing frequency of these drugs to twice yearly, especially if life expectancy is prolonged. If patients deteriorate and develop progressive or symptomatic disease from bone metastases, then it makes sense to ratchet up the dosing frequency to every 1–3 months depending on the clinical severity.

This paradigm represents our best judgment and personal approach on how to manage thyroid cancer bone metastases based on an extrapolation of data derived from clinical trials of patients with breast cancer, prostate cancer, and other solid malignancies. While these recommendations differ somewhat from those with bone metastases from other solid tumors, since patients with thyroid cancer may live many years even with osseous metastases, it seems a reasonable compromise between the potential advantages bisphosphonates and denosumab may offer and the potential adverse effects that could be linked to their long-term use, specifically atypical femoral shaft fractures and osteonecrosis of the jaw.

## Palliative Treatment

Surgery and percutaneous ablation may be used for palliative treatment in selected patients. In a retrospective review at a single institution, 41 patients underwent surgery for thyroid carcinoma bone metastasis from 1988 to 2011. Overall patient survival probability was 72 % at 1 year, 29 % at 5 years, and 20 % at 8 years. Disease progression at the surgery site occurred more frequently with a histological diagnosis of follicular carcinoma compared with other subtypes ($p=0.023$). Patients who had their tumor excised ($p=0.001$) or presented with solitary bone involvement had a lower risk of death following surgery adjusting for age and gender.

External beam radiotherapy (EBRT) is used to palliate pain in some individuals. EBRT should be used only when there is significant pain, risk of fracture, and risk of spinal cord compression. It is more useful in radioiodine refractory disease. When used with debulking surgery, it is more successful in achieving the goals of pain improvement and reducing risk of neurological sequelae than either therapeutic option alone. In a recent trial by Howell et al. comparing single fraction radiation therapy to conventional multifraction radiation therapy in patients with vertebral bone metastases, it was shown that both treatment schedules give equivalent pain relief without any increased risk of compressive myelopathy from radiation.

## New Directions: Tyrosine Kinase Inhibitors

Tyrosine kinase is involved in the activation of cell growth and proliferation through a number of pathways which include RET and MAP kinases. Tyrosine kinase inhibitors are competitive inhibitors of tyrosine kinase receptors. They also act on VEGF receptors to inhibit vascular proliferation. Since the tyrosine kinase receptors and VEGF receptors are widely distributed, tyrosine kinase inhibitors target multiple tissues.

Sorafenib has been approved by the Food and Drug Administration for the treatment of progressive, metastatic well-differentiated thyroid carcinoma refractory to radioactive iodine (RAI) treatment. A phase-3 trial of sorafenib in metastatic differentiated thyroid cancer not responsive to RAI treatment increased the progression free survival to 10.8 months compared with 5.8 months in patients receiving placebo. Phase-2 trials of sorafenib in iodine refractory metastatic well-differentiated thyroid cancer have shown partial response rates in 15–23 % of patients and stable disease in 53–56 %.

While the general response of patients to these compounds has been encouraging with significant increases in progression free survival, the specific value of these agents for bone metastases has not yet been elucidated. In one study, 62 patients with various subtypes of thyroid cancer were treated with sorafenib (62 %), sunitinib (22 %), and vandetanib (16 %) outside of clinical trials. Most were treated with a single TKI, but a few were exposed to several lines of TKI therapy.

Of those treated with sorafenib and sunitinib, the partial response (PR) rate was 15 % and 8 %, respectively. Unfortunately, however, bone and pleural lesions were the most refractory sites to treatment, suggesting TKIs might not be an optimal therapy for those with osseous metastases as the only site of distant disease.

Patients taking tyrosine kinase inhibitors need to be monitored for development of hypertension, prolongation of QTc interval, elevation of liver enzymes, bone marrow suppression, and heart failure. The most common skin reaction associated with use of these agents is hand–foot skin disease, a blistering skin toxicity. Contraindications to their use include healing surgical wounds, QTc interval >450 ms, recent radiotherapy treatment, and history of cerebral or gastrointestinal bleeding within the 6 months prior to use of TKI therapy.

## Monitoring and Follow-Up

Thyroglobulin is a sensitive and specific marker for follow-up of thyroid cancer patients especially after total thyroidectomy and radioactive iodine ablation. It is usually measured by immunoradiometric assay (IRMA) and to improve accuracy with this technique, one must rule out the presence of anti-Tg antibodies in the serum. It is usually <0.2 ng/ml after total thyroidectomy and RAI ablation. A value of more than 2 ng/ml should prompt further investigation with diagnostic radioiodine whole body scan and neck sonogram. If these are negative, PET/CT scan, CT chest and bone imaging should be considered.

Suppressive levothyroxine therapy should be used in all intermediate to high-risk thyroid cancer patients with a goal TSH <0.1 µU/ml. Treatment with RAI ablation should be followed by post-therapy scans especially in patients with metastatic disease. If patients are being considered for inclusion in a clinical trial, patients must meet RECIST criteria (Response Evaluation Criteria in Solid Tumors). According to these criteria, lytic bone lesions with an identifiable soft tissue component evaluated by CT or MRI can be considered as measurable lesions when the soft tissue component meets the definition of measurability.

## Back to Our Patient

Our patient is a 47-year-old man with papillary thyroid carcinoma with progressive lung and bone metastases. He no longer has disease responsive to radioiodine therapy. He has been receiving monthly subcutaneous denosumab and has not experienced a skeletal related event since being on this therapy. He is also enrolled in a clinical trial of lenvatinib and has stable disease more than 6 months into treatment with this agent. He has not experienced any significant drug-related toxicities while on lenvatinib.

## Questions

1. A 56-year-old woman is found to have a thyroid nodule on routine physical examination. FNA shows papillary thyroid cancer. She undergoes a total thyroidectomy and pathology confirmed multifocal papillary thyroid cancer with the largest lesion on the right being 1.6 cm with involvement of right central lymph nodes—10/16 lymph nodes positive. She undergoes therapy with 125 mCi of I-131. Six month follow-up shows a Tg level of 5 ng/ml with negative Tg antibodies, stimulated Tg level is 40 mg/ml, neck sonogram is negative for pathologic lymph nodes or neck masses. A Thyrogen stimulated diagnostic I-123 whole body scan shows three areas of increased uptake in lumbar and thoracic spine and the left 12th posterior rib. The patient is asymptomatic. Which of the following is the next best step in her management?

    (a) External beam radiotherapy
    (b) Treat with radioactive iodine
    (c) Cryotherapy
    (d) Radiofrequency ablation

2. How should one follow this patient after treatment with I-131?

    (a) Serial x-rays
    (b) Serial diagnostic whole body-scans
    (c) Thyroglobulin levels
    (d) Measurement of alkaline phosphatase levels

3. A 60-year-old man presents with right hip pain. MRI shows a lytic lesion in the right femoral head that on biopsy reveals cells of thyroid origin. He undergoes a total thyroidectomy which shows a 5 cm focus of follicular thyroid cancer followed by 200 mCi I-131 therapy. Post-therapy scan shows uptake in the thyroid bed, right femur, and lungs. What is the next step in management?

    (a) Nothing further can be done
    (b) Sorafenib
    (c) I-131 treatment
    (d) Denosumab

## Answers to Questions

1. b: Treatment with radioactive is the treatment of choice for iodine avid lesions. Responsiveness to radioactive iodine is the single most important factor associated with good prognosis in these patients. Bisphosphonates and denosumab are indicated to prevent secondary complications of metastases in these patients and denosumab has been shown to prevent skeletal-related events for a longer time compared to bisphosphonates. Surgery is only indicated for progressive neural deficits and palliation of pain.

2. c: Thyroglobulin levels. Our approach is to follow Tg levels while on levothyrox-ine suppression in these patients closely for a year, then at 6 month intervals for 5 years followed by yearly assessments. Stimulated Tg levels can be checked periodically if needed. Any suspicion of metastases should be followed by a work-up that should include neck ultrasound, diagnostic radioiodine whole body scan, and cross-sectional imaging studies, including PET/CT when indicated.
3. d: Denosumab. Denosumab is indicated for use in the prevention of skeletal-related events in patients with bone metastases from breast cancer, prostate cancer, and other solid malignancies.

# References

1. Wexler JA. Approach to thyroid cancer patient with bone metastases. J Clin Endocrinol Metab. 2011;96(8):2296–307.
2. Muresan MM, Olivier P, Leclère J, Sirveaux F, Brunaud L, Klein M, Zarnegar R, Weryha G. Bone metastases from differentiated thyroid carcinoma. Endocr Relat Cancer. 2008;15(1): 37–49.
3. Schlumberger M, Challeton C, De Vathaire F, Travagli J-P, et al. Radioactive iodine treatment and external radiotherapy for lung and bone metastases from thyroid carcinoma. J Nucl Med. 1996;37(4):598–605.
4. Carhill AA, Cabanillas ME, Jimenez C, Waguespack SG, et al. The noninvestigational use of tyrosine kinase inhibitors in thyroid cancer: establishing a standard for patient safety and moni-toring. J Clin Endocrinol Metab. 2013;98:31–42.
5. Lipton A, Fizazi K, Stopeck AT, Henry DH, et al. Superiority of denosumab to zoledronic acid for prevention of skeletal-related events: a combined analysis of 3 pivotal, randomised, phase 3 trials. Eur J Cancer. 2012;48:3082–92.
6. Ramadan S, Ugas MA, Berwick RJ, Notay M, Cho H, Jerjes W, Giannoudis PV. Spinal metas-tases in thyroid cancer. Head Neck Oncol. 2012;4:39.

# Part V
# Adrenal

# Chapter 20
# Introduction

Alice C. Levine

Over 150 years ago, Brown-Sequard demonstrated that the adrenal glands are essential for life. In the late nineteenth and twentieth centuries, the hormones secreted by the adrenal cortex and medulla were isolated, purified, and synthesized for therapeutic use. In addition, their receptors, stimulators, inhibitors, co-activators, co-repressors, intracellular signaling cascades, and downstream effectors have been delineated. In the twenty-first century, the molecular genetics underlying many adrenal disorders have been uncovered.

Although physiologic levels of adrenal hormones are necessary for the proper functioning of all tissues and organs and critical for the stress response, pharmacologic levels of these hormones have devastating effects on multiple organ systems. Clinical studies over the past 20 years have revealed that many cases of so-called "idiopathic" hypertension are due to aldosterone hypersecretion and furthermore that these disorders often have an underlying genetic basis. Very recently, a number of retrospective studies indicate that any degree of hypercortisolism is deleterious to bone, metabolic, and cardiovascular health. Advances in radiologic imaging, particularly the introduction of the CT scan in the early 1970s, led to the epidemic of "adrenal incidentalomas"—incidentally discovered adrenal masses, an entity that is particularly prevalent in older individuals. Detailed hormonal testing of patients with adrenal incidentalomas has revealed that many are associated with mild hypercortisolism. Excessive catecholamine secretion from pheochromocytomas, even if only episodic, can result in sudden death. Pheochromocytomas are considered "ticking time bombs" and once discovered need careful preoperative and perioperative management in order to insure a safe outcome.

A.C. Levine (✉)
Medicine, Division of Endocrinology, Diabetes and Bone Diseases,
Mount Sinai (Icahn School of Medicine at Mount Sinai Hospital), New York, NY, USA
e-mail: Jason.a.wexler@medstar.net

© Springer Science+Business Media New York 2015
T.F. Davies (ed.), *A Case-Based Guide to Clinical Endocrinology*,
DOI 10.1007/978-1-4939-2059-4_20

In this section, three cases of adrenal hormonal hypersecretion are presented. The case of primary aldosteronism underscores the recent epidemiologic data demonstrating the relatively high prevalence in patients with resistant hypertension with or without hypokalemia, the appropriate diagnostic algorithms, therapeutic options, and genetic forms of the disease. The case of an adrenal incidentaloma describes the necessary workup to rule out malignancy and adrenal hypersecretion. This case also focuses on the controversies surrounding the diagnosis of mild hypercortisolism as well as the current medical and surgical therapies. Finally, the case of pheochromocytoma illustrates the biochemical and radiologic tools available to identify adrenal medullary tumors as well as the best available approaches for their management.

# Chapter 21
# Primary Aldosteronism

**Sandi-Jo Galati and Alice C. Levine**

## Case Description

A 50-year-old woman was referred to endocrinology by her primary care physician for complaints of fatigue and hair loss. Her past medical history was notable for hypertension diagnosed 1 year prior with several blood pressure recordings of 160/100. Her blood pressure (BP) was effectively managed with the angiotensin-converting enzyme inhibitor (ACEi) ramipril 10 mg daily and the β-blocker biso-prolol 10 mg daily. She reported a family history of essential hypertension in both parents and two of her siblings.

On physical examination she was a thin woman with no stigmata of Cushing's disease. Her blood pressure was 140/80 with pulse 72. She had mild diffuse scalp hair thinning. She had no thyromegaly or palpable nodules. Lungs were clear to auscultation and cardiac exam was normal. Abdomen was soft, and there was no peripheral edema.

Laboratory evaluation revealed a serum sodium of 140 mEq/L, potassium 4.1 mEq/L, and creatinine 0.8 mg/dL. Plasma aldosterone concentration (PAC) was 18 ng/dL with plasma renin activity (PRA) 0.23 ng/mL/h (0.25–5.82). The aldosterone/renin ratio (ARR) was 78 ng/dL per ng/L/h, suggesting primary aldosteronism (PA) as the underlying cause of her hypertension.

S.-J. Galati, M.D. (✉)
Endocrine and Diabetes Specialists of CT, 112 Quarry Road, Ste 250,
Trumbull, CT 06611, USA
e-mail: sandijo.galati@gmail.com

A.C. Levine, M.D.
Division of Endocrinology, Diabetes and Bone Diseases, Department of Medicine,
Icahn School of Medicine at Mount Sinai Hospital, 1 Gustave L. Levy Place,
Box 1055, New York, NY 10029, USA

© Springer Science+Business Media New York 2015                                   187
T.F. Davies (ed.), *A Case-Based Guide to Clinical Endocrinology*,
DOI 10.1007/978-1-4939-2059-4_21

The patient underwent confirmatory testing with a 2 L intravenous saline infusion. Pre-infusion PAC was 16 ng/dL, post-infusion was 11 ng/dL, indicating lack of appropriate suppression and confirming the diagnosis of PA.

CT abdomen was performed and demonstrated thickening in the medial limb of the left adrenal, but no adenoma. She then underwent adrenal venous sampling (AVS), which did not demonstrate lateralization, suggesting bilateral adrenal hyperplasia (BAH) as the underlying pathophysiologic mechanism driving her PA.

She was started on the mineralocorticoid receptor antagonist spironolactone at a dose of 25 mg daily and ramipril was stopped. She tolerated spironolactone without side effects. Bisoprolol was subsequently discontinued and spironolactone was ultimately titrated to 100 mg daily, resulting in control of her blood pressure.

## How Does PA Cause Hypertension?

Aldosterone exerts its main effect at the distal tubule of the nephron where it binds to the mineralocorticoid receptor (MR) and promotes gene expression of epithelium sodium channels (ENaC). Increased ENaC expression results in sodium and water absorption, volume expansion with renin suppression, reflexive vasoconstriction, and ultimately hypertension in states of aldosterone excess, such as PA [1].

## What Is the Prevalence of PA in Hypertensive Patients *Without Hypokalemia?*

Jerome Conn described the initial patient with PA in 1954, a young woman with intractable hypertension, tetany, and hypokalemia in which bilateral adrenalectomy was planned in order to control her symptoms. Fortunately, an adrenal adenoma was identified and resected in the operating room, sparing the patient from bilateral adrenalectomy, and resolving her metabolic abnormalities, tetany, and hypertension [2].

Classical teaching recommends screening patients for PA only if they have hypertension and hypokalemia. And, in fact, patients with concomitant hypertension and potassium less than 3.2 mEq/L have a 11-fold increase in the incidence of PA compared to normokalemic (potassium greater than 3.5 mEq/L) patients [3]. However, recent prevalence studies have demonstrated only a 9–37 % incidence of hypokalemia in patients with documented PA, indicating the absence of hypokalemia should not be used as exclusion criteria for PA [4].

Current guidelines recommend screening all patients with moderate or severe hypertension, spontaneous or diuretic-induced hypokalemia, or hypertension with an adrenal adenoma [5].

## What Is the *Prevalence* of Primary Aldosteronism in Outpatient Hypertensive Patients?

After 10 years of studying and treating patients with PA, Conn postulated the prevalence in hypertensive patients to be high, potentially 20 %. He later modified this estimate to 10 %, however, a 1967 study by Fishman et al. suggested disease presence in <1 % of hypertensive patients screened [6], a statistic that debunked the estimates of Conn and has persisted in the medical literature until recently.

Since the widespread use and validation of the ARR in the early 1990s, worldwide prevalence studies in patients with hypertension have demonstrated a much higher prevalence, closer to Conn's original estimates. Prevalence studies in Australia, Singapore, and Italy demonstrated a prevalence of 5–12 % [7–9]. Even higher prevalence rates have been described in specific populations, such as patients with resistant hypertension (20 %), diabetes and hypertension (13–14 %), and hypertension with obstructive sleep apnea (34 %) [10–16].

## Why Is Early Screening and Detection Beneficial?

In addition to its role in salt and water homeostasis, aldosterone has effects at the local tissue level, mediating expression of tissue growth factors and collagen, and increasing oxidative stress and endothelial dysfunction. Ultimately, this results in the deposition of collagen within arterial walls, leading to increased stiffness and increased intima to media thickness [17].

Independent of blood pressure control, aldosterone excess in patients with PA results in left ventricular remodeling and hypertrophy [18–20]. In a retrospective study of patients with PA, Milliez et al. demonstrated in increased risk of cardiovascular events including nonfatal myocardial infarction (MI), cerebrovascular accidents, and atrial fibrillation independent of blood pressure control [21]. These finding were subsequently recapitulated in a prospective study by Catena et al., in which coronary artery disease, cerebrovascular disease, and sustained arrhythmias were more prevalent in patients with untreated PA compared to age, sex, and blood pressure-matched controls [22]. Aldosterone excess has also been implicated in obstructive sleep apnea, insulin resistance and the metabolic syndrome, osteoporosis, and renal insufficiency.

## What Is the Best *Screening Test* for Primary Aldosteronism?

The aldosterone–renin ratio (ARR) is the most sensitive and specific screening tool for PA. It relies on the known pathophysiology of PA, in which aldosterone levels are disproportionately high in comparison to renin concentration. Screening with

ARR is generally accepted as positive if ARR exceeds 20 ng/dL per ng/mL/h and PAC exceeds 10 ng/dL [23]. Aldosterone elevation is crucial to interpreting the ARR, as false positives can occur if renin is sufficiently suppressed, as seen in patients with low-renin hypertension.

The ARR is affected by most anti-hypertensive medications; however, it can be reliably interpreted if patients are on any agent except the MR-receptor antagonists (spironolactone and eplerenone) with the knowledge of how these agents affect the ratio [5]. For example, a patient with essential hypertension on an ACEi or angiotensin receptor blocker (ARB) would be expected to have elevated renin with compensatory decrease in aldosterone due to downstream inhibition of the renin–angiotensin system. If the patient had PA, aldosterone synthesis and release would escape regulation by the renin–angiotensin system and would be elevated. Furthermore, elevated aldosterone and volume expansion would suppress renin levels despite the expected renin elevation with ACEi or ARB use.

Patients with suspected PA on MR-receptor antagonist require a 6-week medication washout prior to screening. Alternative medications that do not significantly affect the ARR include the nondihydropyridine calcium channel blockers (verapamil and diltiazem), hydralazine, or the peripheral α-blockers (prazosin, doxazosin, or terazosin) [5, 23].

Finally, even in the setting of a negative ARR screen, knowledge of renin and aldosterone levels are useful tools in selecting appropriate antihypertensive therapy for any patient. For instance, an agent that interferes with the renin–angiotensin system such as an ACEi or ARB may be ineffective in patients with low-renin hypertension.

## How Is the Diagnosis *Confirmed*?

Confirmatory testing must be performed in all patients who screen positive with the ARR for PA. Current clinical guidelines support confirmation with oral sodium loading, saline infusion, fludrocortisone suppression, or captopril challenge testing. Using any of the four modalities, failure to suppress aldosterone secretion is diagnostic of PA. There is no consensus on the optimal test due to insufficient evidence [5]; therefore, the selection of a confirmatory test should be based on patient preference and institution capabilities.

## What Is the *Molecular Pathophysiology* of Primary Aldosteronism?

Aldosterone synthesis and secretion is mediated by renin-dependent angiotensin II. Hyperkalemia and, to a lesser extent, adrenocorticotroph hormone (ACTH) also stimulate aldosterone secretion. PA is a high aldosterone, low renin state resulting from constitutive aldosterone synthesis and release from one or both adrenal glands.

The most common etiology of aldosterone excess, accounting for two-thirds of cases, is bilateral adrenal hyperplasia (BAH). Aldosterone-producing adenomas (APAs) account for one-third of cases. Unilateral hyperplasia, adrenocortical carcinoma, ectopic aldosterone production, and familial hyperaldosteronism 1, 2, and 3 (FH 1, 2, 3) are rare causes.

The underlying molecular changes that result in PA are largely unknown; however, recent descriptions of the germline mutations underlying FH 3 has yielded some insight into sporadic disease. The index family with FH 3 presented with severe hypertension and hypokalemia during childhood requiring bilateral adrenalectomies for management [24]. Pathologic analysis of the adrenals demonstrated massive hyperplasia. The underlying genetic mutation was located to the *KCNJ5* gene, which encodes a component of the Kir3.4 potassium channel. Abnormal function of Kir3.4 decreases its selectivity for potassium and allows sodium entry into the cell, prolonged depolarization, and resultant constitutive aldosterone synthesis and release [25]. Several mutations within the *KCNJ5* sequence have been identified, resulting in variable phenotypes. Further, genetic analysis of presumed sporadic APAs has demonstrated somatic mutations in *KCNJ5* suggesting acquired genetic abnormalities have a significant contributing factor in the development of PA [25–30].

## Once PA Is Confirmed Should You Proceed with *Subtype Differentiation*?

Once the diagnosis of PA is confirmed, it is crucial to adapt a patient-centered approach in the final diagnostic steps, taking into consideration the age, comorbid conditions, and treatment goals of the patient. Abdominal computed tomography (CT) is typically the first localization study performed once the diagnosis of PA is confirmed. CT enables the identification of adrenal enlargement, adenomas, or rarely carcinomas [5]. In patients who ultimately do not desire or would not be candidates for surgery, the requirement for any localization study is questionable. Current guidelines recommend CT in all patients to exclude the possibility of an adrenocortical carcinoma (ACC) [5]. However, in practice, ACC is very rare, and also typically cosecretes other adrenocortical hormones. In patients with mild disease or long-standing hypertension desiring medical therapy, our practice is to not pursue CT.

Adrenal venous sampling (AVS) is an invasive diagnostic test used for localization that must be pursued in all patients in which surgery is the planned treatment modality. CT alone is insufficient for presurgical localization as concordance between CT and AVS is approximately 50 %, placing 25 % of patients at risk for unilateral adrenalectomy of the wrong side.

AVS technique and interpretation varies by institution. In our center, the bilateral adrenal veins are accessed via femoral puncture and catheterization, and ACTH is infused via peripheral IV. ACTH-stimulated adrenal vein and inferior vena cava (IVC) cortisol levels are compared to confirm proper catheter placement in the adrenal veins. Adrenal vein aldosterone values are then corrected for cortisol to account for venous dilution by the phrenic vein. The bilateral cortisol-corrected aldosterone values are compared, and a 4:1 ratio favoring one side is suggestive of unilateral disease. More importantly however, adrenal vein aldosterone secretion must be suppressed from the contralateral side to confirm the diagnosis of unilateral disease.

AVS is 95 % sensitive and 100 % specific for localizing unilateral APAs, however, success of this procedure and complication rate is practitioner dependent, mainly due to the technical difficulty of catheterizing the right adrenal vein [31, 32]. Because of these risks, AVS should only be pursued for patients in whom surgical intervention would be considered.

## What Is the Preferred Treatment for Each Subtype?

The majority of patients with PA have BAH which is amenable to medical therapy with MR-antagonists such as spironolactone or eplerenone. Spironolactone at doses of 25–400 mg daily is the initial agent of choice and results in a 25 % systolic blood pressure reduction and a 22 % diastolic reduction [5]. Spironolactone is inexpensive and may decrease polypharmacy. In a study of patients with PA and uncontrolled hypertension, addition of spironolactone improved blood pressure to goal in 50 % of patients studied and was the sole agent required to maintain control in 50 % of these responders [33].

In addition to its actions at the MR, spironolactone has antagonistic properties at the androgen receptor and agonistic properties at the progesterone receptor, which result in its main side effects of gynecomastia in men and mastodynia in women. Although these side effects are dose- dependent, patients with PA often require high doses, and as a result eplerenone may be a more tolerable agent [5].

Eplerenone is a selective MR antagonist and, as a result, lacks the progesterone receptor-stimulating and anti-androgen properties of spironolactone that result in its side effects [34]. However, in a head-to-head trial comparing effectiveness of the two agents, spironolactone resulted in more potent blood pressure reduction [35].

Amiloride and triamterene target blood pressure at the level of the ENaC receptor, which is increased as a result of aldosterone action at the distal renal tubule. These agents are less potent than MR antagonists in achieving blood pressure control in patients with PA and should be reserved for second-line use.

Surgery should be pursued in all patients with APAs in which the benefit outweighs the risk of unilateral adrenalectomy. Laparoscopic unilateral adrenalectomy is the preferred procedure. Postoperatively, BP and hypokalemia improve in 100 % of patients [5], and myocardial fibrosis improves within 1 year [36]. However, long-term hypertension cure rate is only 30–60 % [37–39]. Persistent postoperative hypertension is likely related to underlying essential hypertension and correlates to duration of disease, increased creatinine, older age, family history of essential hypertension, and use of more than two antihypertensive agents preoperatively [37, 39]. Patients with APAs who are not surgical candidates due to comorbid conditions or those who are unlikely to be cured can be managed medically, although higher doses of MR antagonists are typically required.

## What Are the Expected Long-Term Cardiovascular Outcomes in Patients with Treated PA?

The risk of excess cardiovascular and cerebrovascular disease in untreated patients with PA has been established [21, 22]. Unfortunately, there is limited prospective outcome data in patients treated either medically or surgically for PA. Catena et al. reported that *either* medical or surgical treatment of PA resulted in a reversal of the increased risk of MI, sustained arrhythmias, revascularization procedures, or cerebrovascular events in patients with PA after 7.4 years of follow-up [22].

A subsequent study by Bernini et al. following patients with PA over 2.5 years demonstrated significantly improved blood pressure control in patients treated with MR-antagonist or surgery, but significant decreases in left-ventricular mass were appreciated only in the surgically treated group [40]. This discrepancy compared to the studies by Catena et al. suggests an immediate improvement in cardiometabolic parameters occurring in patients who undergo surgery. However, in patients treated with medical management, a longer duration of treatment may be required for appreciable outcomes.

Mortality data for patients with PA is limited to one retrospective analysis of 337 patients treated for PA either medically or surgically. When compared to controls matched for age, sex, body mass index, and blood pressure, there was no difference in all-cause mortality in the patients treated for PA after 10 years, indicating a beneficial effect of treatment. However, among the deaths in the PA patients, significantly more were attributed to cardiovascular causes compared to controls [41].

## Lessons Learned

Our patient had moderate HTN at diagnosis, and, despite being normokalemic, screening was pursued based on the knowledge that PA is more prevalent than previous estimates, and that patients with PA often are normokalemic. She had an elevated ARR with elevated PAC and suppressed PRA, suggesting PA. She was using an ACEi at the time of screening, which would be expected to raise PRA and suppress PAC, rendering the observed PAC, PRA, and ARR more convincing of PA.

The decision to treat patients medically or surgically varies depending on disease subtype, duration of disease, medical comorbidities, and patient preference. In the case of our patient, she is young with a fairly recent diagnosis of HTN. Therefore, surgery was a reasonable consideration. Abdominal CT demonstrated a thickened left adrenal gland, however CT is unreliable for APA localization, so AVS was pursued and, ultimately, did not lateralize, suggesting BAH. The results of AVS in our patient underscore the importance of performing AVS in all surgical candidates. Our patient would have undergone an unnecessary unilateral adrenalectomy with no improvement in her blood pressure if surgery had been performed without AVS. Instead, she was treated with spironolactone, enabling cessation of her other antihypertensive agents with blood pressure control on one agent.

## Questions

1. A 50-year-old man is referred for evaluation of primary aldosteronism (PA). He has a 4-year history of hypertension that has become difficult to control over the last 6 months. He is treated currently with hydrochlorothiazide, lisinopril, atenolol, and amlodipine. His blood pressure at the time of initial consultation is 150/96. Serum creatinine is 1 mg/dL, and serum potassium is 3.8 mEq/L. His serum aldosterone is 18 ng/dL with plasma renin activity of 0.1 ng/mL/h [aldosterone-to-renin ratio (ARR) 180 ng/dL per ng/(mL×h)]. He had an abdominal CT scan 1 year ago that demonstrated an incidental 1 cm left adrenal adenoma. What is the next best step?

(A) Left adrenalectomy
(B) A confirmatory test such as an oral salt loading test
(C) Add spironolactone to his treatment regimen
(D) Repeat abdominal CT to see if the adenoma has grownAnswer: (b) A confirmatory test. The patient has an elevated ARR, which is suggestive of PA, but not diagnostic. The ARR is a screening test that must be confirmed by an oral salt loading test, and intravenous saline loading test, a captopril challenge test, or a fludrocortisone suppression test. Only following a positive confirmatory test can a diagnosis of PA be made. Adrenalectomy should not be performed without (1) confirming disease and (2) performing adrenal vein sampling to localize the side of the adenoma. Starting spironolactone is a reasonable future treatment option, but again, the presence of PA must be made with a confirmatory test. Further, confirmatory tests cannot be performed while a patient is on spironolactone. Repeating the abdominal CT would not provide any further diagnostic information.

2. The above patient undergoes an oral salt loading test. His 24-h urine aldosterone is elevated, confirming PA. Since his last visit 2 weeks ago, he has become strict with his diet and exercise regimen and has lost 10 lbs. His blood pressure is now 138/88 on the above medications. You suggest proceeding with adrenal vein sampling. He states since his blood pressure is at goal, he does not think further

testing is worthwhile. What information can you provide that will encourage him to complete the evaluation?

(A) Aldosterone excess results in increased cardiovascular and renal disease even if blood pressure is controlled, and treatment of PA reverses these complications
(B) Medical treatment with spironolactone may improve his blood pressure further and allow him to stop some of his other blood pressure medications
(C) If he is a surgical candidate, unilateral adrenalectomy may cure his hypertension
(D) All of the aboveAnswer: (d) All of the above. Excess aldosterone confers increased cardiovascular and renal morbidity regardless of blood pressure control. Treatment, either medical or surgical, reduces these excess complications as well as improves blood pressure control.

3. The patient agrees to proceed with adrenal vein sampling and is ultimately diagnosed with PA secondary to bilateral adrenal hyperplasia. You start spironolactone and titrate to a dose of 100 mg daily. He is able to stop his hydrochlorothiazide, lisinopril, and amlodipine. At his 1-month follow-up visit, his blood pressure is 118/78 on spironolactone and atenolol alone. He is pleased with his blood pressure control, but reports the development of painful gynecomastia that is impairing his quality of life. What other options do you have?

(A) Stop spironolactone and restart his old blood pressure medications
(B) Replace spironolactone with eplerenone
(C) Proceed with bilateral adrenalectomy
(D) There are no other options; he should continue spironolactoneAnswer: (b) Replace spironolactone with eplerenone. In addition to being a mineralocorticoid receptor blocker, spironolactone acts as an androgen receptor antagonist and a progesterone agonist. As a result, potential side effects include gynecomastia, mastodynia, and increased menstrual bleeding. These potential complications are more common as the dose of spironolactone increases. Eplerenone is a mineralocorticoid receptor blocker that does not interact with the androgen or progesterone receptor and therefore does not have the same side effects. In some studies, eplerenone is not as potent of a blood pressure lowering agent as spironolactone. But, in a patient suffering from side effects of spironolactone, it is an appropriate choice. He should be on targeted therapy to minimize cardiovascular and renal disease, so returning to his old blood pressure medications is not appropriate, nor is bilateral adrenalectomy.

# References

1. Funder JW. Aldosterone and mineralocorticoid receptors in the cardiovascular system. Prog Cardiovasc Dis. 2010;53(5):393–400.
2. Young WF. Primary aldosteronism: renaissance of a syndrome. Clin Endocrinol. 2007;669(5):607–18.

3. Goldenberg K, Snyder DK. Screening for primary aldosteronism: hypokalemia in hypertensive patients. J Gen Int Med. 1986;1(6):368–72.
4. Mulatero P, Stowasser M, Loh KC, Fardella CE, Gordon RD, Mosso L, Gomez-Sanchez CE, Veglio F, Young Jr WF. Increased diagnosis of primary aldosteronism, including surgically correctable forms, in centers from five continents. J Clin Endocrinol Metab. 2004;89(3): 1045–50.
5. Funder JW, Carey RM, Fardella C, Gomez-Sanchez CE, Mantero F, Stowasser M, Young Jr WF, Montori VM. Case detection, diagnosis, and treatment of patients with primary aldosteronism: an endocrine society clinical practice guideline. J Clin Endocrinol Metab. 2008; 93(9):3266–81.
6. Fishman LM, Küchel O, Liddle GW, Michelakis AM, Gordon RD, Chick WT. Incidence of primary aldosteronism uncomplicated "essential" hypertension. A prospective study with elevated aldosterone secretion and suppressed plasma renin activity used as diagnostic criteria. JAMA. 1968;205(7):497–502.
7. Gordon RD, Stowasser MD, Tunny TJ, Klemm SA, Rutherford JC. High prevalence in primary aldosteronism in 199 patients referred with hypertension. Clin Exp Pharmacol Physiol. 1994;21(4):315–8.
8. Loh KC, Koay ES, Khaw MC, Emmanuel SC, Young Jr WF. Prevalence of primary aldosteronism among Asian hypertensive patients in Singapore. J Clin Endocrinol Metab. 2000;85:2854–9.
9. Rossi GP, Bernini G, Caliumi C, Desideri G, Fabris B, Ferri C, Ganzaroli C, Giacchetti G, Letizia C, Maccario M, Mallamaci F, Mannelli M, Mattarello MJ, Moretti A, Palumbo G, Parenti G, Porteri E, Semplicini A, Rizzoni D, Rossi E, Boscaro M, Pessina AC, Mantero F, PAPY Study Investigators. A prospective study of the prevalence of primary aldosteronism in 1,125 hypertensive patients. J Am Coll Cardiol. 2006;48(11):2293–300.
10. Calhoun DA, Nishizaka MK, Zaman MA, Thakkar RB, Weissmann P. Hyperaldosteronism among black and white subjects with resistant hypertension. Hypertension. 2002;40(6): 892–6.
11. Gallay BJ, Ahmad S, Xu L, Toivola B, Davidson RC. Screening for primary aldosteronism without discontinuing hypertensive medications: plasma aldosterone- renin ratio. Am J Kidney Dis. 2001;37(4):699–705.
12. Strauch B, Zelinka T, Hampf M, Bernhardt R, Widimsky Jr J. Prevalence of primary aldosteronism in moderate to severe hypertension in the Central Europe region. J Hum Hypertens. 2003;17(5):349–52.
13. Mukherjee JJ, Khoo CM, Thai AC, Chionh SB, Pin L, Lee KO. Type 2 diabetic patients with resistant hypertension should be screened for primary aldosteronism. Diab Vasc Dis Res. 2010;7(1):6–13.
14. Umpierrez GE, Cantey P, Smiley D, Palacio A, Temponi D, Luster K, Chapman A. Primary aldosteronism in diabetic subjects with resistant hypertension. Diabetes Care. 2007;30(7): 1699–703.
15. Li N, Wang M, Wang H, Zhang D, Wang X, Zu F, Chang G, Zhou K. Prevalence of primary aldosteronism in hypertensive subjects with hyperglycemia. Clin Exp Hypertens. 2013;35(3):175–82.
16. Di Murro A, Petramala L, Cotesta D, Zinnamosca L, Crescenzi E, Marinelli C, Saponara M, Letizia C. Renin-angiotensin-aldosterone system in patients with sleep apnoea: prevalence of primary aldosteronism. J Renin Angiotensin Aldosterone Syst. 2010;11(3):165–72.
17. Widimsky Jr J, Strauch B, Petrák O, Rosa J, Somloova Z, Zelinka T, Holaj R. Vascular disturbances in primary aldosteronism: clinical evidence. Kidney Blood Press Res. 2012; 35(6):529–33.
18. Rossi GP, Sacchetto A, Visentin P, Canali C, Graniero GR, Palatini P, Pessina AC. Changes in left ventricular anatomy and function in hypertension and primary aldosteronism. Hypertension. 1996;27(5):1039–45.
19. Rossi GP, Sacchetto A, Pavan E, Palatini P, Graniero GR, Canali C, Pessina AC. Remodeling of the left ventricle in primary aldosteronism due to Conn's adenoma. Circulation. 1997;95(60):1471–8.

20. Matsumura K, Fujii K, Oniki H, Oka M, Iida M. Role of aldosterone in left ventricular hypertrophy in hypertension. Am J Hypertens. 2006;19(1):13–8.
21. Milliez P, Girerd X, Plouin PF, Blacher J, Safar ME, Mourad JJ. Evidence for an increased rate of cardiovascular events in patients with primary aldosteronism. J Am Coll Cardiol. 2005;45(8):1243–8.
22. Catena C, Colussi G, Nadalini E, Chiuch A, Baroselli S, Lapenna R, Sechi LA. Cardiovascular outcomes in patients with primary aldosteronism after treatment. Arch Intern Med. 2008;168(1):80–5.
23. Stowasser M, Ahmed AH, Pimenta E, Taylor PJ, Gordon RD. Factors affecting the aldosterone/renin ratio. Horm Metab Res. 2012;44(3):170–6.
24. Geller DS, Zhang J, Wisgerhof MV, Kashgarian M, Lifton RP. A novel form of human mendelian hypertension featuring nonglucocorticoid-remediable aldosteronism. J Clin Endocrinol Metab. 2008;93(8):3117–23.
25. Choi M, Scholl UI, Yue P, Björklund P, Zhao B, Nelson-Williams C, Ji W, Cho Y, Patel A, Men CJ, Lolis E, Wiserhof MV, Geller DS, Mane S, Hellman P, Westin G, Åkerström G, Wang W, Carling T, Lifton RP. K+ Channel mutations in adrenal aldosterone-producing adenomas and hereditary hypertension. Science. 2011;331(6018):768–72.
26. Boulkroun S, Beuschlein F, Rossi GP, Golib-Dzib JF, Fischer E, Amar L, Mulatero P, Samson-Couterie B, Hahner S, Quinkler M, Fallo F, Letizia C, Allolio B, Ceolotto G, Cicala MV, Lang K, Lefebvre H, Lenzini L, Maniero C, Monticone S, Perrocheau M, Pilon C, Plouin PF, Rayes N, Seccia TM, Veglio F, Williams TA, Zinnamosca L, Mantero F, Benecke A, Jeunemaitre X, Reincke M, Zennaro MC. Prevalence, clinical and molecular correlates of KCNJ5 mutations in primary aldosteronism. Hypertension. 2012;59(3):592–8.
27. Azizan EA, Murthy M, Stowasser M, Gordon R, Kowalski B, Xu S, Brown MJ, O'Shaughnessy KM. Somatic mutations affecting the selectivity filter of KCNJ5 are frequent in 2 large unselected collections of adrenal aldosteronomas. Hypertension. 2012;59(3):587–91.
28. Taguchi R, Yamada M, Nakajima Y, Satoh T, Hashimoto K, Shibusawa N, Ozawa A, Okada S, Rokutanda N, Takata D, Koibuchi Y, Horiguchi J, Oyama T, Takeyoshi I, Mori M. Expression and mutations of KCNJ5 mRNA in Japanese patients with aldosterone-producing adenomas. J Clin Endocrinol Metab. 2012;97(4):1311–9.
29. Azizan EA, Lam BY, Newhouse SJ, Zhou J, Kuc RE, Clarke J, Happerfield L, Marker A, Hoffman GJ, Brown MJ. Microarray, qPCR, and KCNJ5 sequencing of aldosterone-producing adenomas reveal differences in genotype and phenotype between zona glomerulosa- and zona fasciculate-like tumors. J Clin Endocrinol Metab. 2012;97(5):E819–29.
30. Monticone S, Hattangady NG, Nishimoto K, Mantero F, Rubin B, Cicala MV, Pezzani R, Auchus RJ, Ghayee HK, Shibata H, Kurihara I, Williams TA, Giri JG, Bollag RJ, Edwards MA, Isales CM, Rainey WE. Effect of KCNJ5 mutations on gene expression in aldosterone-producing adenomas and adrenocortical cells. J Clin Endocrinol Metab. 2012;97(8):E1567–72.
31. Young WF, Stanson AW, Thompson GB, Grant CS, Farley DR, van Heerden JA. Role for adrenal venous sampling in primary aldosteronism. Surgery. 2004;136(6):1227–35.
32. Nwariaku FE, Miller BS, Auchus R, Holt S, Watumull L, Dolmatch B, Nesbitt S, Vongpatanasin W, Victor R, Wians F, Livingston E, Snyder III WH. Primary hyperaldosteronism: effect of adrenal venous sampling on surgical outcome. Arch Surg. 2006;141(5):497–502.
33. Lim PO, Jung RT, MacDonald TM. Raised aldosterone to renin ratio predicts antihypertensive efficacy of spironolactone: a prospective cohort. Br J Clin Pharmacol. 1999;48(5):756–60.
34. de Gasparo M, Joss U, Ramjoue HP, Whitebread SE, Haenni H, Schenkel L, Kraehenbuehl C, Biollaz M, Grob J, Schmidlin J, et al. Three new epoxy-spirolactone derivatives: characterization in vivo and in vitro. J Pharmacol Exp Ther. 1987;240(2):650–6.
35. Parthasaathy HK, Menard J, White W. A double-blind, randomized study comparing the antihypertensive effect of eplerenome and spironolactone in patients with hypertension and evidence of primary aldosteronism. J Hypertens. 2011;29(5):980–90.
36. Lin YH, Wu XM, Lee HH. Adrenalectomy reverses myocardial fibrosis in patients with primary aldosteronism. J Hypertens. 2012;30(8):1606–13.

37. Sawka AM, Young WF, Thompson GB, Grant CS, Farley DR, Leibson C, van Heerden JA. Primary aldosteronism: factors associated with normalization of blood pressure after surgery. Ann Intern Med. 2001;135(4):258–61.
38. Meyer A, Brabant G, Behrend M. Long-term follow-up after adrenalectomy for primary aldosteronism. World J Surg. 2005;29(2):155–9.
39. Celen O, O'Brien MJ, Melby JC, Beazley RM. Factors influencing outcome of surgery for primary aldosteronism. Arch Surg. 1996;131(6):646–50.
40. Bernini G, Bacca A, Carli V, Carrara D, Materazzi G, Berti P, Miccoli P, Pisano R, Tantardini V, Bernini M, Taddei S. Cardiovascular changes in patients with primary aldosteronism after surgical or medical treatment. J Endocrinol Invest. 2012;35(3):274–80.
41. Reincke M, Fischer E, Gerum S, Merkle K, Schulz S, Pallauf A, Quinkler M, Hanslik G, Lang K, Hahner S, Allolio B, Meisinger C, Holle R, Beuschlein F, Bidlingmaier M, Endres S, German Conn's Registry-Else Kröner-Fresenius-Hyperaldosteronism Registry. Observational study mortality in treated primary aldosteronism. Hypertension. 2012;60(3):618–24.

# Chapter 22
# Adrenal Incidentaloma and Subclinical Hypercortisolism

Gillian M. Goddard and Eliza B. Geer

## Case Description

A 68-year-old woman was referred to an Endocrinologist by her primary care physician after a 1.5 cm adrenal mass was incidentally noted on an abdominal CT urogram of the abdomen performed for the work-up of persistent hematuria. It measured 3 Hounsfield units before contrast was given, consistent with adrenal adenoma.

The patient's past medical history was significant for hypertension controlled on a single anti-hypertensive agent, hyperlipidemia, and osteopenia. Upon further questioning the patient noted that she had gained 25 pounds in the previous 18 months. She had undergone menopause at 50 years of age.

On physical exam the patient was well appearing and obese. Her blood pressure was 158/88 mmHg and her pulse was 80 beats/min. She had no scalp hair loss, hirsutism, or acne. She did have an increase in the size of her dorsocervical fat pad. Cardiovascular exam revealed regular heart rate and rhythm, with no extra heart sounds. Lung exam was clear to auscultation with no wheezes. Abdomen was obese and soft. She did not have abdominal striae, lower extremity edema, or proximal muscle weakness or wasting.

Biochemical work-up revealed a fasting glucose of 78 mg/dl, creatinine if 0.7 mg/dl, BUN of 16 mg/dl, AST 19 U/l, and ALT of 15 U/l. The patient's late afternoon serum cortisol level was 6.5 mcg/dl, ACTH was <10 pg/ml and DHEA-S was 31 mcg/dl (normal 35–430 mcg/dl). Midnight salivary free cortisol concentrations were 1.4 nmol/l and 1.6 nmol/l (normal range <0.3–4.3 nmol/l). Serum cortisol concentration after a 1 mg dexamethasone suppression test was 6.1 mcg/dl. 24-h urine free cortisol levels were 55 mcg/24 h and 32 mcg/24 h (normal <50 mcg/24 h).

G.M. Goddard, M.D. (✉) • E.B. Geer, M.D.
Division of Endocrinology, Diabetes and Bone Diseases, Department of Medicine, Icahn School of Medicine at Mount Sinai Hospital, 1 Gustave L. Levy Place, Box 1055, New York, NY 10029, USA
e-mail: gillianmgoddard@yahoo.com; eliza.geer@mssm.edu

© Springer Science+Business Media New York 2015
T.F. Davies (ed.), *A Case-Based Guide to Clinical Endocrinology*,
DOI 10.1007/978-1-4939-2059-4_22

Serum aldosterone was 7.0 ng/dl and renin was 0.40. Serum catecholamine and 24-h urine catecholamine levels were normal.

Based on the partial serum cortisol suppression after 1 mg dexamethasone and mild elevation in urinary-free cortisol in the setting of a suppressed plasma ACTH concentration, the diagnosis of subclinical hypercortisolism was made. Treatment options were discussed with the patient including surgical removal of the adenoma or conservative management. The patient opted for conservative management with serial imaging and biochemical evaluation.

## What Is the Prevalence of Incidentally Identified Adrenal Nodules?

Incidentally identified adrenal nodules, adrenal "incidentalomas," are becoming more commonly identified as the frequency of abdominal imaging has increased. An incidentaloma is defined as an adrenal mass of 1 cm or greater identified on imaging performed for indications other than the work-up or diagnosis of diseases of the adrenal gland [1].

Autopsy data report an overall prevalence of 1.0–8.7 % (mean 2.0 %). Prevalence varies significantly with age, with fewer than 1.0 % of patients less than 30 years of age having incidentalomas compared to 7.0 % of patients over 70 years of age [2]. The greatest rates of incidence appear to be in the fifth to seventh decades of life. Prevalence of incidentalomas identified by CT appears similar to autopsy data, with reports of <1.0 % prevalence to as great as 4.4 %. Some authors argue that the prevalence of incidentaloma on CT scan is increasing as these imaging techniques improve [2].

## Is the Nodule Malignant?

Malignant disease is always a concern in patients with adrenal incidentaloma. Adrenal cortical carcinoma (ACC) and metastatic disease comprise the majority of malignant disease in these patients. In populations with no history of cancer, two-thirds of clinically inapparent adrenal lesions are labeled benign [3]. To date there is no evidence suggesting that benign adenomas degenerate into malignant lesions [4].

ACC is rare, with an estimated incidence of 0.6–2 cases per million in the general population. In one case series ACC was found in 4.7 % of incidentally found adrenal masses [1]. The prevalence of ACC in incidentalomas may increase with size, with the greatest frequency in masses greater than 6 cm in diameter [4]. Metastatic disease is identified in approximately 2 % of incidentally identified adrenal masses, with the most commonly identified primary sites being breast, lung, lymphoma and melanoma [1, 4]. Most patients with adrenal metastases have a known primary malignancy and widespread disease.

Size and imaging characteristics can be used to help distinguish benign from malignant lesions. A diameter of greater than 4 cm has a 90 % sensitivity for detection of ACC, but only 24 % of lesions larger than 4 cm are malignant [5]. Retrospective analyses suggest that benign adenomas range in size from 1.0 to 9.0 cm in diameter, with a mean diameter of 3.3–3.5 cm [3]. Benign lesions are typically lipid rich, which results in a hypodense lesion on CT with low Hounsfield units, typically less than 10. Pheochronocytoma and malignant disease (both ACC and metastases) are lipid poor lesions and thus have high Hounsfield units, often greater than 25 [1]. Additionally, on delayed contrast-enhanced CT, adenomas show rapid washout (greater than 50 % at 10 min) while nonadenomas show delayed washout (less than 50 % at 10 min) [6].

## Is the Nodule Hormonally Active?

The vast majority of incidentally identified adrenal nodules are benign adenomas and most are non-functional [7]. Work-up of these nodules should focus on finding the few that are hormonally active. This should include a careful history and physical exam focusing in particular on possible signs of hypercortisolism, elevated catecholamines, hyperaldosteronism, and hyperandrogenism. Biochemical testing should focus on evaluation for pheochromocytoma, subclinical hypercortisolism, and hyperaldosteronism. Hormonal work-up should be performed regardless of imaging phenotype or lesion size [1]. Incidental adenomas that secrete androgens or estrogens are quite rare and biochemical testing need only be performed if signs and symptoms are present [4].

Plasma free metanephrines have high sensitivity and are simpler to perform than 24-h urine testing and thus are an excellent initial test for the identification of pheochromocytoma [8]. Confirmatory testing in the form of a 24-h urine fractionated metanephrines and normetanephrines should be performed if the initial screening test is positive. Estimates of the frequency of pheochromocytoma in patients with adrenal incidentaloma are variable. Retrospective analyses report a prevalence of 1.5–23 % [4]. Most estimate that approximately 5 % of adrenal incidentalomas are clinically silent pheochromocytoma [1].

The initial screening test for adrenal hypercortisolism should include a 1 mg overnight dexamethasone suppression test. There is on-going debate regarding the appropriate cut-off for this test, though a serum cortisol concentration at 8 AM of >5 mcg/dl is currently considered consistent with autonomous cortisol production [1, 4, 8]. A post-dexamethasone serum cortisol concentration of >5 mcg/dl will identify hypercortisolism with a specificity of 83–100 % but a sensitivity of only 44–58 %. Thus, one might adopt the lower serum cortisol cut-off of >1.8 mcg/dl after 1 mg overnight dexamethasone suppression, which is used in the diagnosis of overt Cushing's syndrome, if the clinical suspicion for hypercortisolism is high. This cut-off will identify hypercortisolism with a sensitivity of 75–100 %, but with a specificity of only 67–72 %. A serum cortisol level of >5 mcg/dl after 1 mg overnight dexamethasone suppression should trigger confirmatory testing which will be discussed later in this chapter. Approximately 5 % of incidentalomas secrete cortisol [4].

Work-up for hyperaldosteronism should only be performed in patients with hypertension [1]. While many patients with hyperaldosteronism have hypokalemia, normokalemic hyperaldosteronism is much more common than previously thought. Thus, serum potassium cannot be used for screening in these patients. Plasma aldosterone to plasma renin activity ratio is recommended for screening. If this ratio is elevated confirmatory testing should be performed [9]. Approximately 1 % of incidentalomas secrete aldosterone.

## What Follow-Up Should Patients Receive for Adrenal Nodules That Are Not Surgically Resected?

There is little prospective data regarding the follow-up of patients with adrenal incidentalomas. Retrospective studies suggest that the majority of patients will not experience significant growth of their benign appearing incidentaloma or new hyperfunction up to 10 years after initial identification of a nodule [10]. In contrast, one case series of nine patients who underwent serial imaging with pheochromocytoma and adrenal cortical carcinoma suggest that these masses grow at a rate of 1.0 cm/year and 2.0 cm/year, respectively [1]. However, the majority of adrenal masses that grow have benign pathology when surgically removed.

Current recommendations suggest repeat imagining with contrast CT scan at 6, 12, and 24 months, though imaging can be repeated earlier for nodules with suspicious imaging characteristics as previously mentioned [1]. Annual hormonal evaluation is recommended for 4 years after the initial evaluation. A change in size of >1.0 cm or a change in hormonal activity should prompt referral for surgical evaluation [8].

## What Is Subclinical Hypercortisolism?

Subclinical hypercortisolism, also referred to as preclinical Cushing's syndrome or subclinical Cushing's syndrome, is the condition of autonomous cortisol production with or without mild cortisol hypersecretion. By definition these patients do not develop classic symptoms of Cushing's syndrome such as pigmented striae, muscle weakness, and easy bruising, but they may develop diabetes, hypertension, or osteoporosis resulting from long-term mild cortisol excess [11]. As a result the term "subclinical" may be inaccurate given that patients often have clinically apparent sequelae of hypercortisolism, if not classic Cushing's syndrome.

There is little agreement regarding the biochemical definition of subclinical hypercortisolism, which makes diagnosis challenging. As previously mentioned, the 1 mg overnight dexamethasone suppression test is generally considered to be the best choice for initial work-up, although the appropriate serum cortisol cut-off to make the diagnosis is controversial [11]. A post-dexamethasone cortisol of >1.8 mcg/dl has a sensitivity of nearly 100 % for overt Cushing's syndrome but specificity for subclinical hypercortisolism is as low as 44 % [12]. A cutoff of 5 mcg/dl may be more appropriate in patients with suspected subclinical disease including those undergoing work-up of an adrenal incidentaloma. While it is counterintuitive to set the cutoff higher for subclinical compared to overt disease, considering that the probability of hypercortisolism is lower in patients without symptoms, a post-dexamethasone serum cortisol of >1.8 mcg/dl would result in more false positive than true positive results [13].

Other diagnostic tests have been assessed in the diagnosis of subclinical hypercortisolism, including measurement of 24-h urinary-free cortisol (UFC) and midnight salivary-free cortisol concentrations. However, 24-h UFC concentrations are frequently normal in patients with subclinical disease. The sensitivity of UFC for the diagnosis of subclinical hypercortisolism is 32–76 % [11]. As UFC levels are variable from sample to sample, this test is insensitive for detecting mild elevations in cortisol concentrations as seen in patients with subclinical disease. Lack of sensitivity makes this a poor screening test for subclinical hypercortisolism [13].

Several studies have reported altered circadian cortisol secretion in subclinical disease [14, 15]. As a result, and due to the ease with which midnight salivary cortisol testing can be performed, this test has been assessed for the diagnosis of subclinical Cushing's syndrome. However most studies show no difference in midnight salivary free cortisol concentrations between patients with and without subclinical hypercortisolism [14–16].

## What Are the Clinical Consequences of Subclinical Hypercortisolism?

By definition patients with subclinical hypercortisolism do not have classic symptoms of Cushing's. Possible manifestations of subclinical disease include type-2 diabetes, obesity, dyslipidemia, and hypertension, all of which are common in the general population [17–19]. Only a few studies have investigated the prevalence of these metabolic derangements in patients with adrenal incidentaloma and/or subclinical hypercortisolism [17–19]. These studies suggest that subclinical hypercortisolism is not really subclinical.

In fact, women with adrenal incidentaloma may be overweight with a central fat distribution and higher total body fat as compared to controls [19]. While these body composition changes are not as dramatic as those seen in overt Cushing's syndrome, they are statistically significant [19]. Patient's with subclinical hypercortisolism also appear to develop other aspects of the metabolic syndrome including elevations in triglycerides by as much as 75 % and impaired glucose tolerance as measured by oral glucose tolerance testing, though fasting glucose concentrations were not significantly different from controls [18].

A limited number of studies have assessed whether more features of metabolic syndrome translate to an increase in cardiovascular disease in patients with subclinical hypercortisolism. Compared to age matched controls, patients with subclinical hypercortisolism had more evidence of atherosclerotic plaques, and 60 % of patients had clinical, electrocardiographic, or sonographic evidence (i.e., carotid artery plaques) of cardiovascular disease [17].

## Does Treatment Improve the Clinical Manifestations of Subclinical Hypercortisolism?

Efforts to treat subclinical hypercortisolism have largely focused on surgical intervention (unilateral adrenalectomy). To date studies are all small and few prospectively compare surgical intervention and conservative management [11]. Outcomes focus primarily on improvement in hypertension, diabetes, dyslipidemia, and obesity. Several studies demonstrate improvement in blood pressure, dyslipidemia, and diabetes in surgically treated patients [12, 20]. Retrospective studies suggest that patients who benefit most from surgery are those with an adrenal incidentaloma and post-1 mg dexamethasone suppression serum cortisol greater than 5 mcg/dl [21].

There are no clinical studies of medical treatment of subclinical hypercortisolism including the use of cortisol biosynthesis inhibition with ketoconazole or glucocorticoid receptor blockade with mifepristone.

## Summary

Incidentally identified adrenal masses are a common clinical quandary as the number of imaging tests for other indications grows and as imaging techniques improve. Most incidentalomas are benign, nonfunctioning adrenal adenomas. Increasingly, patients with incidentalomas are managed conservatively, which provokes the question of what appropriate follow-up should be for these patients. Current recommendations suggest that follow-up imaging at 6, 12, and 24 months is advised and that biochemical work-up should be performed at the time the mass is identified and annually for 4 years. Biochemical evaluation should focus on excluding pheochromocytoma and Cushing's syndrome, as well as hyperaldosteronism in patients with hypertension.

Increasing identification of adrenal incidentalomas has resulted in a growth in incidence and interest in subclinical hypercortisolism—that is autonomous cortisol production in the absence of classic signs or symptoms of Cushing's syndrome. At present this disease entity is poorly defined and incompletely characterized. Mild hypercortisolism may cause obesity and derangements in metabolic parameters including impaired glucose tolerance, hypertension, and dyslipidemia. While recent data suggest surgical removal results in clinical benefit, results are conflicting, in part due to lack of consensus on the definition of subclinical hypercortisolism. To date, there are little data to support surgical intervention for the treatment of subclinical hypercortisolism, and medical therapies for this condition have not yet been explored.

## Multiple Choice Questions

1. Which of the following characteristics would be consistent with a malignant adrenal nodule?

   (a) Diameter greater than 4 cm
   (b) High Hounsfield units on CT
   (c) Delayed contrast washout on CT
   (d) All of the above

2. What is the initial screening test for adrenal hypercortisolism?

   (a) 24 h urine free cortisol collection
   (b) Midnight salivary cortisol collection
   (c) 1 mg overnight dexamethasone suppression test
   (d) Plasma ACTH level

3. In a patient with Cushing's syndrome due to an adrenal cortisol producing adenoma, what level is the plasma ACTH?

   (a) Normal
   (b) High
   (c) Low
   (d) None of the above

4. What are the clinical consequences of hypercortisolism?

   (a) Type 2 diabetes
   (b) Obesity
   (c) Hypertension
   (d) Dyslipidemia
   (e) All of the above

## Answers to Questions

1. (d)
2. (c)
3. (c)
4. (e)

## References

1. Young WF. Management approaches to adrenal indicentalomas: a view from Rochester, Minnesota. Endocrinol Metab Clin North Am. 2000;29:159–85.
2. Bovio S, Cataldi A, Reimondo G, Sperone P, Novello S, Berruti A, Borasio P, Fava C, Dogliotti L, Scagliotti GV, Angeli A, Terzolo M. Prevalence of adrenal incidentaloma in a contemporary computerized tomography series. J Endocrinol Invest. 2006;29:298–302.

3. Mantero F, Terzolo M, Arnaldi G, Osella G, Masini AM, Ali A, Giovagnetti M, Opocher G, Angeli A. A survey on adrenal indicentaloma in Italy. Study Group on Adrenal Tumors of the Italian Society of Endocrinology. J Clin Endocrinol Metab. 2000;85:637–44.
4. Mansmann G, Lau J, Balk E, Rothberg M, Yukitaka M, Bornstein SR. The clinically inapparent adrenal mass: update in diagnosis and management. Endocr Rev. 2004;25:309–40.
5. Angeli A, Osella G, Ali A, Terzolo M. Adrenal incidentaloma: an overview of clinical and epidemiological data from the National Italian Study Group. Horm Res. 1997;47:279–83.
6. Lenert JT, Barnett Jr CC, Kudelka AP, Sellin RV, Gagel RF, Prieto VG, Skibber JM, Ross MI, Pisters PWT, Curley SA, Evans DB, Lee JE. Evaluation and surgical resection of adrenal masses in patients with a history of extra-adrenal malignancy. Surgery. 1998;130:1060–7.
7. Kloos RT, Groos MD, Francis IR, Korobkin M, Shapiro B. Incidentally discovered adrenal masses. Endocr Rev. 1995;16:460–84.
8. Zeiger M, Thompson G, Duh QY, Hamrahian A, Angelos P, Elaraj D, Fishman E, Kharlip J. American Association of Clinical Endocrinologists and American Association of Endocrine Surgeons medical guidelines for the management of adrenal incidentalomas. Endocr Pract. 2009;15 Suppl 1:450–3.
9. Mulatero P, Stowasser M, Loh KC, et al. Increased diagnosis of primary aldosteronism, including surgically correctable forms, in centers from five continents. J Clin Endocrinol Metab. 2004;89:1045–50.
10. Barzon L, Scaroni C, Sonino N, Fallo F, Paoletta A, Boscaro M. Risk factors and long-term follow-up of adrenal incidentalomas. J Clin Endocrinol Metab. 1999;84:520–6.
11. Chiodini I. Diagnosis and treatment of subclinical hypercortisolism. J Clin Endocrinol Metab. 2011;96:1223–36.
12. Chiodini I, Torlontano M, Carnevale V, Gugglielmi G, Cammisa M, Trischitta V, Scillitani A. Bone loss rate in adrenal indicentalomas: a longitudinal study. J Clin Endocrinol Metab. 2001;144:401–8.
13. Terzolo M, Bovio S, Reimondo G, Pia A, Osella G, Boretta G, Angeli A. Subclinical Cushing's syndrome in adrenal incidentalomas. Endocrinol Metab Clin North Am. 2005;34:423–39.
14. Nunes ML, Vattaut S, Corcuff JB, Rault A, Loiseau H, Gatta B, Valli N, Letenneur L, Tabarin A. Late-night salivary cortisol for the diagnosis of overt and subclinical Cushing's syndrome in hospitalized and ambulatory patients. J Clin Endocrinol Metab. 2009;94:456–62.
15. Masserini B, Morelli V, Bergamaschi S, Ermetici F, Eller-Vainicher C, Barbieri AM, Maffini MA, Scillitani A, Ambrosi B, Beck-Peccoz P, Chiodini I. The limited role of midnight salivary cortisol in the diagnosis of subclinical hypercortisolism in patients with adrenal incidentalomas. Eur J Endocrinol. 2009;160:87–92.
16. Kidambi S, Raff H, Findling JW. Limitations of nocturnal salivary cortisol and urine free cortisol in the diagnosis of mild Cushing's syndrome. Eur J Endocrinol. 2007;157:725–31.
17. Tauchmanova L, Rossi R, Biondi B, Pulcrano M, Nuzzo V, Palmieri E, Fazio S, Lombardi G. Patients with subclinical Cushing's syndrome due to adrenal adenoma have increased cardiovascular risk. J Clin Endocrinol Metab. 2002;87:4872–8.
18. Terzolo M, Pia A, Ali A, Osella G, Reimondo G, Bovio S, Daffara F, Procopio M, Paccotti P, Borretta G, Angeli A. Adrenal incidentaloma: a new cause of the metabolic syndrome? J Clin Endocrinol Metab. 2002;87:998–1003.
19. Gabriella GM, Garrapa G, Pantanetti P, Arnaldi G, Mantero F, Faloia E. Body composition and metabolic features of women with adrenal incidentaloma or Cushing's syndrome. J Clin Endocrinol Metab. 2001;86:5301–6.
20. Rossi R, Tauchmanova L, Luciano A, Di Martino M, Battista C, Del Viscovo L, Nuzzo V, Lombardi G. Subclinical Cushing's syndrome in patients with adrenal indicentalomas: clinical and biochemical features. J Clin Endocrinol Metab. 2000;85:1440–8.
21. Eller-Vainicher C, Morelli V, Salcuni AS, Battista C, Torlontano M, Coletti F, Iorio L, Cairoli E, Beck-Peccoz P, Arosio M, Ambrosi B, Scillitani A, Chiodini I. Accuracy of several parameters of hypothalamic-pituitary-adrenal axis activity in predicting before surgery the metabolic effects of removal of an adrenal incidentaloma. Eur J Endocrinol. 2010;163:925–35.

# Chapter 23
# A Case of Pheochromocytoma

**Sandi-Jo Galati and Lawrence R. Krakoff**

A 36-year-old man presented to the emergency department with palpitations and chest pain. His blood pressure was 240/110. One week earlier he had undergone cardiac catheterization at another hospital after presenting with similar symptoms, but no occlusive coronary disease was found. The patient reported several weeks of periodic, transient chest pain and palpitations with headache and diaphoresis that spontaneously resolved. In the past, he had been healthy and took no medications or over the counter remedies. His father was hypertensive and died at age 46 from a cerebral hemorrhage. He denied tobacco or alcohol use. He had occasionally smoked marijuana but never used cocaine. On physical examination his blood pressure was 190/90 on nicardipine, a calcium-channel blocker (CCB), infusion. His skin was warm and dry with no skin lesions. Neck exam is notable for thyromegaly with bilateral nodules. Cardiopulmonary exam was notable only for tachycardia with heart rate of 110. Abdominal and extremity exams were unremarkable.

**Biochemical evaluation**: Elevated serum normetanephrines 1,544 pg/mL (normal <148 pg/mL) with metanephrines 576 pg/mL (normal <57 pg/mL) and elevated 24-h urine metanephrines 13,495 mcg/g creatinine (normal 94–445 mcg/g creatinine), diagnostic of pheochromocytoma. **Subsequent notable labs included**: Elevated calcitonin 2,686 pg/mL, intact parathyroid hormone 56 pg/mL, and serum

S.-J. Galati, M.D. (✉)
Division of Endocrinology, Diabetes and Bone Diseases, Department of Medicine,
Icahn School of Medicine at Mount Sinai Hospital, 1 Gustave L. Levy Place,
Box 1055, New York, NY 10029, USA
e-mail: sandijo.galati@gmail.com

L.R. Krakoff, M.D.
Division of Endocrinology, Diabetes and Bone Diseases, Department of Medicine,
Icahn School of Medicine at Mount Sinai Hospital, 1 Gustave L. Levy Place,
Box 1055, New York, NY 10029, USA

Cardiovascular Institute, Mount Sinai Hospital, New York, NY, USA

© Springer Science+Business Media New York 2015
T.F. Davies (ed.), *A Case-Based Guide to Clinical Endocrinology*,
DOI 10.1007/978-1-4939-2059-4_23

calcium 11.1 mg/dL, concerning for medullary thyroid carcinoma and primary hyperparathyroidism. **CT of the abdomen and pelvis** demonstrated a $7.1 \times 5.6$ cm right adrenal mass.

The patient was transitioned from the nicardipine infusion to the α-adrenergic antagonist phenoxybenzamine 10 mg twice daily and nifedipine, a CCB, for blood pressure control. He was instructed to liberalize salt in his diet as well as maintain adequate hydration. His blood pressure fell to 130/90 with heart rate 105. The β-adrenergic antagonist metoprolol 25 mg twice daily was started. One week later, he underwent laparoscopic left adrenalectomy. Pathology confirmed pheochromocytoma. After surgery his blood pressure normalized without antihypertensive medications.

Biopsy of his neck mass confirmed medullary thyroid carcinoma. He had subsequent total thyroidectomy and subtotal four-gland parathyroidectomy. Gene testing for multiple endocrine neoplasia (MEN) type 2a was positive.

The patient had two daughters, one of whom also tested positive for MEN 2a and underwent prophylactic thyroidectomy at age 2. His mother subsequently accessed his father's autopsy report, which included mention of a pheochromocytoma.

## How Did Pheochromocytoma Result in a Hypertensive Emergency in This Patient?

Hypertension is present in over 80 % of patients with pheochromocytoma due to excess catecholamine release, with approximately half of these presenting with paroxysmal hypertension [1, 2]. Catecholamines, principally norepinephrine and epinephrine, increase heart rate, blood pressure, myocardial contractility, and cardiac conduction by their actions at α- and β-adrenergic receptors.

Catecholamines are stored in vesicles and typically are released in the setting of stressful stimuli. Pheochromocytomas may mirror this secretion with sudden unpredictable release or slow, steady release. Therefore, the resultant hypertension may be paroxysmal, as in our patient, or sustained depending on the pattern of release, the predominant catecholamine, and the duration of excess.

The variable selectivity of adrenergic receptors to norepinephrine and epinephrine results in diverse clinical presentations of catecholamine excess [3]. Sustained hypertension correlates to elevated norepinephrine levels with a continuous pattern of secretion [4, 5], whereas episodic hypertension is associated with tumors with high epinephrine content [5]. Orthostatic hypotension is most common in patients with sustained hypertension (the norepinephrine pattern) due to prolonged vasoconstriction resulting in volume depletion [5]. Finally, patients with early disease may not have hypertension at all. Our patient had markedly elevated plasma epinephrine metabolite concentrations, consistent with his intermittent, dramatic symptoms.

## How Could the Location of the Patient's Pheochromocytoma Be Predicted by the Biochemical Profile?

Pheochromocytomas and paragangliomas are tumors arising from the chromaffin cells of the adrenal medulla and the sympathetic ganglia, respectively. Paragangliomas that secrete catecholamines are also termed extra-adrenal pheochromocytomas. For the sake of simplicity, we will use the term pheochromocytoma to refer to both intra-adrenal and extra-adrenal secreting tumors in this chapter, however, it is important to recognize: (1) not all paragangliomas (extra-adrenal pheochromocytomas) are secretory, and (2) the distinction of paraganglioma, whether secreting or nonsecreting, has important clinical implications, particularly when the potential for metastatic and familial disease is being assessed.

Catecholamines are synthesized from tyrosine, which is converted by tyrosine hydroxylase into dopa as the rate-limiting step of the synthetic cascade. Norepinephrine is the predominant catecholamine synthesized and secreted by the cells of the paraganglia and adrenergic neurons. Epinephrine is synthesized from norepinephrine by the enzyme phenylethanolamine N-methyltransferase (PNMT), which is largely restricted to the chromaffin cells of the adrenal medulla. PNMT is induced by cortisol produced in the neighboring adrenal cortex. Therefore, epinephrine secretion is largely exclusive to intra-adrenal pheochromocytomas, and the predominant epinephrine secretion in our patient was consistent with an adrenal medullary tumor.

## Why Was This Patient Evaluated for Pheochromocytoma? What Is the Danger of Missing the Diagnosis? Who Should Be Screened for the Presence of a Pheochromocytoma?

Pheochromocytoma has been described by the moniker "the great mimicker" because the symptoms are nonspecific and intermittent, occurring in paroxysms or spells. Our patient's presentation was no exception. His intermittent chest pain and palpitations were felt to be consistent enough with acute coronary syndrome to prompt a cardiac catheterization by his healthcare providers. Patients with pheochromocytomas may report sudden onset of chest pain, palpitations, shortness of breath, throbbing headache, diaphoresis with pallor, and nausea. Spells may be unprovoked or precipitated by medications, stress, anxiety, positional change, or valsalva. A lethal paroxysm or pheochromocytoma crisis is the most feared complication of catecholamine excess.

Further complicating the identification of patients with pheochromocytoma is the rarity of the disease. Even in hypertensive populations, the estimated incidence is 2–8 cases per million people with a prevalence of 0.1–0.6 % [6–8]. Conversely, spells are quite common and have a broad differential diagnosis, so most patients with spells will not have a pheochromocytoma. Regardless, despite the rarity of these tumors, identification and treatment of pheochromocytoma is crucial to prevent the morbidity and potential mortality from a crisis. Therefore, all patients with symptoms compatible with pheochromocytoma should be screened, even in the absence of sustained hypertension.

The sustained effects of catecholamine excess include orthostatic hypotension, resistant hypertension and the sequelae of untreated hypertension, such as retinopathy, congestive heart failure with hypertrophic or dilated cardiomyopathy, and hyperglycemia or diabetes. Therefore, patients with resistant hypertension, unexplained cardiomyopathy, or diabetes should be screened as well [9, 10].

The clinically silent pheochromocytoma is an entity more recently appreciated with the increased incidental detection of adrenal masses, and, in fact, represents approximately half of all pheochromocytomas diagnosed [11]. Of note, the prevalence of pheochromocytoma is higher, from 4.2 % to 6.5 % in patients with a known adrenal mass, regardless of the presence of symptoms [12, 13]. Therefore, screening for pheochromocytoma must be performed in all patients with incidentalomas discovered on adrenal imaging due to the risk of silent pheochromocytoma.

Several heritable syndromes including neurofibromatosis type 1, von Hippel-Lindau, MEN 2a and 2b, and paraganglioma syndromes types 1–5 have an increased incidence of pheochromocytoma. Patients with these diagnoses should be screened annually for pheochromocytoma [9, 10]. Further, pheochromocytoma may be the initial manifestation of any of these syndromes. At least one-quarter of apparently sporadic pheochromocytomas are actually the result of familial diseases [14], so identification of index cases is essential for screening relations.

## How Are Patients with Suspected Pheochromocytoma Diagnosed?

Plasma or urinary metanephrines are the recommended initial approach in screening for pheochromocytoma; however, no consensus exists regarding which is preferred [15]. Catecholamines are stored within vesicles in the chromaffin cells; however, there is continual leakage into the cell cytoplasm where norepinephrine, epinephrine, and dopamine are metabolized by catechol-*O*-methyltransferase into their plasma metabolites, normetanephrine, metanephrine, and methoxytyramine, respectively. Normetanephrine and metaneprine undergo further sulfate conjugation prior to excretion in the urine. These processes account for the majority of measured metabolites in the blood and the urine. Because catecholamine secretion tends not to be continuous and even venipuncture can quickly raise blood catecholamine levels, measurement of metabolites is a more sensitive and specific marker of catecholamine excess [16, 17]. Our approach is to measure plasma metanephrines first given the ease of collection and high sensitivity, such that a negative value excludes pheochromocytoma. In 80 % of patients with pheochromocytoma, plasma metanephrines are elevated fourfold over the upper limit of normal, and localization of the tumor is the next diagnostic step [18].

Measurement of plasma free metanephrines is 96–100 % sensitive and 89–98 % specific for disease detection [9, 17]. Renal dysfunction does not influence plasma metanephrines measurement [19]; however, false positive results may occur with use of tricyclic anti-depressants, monoamine oxidase inhibitors, buspirone, phenoxyben-zamine, or sympathomimetics such as pseudoephedrine, and weight-loss medications. False positives may also occur due to recent abrupt clonidine or benzodiazepine discontinuation, alcohol excess or withdrawal, untreated obstructive sleep apnea, or if samples are drawn in the seated rather than supine position [9]. Use of gas chromatography with mass spectrometry or liquid chromatography-tandem mass spectrometry has increased the diagnostic accuracy of plasma metanephrines [20]. Urinary fractionated metanephrines are less sensitive (86–97 %) and slightly less specific (86–95 %) than plasma metanephrines, and require 24-h urine collection. Renal dysfunction and diets rich in biogenic amines may alter interpretation [9].

## Once Confirmed Biochemically, What Is the Best Tumor Localization Study?

Imaging should only be pursued in cases with biochemical evidence of catecholamine excess or for surveillance in patients with hereditary syndromes predisposing them to the development of pheochromocytoma. 85 % of tumors arise from the adrenal glands and 95 % are located within the abdomen [10]. Computed tomography (CT) or magnetic resonance imaging (MRI) of the abdomen and pelvis are the preferred initial imaging techniques in localizing pheochromocytoma, with subsequent imaging of the neck and chest if a tumor is not located. There is no consensus regarding the choice of imaging modality [15]. MRI may be useful in indeterminate cases, as pheochromocytomas tend to have high signal uptake on T2-weighted images. This modality is especially useful in the evaluation of adrenal incidentalomas in which there is concern for silent a pheochromocytoma.

[123]I-labeled meta-iodobenzylguanide (MIBG) scintigraphy provides functional information about pheochromocytoma because MIBG is taken up into the secretory granules of chromaffin cells via the norepinehrine transporter [21]. MIBG lacks the sensitivity of CT and MRI and should only be used when CT and MRI imaging are negative, in cases where metastatic disease is suspected, or for surveillance in patients with hereditary diseases [11]. Positron-emitted tomography can also be used to detect pheochromocytoma, but should be reserved for detection of metastatic disease when MIBG is negative [11, 15]. Our case patient had biochemically confirmed disease with a large adrenal tumor identified on CT; therefore, there was no indication to pursue further imaging prior to surgical resection.

## How Should the Patient Be Managed Preoperatively?

A multidisciplinary approach among the patient, endocrinologist, anesthesiologist, and surgeon is been regarded as essential to prevent an intraoperative hypertensive crisis. There is argument that with close intraoperative monitoring by an anesthesiologist familiar with the nuances of pheochromocytoma management, preoperative medical treatment is unnecessary, particularly in patients who do not have hypertension [22]. However, due to lack of sufficient evidence, most centers institute a preoperative treatment plan preceding surgery aimed at blood pressure-control and volume expansion [10, 23].

α-blockers lower blood pressure by antagonizing catecholamine-stimulated vasoconstriction. They are the agents of choice in preoperative blood pressure management, although there is no data on dose, agent selection, duration of therapy, or BP goal [24]. Several α-blockers are available for use. Phenoxybenzamine is a nonselective, irreversible antagonist, and, because of its long duration of action and irreversibility, it is the preferred initial choice. The side effects, which include nasal congestion, severe fatigue and orthostatic hypotension, can limit dose titration or use of this agent [23]. Alternatively, the selective α1-adrenergic antagonists such as doxazosin, prazosin, or terazosin can be used in patients that cannot tolerate phenoxybenzamine, particularly in patients requiring long-term treatment [25].

β-adrenergic blockade is indicated for management of tachycardia or arrhythmias induced by catecholamine excess with α-antagonist use. It is essential to ensure blood pressure control with α-adrenergic blockage as was done with our patient prior to initiation of β-blocker use to prevent unopposed α-adrenergic stimulation and worsening hypertension. β1 selective drugs, such as atenolol, metoprolol, or bisoprolol are generally preferred to avoid antagonism of β2 vasodilator action [26].

CCBs may be added to existing α- and β-adrenergic blockade when blood pressure control is inadequate or used as alone for blood pressure control [25]. Agents acting on the renin–angiotensin system, such as angiotensin-converting enzyme inhibitors (ACEi) and angiotensin receptor blockers (ARB) may improve blood pressure control in patients with elevated renin due to β-adrenergic-stimulated release, although renin elevation is not present in all patients with pheochromocytoma (Table 23.1) [27]. Following initiation of antihypertensive therapy and BP improvement, a liberalized salt diet should be instituted for volume expansion, although little data exists for this practice [10].

## What Is the Expected Intraoperative Course?
## What Precautions Are Required?

Laparoscopic unilateral adrenalectomy is the procedure of choice for most pheochromocytomas [15]. Hypertensive crisis from catecholamine release during tumor manipulation is the feared complication [10]. Intravenous infusion of nicardipine or nitroprusside, a vasodilating agent, is the preferred intraoperative BP agents. In patients who may not have adequate pre-operative α-adrenergic blockage, the intravenous α-adrenergic antagonist phentolamine may be used (Table 23.1) [24].

Anesthetic agents known to stimulate catecholamine secretion such as fentanyl, morphine, ketamine, halothane, and desflurane must be avoided, whereas propofol, barbiturates, synthetic opioids, etomidate, and the other anesthetic gases are safe [23]. Intravenous volume expansion is often begun preoperatively provided cardiac

**Table 23.1** Pharmacologic management of pheochromocytoma

| | Class | Drug and dosing | Clinical pearls |
|---|---|---|---|
| Preoperative management | Adrenergic blockade | Nonselective α-blockade<br>• Phenoxybenzamine: 10–20 mg 2–3 times/day (100 mg max daily)<br>Selective α-blockade<br>• Doxazosin: 1 mg daily[a]<br>• Terazosin: 1 mg 2 times/day[a]<br>• Prazosin: 1 mg 3 times/day[a]<br>β-blockade | • Phenoxybenzamine, preferred due to long-acting nonselective α-blockade.<br>• Side effects include extreme fatigue, nasalcongestion, and orthostasis, all less pronounced in selective blockade.<br>• β-blockade instituted *after* α-blockade for tachycardia.<br>• β1 selective blockade preferred (metoprolol, bisoprolol, and atenolol).<br>• Combined α- and β-blockade with labetalol not recommended. |
| | Calcium channel blockade | Nifedipine: SR 30–120 mg daily<br>Nicardipine: 30 mg 2 times/day (120 mg max daily) | • Blocks NE-mediated calcium transport into the vascular smooth muscle.<br>• Adjunctive agent to α- and β-blockade or in patients who cannot tolerate α-blockade. |
| | Catecholamine synthesis inhibition | Metyrosine 250 mg 3–4 times/day, 4 g max daily) | • Not routinely used preoperatively unless for short-course due to severe symptoms.<br>• Main short-term side effect is somnolence. |
| Intraoperative or crisis management | Adrenergic blockade | Phentolamine: 1–5 mg IV boluses or infusion<br>Esmolol: 0.5 mg/kg over 1 min then 0.05 mg/kg/min infusion | • Phentolamine is a nonselective α-blocking agent.<br>• Esmolol is a β-blocker that should be used for tachyarrhythmias<br>• Thiocyanate levels must be measured with nitroprusside use. |
| | Calcium channel blockade | Nicardipine: 5 mg/h infusion titratable to 15 mg/h | |
| | Vasodilators | Nitroprusside: 2 μg/kg/min, not to exceed 800 μg/h | |
| Postoperative management[b] | Adrenergic blockade | Phenoxybenzamine, doxazosin, terazosin, prazosin | • Continued α-blocker use should be employed for residual or metastatic disease.<br>• Selective agents are preferred to minimize side effects. |
| | Catecholamine synthesis inhibition | Metyrosine | • Indicated for residual or metastatic disease.<br>• Side effects with long term use include diarrhea, anxiety, nightmares, crystalluria, galactorrhea, extrapyrimidal symptoms in addition to sedation. |

[a]Max daily dose 20 mg
[b]Most residual hypertension postoperatively is essential hypertension and should be managed following JNC 7 guidelines

and renal function will tolerate. Intravenous insulin may also be required for catecholamine-induced hyperglycemia.

Immediately postoperative, approximately 50 % of patients have sustained hypertension [28], whereas others experience hypotension, usually a multifactorial response to sudden catecholamine depletion, hypovolemia, and persistence of α-adrenergic blockade. Intravascular volume replacement followed by pressor support is the cornerstone of management.

## What Postoperative Monitoring Is Required for the Patient?

Complete tumor resection should be assessed 2–6 weeks postoperatively with collection of plasma or urine metanephrines [15, 23]. Normal values do not exclude the possibility of remaining microscopic disease; therefore, biochemical screening must be performed annually, although no further imaging is required. Residual essential hypertension should be managed following the seventh report of the Joint National Committee (JNC 7) hypertension guidelines [29].

Persistent metanephrine elevations may signal residual tumor, multifocal disease, or metastatic disease and must be followed by CT, MRI, or functional imaging. Hypertension and symptoms of catecholamine excess should be managed as they were preoperatively, primarily with α-adrenergic blockade; however, the selective α-blocking agents are typically employed in these cases to minimize the side effects of expected long-term use.

In patients with refractory disease, such as those with residual or metastatic disease, metyrosine, a tyrosine hydroxylase inhibitor, can be used [23]. The side effects of metyrosine can be disabling, including extrapyramidal symptoms, depression, galactorrhea, and sedation, particularly with long-term use. Therefore, its use should be reserved for widespread disease with intractable symptoms despite α-adrenergic blockade (Table 23.1).

Finally, genetic testing should be discussed at the initial postoperative visit in any patient with a family history of pheochromocytoma, a paraganglioma, younger than 45 years, a malignant tumor, bilateral or multicentric disease, or clinical presentation consistent with one of the known hereditary syndromes [30, 31]. Our patient's presentation with pheochromocytoma, medullary thyroid cancer, and primary hyperparathyroidism was consistent with MEN 2a, which was ultimately confirmed with gene testing. His diseased father, who had a pheochromocytoma at autopsy, was likely affected as well. Prior knowledge of his father's medical history may have prompted increased screening in our patient with early detection of pheochromocytoma. The health of the patient's affected daughter, however, has benefited. She underwent prophylactic thyroidectomy within weeks of diagnosis at age 2 and the pathology revealed C-cell hyperplasia. She will undergo annual screening for pheochromocytoma in hopes of preventing the complications suffered by her father and grandfather.

## Lessons Learned

Pheochromocytomas are rare, potentially fatal tumors that may be clinically silent or present with hypertensive emergencies, sustained arrhythmias, or sudden death. The manifestations of pheochromocytoma result from catecholamine excess, which is variable based on the predominant catecholamine released and the adrenergic receptor affected. Our patient experienced episodic hypertension, which was consistent with the markedly elevated epinephrine secretion of his tumor, and ultimately presented with a hypertensive emergency. His tumor was identified immediately on presentation, and blood pressure control was achieved with α-blockade, followed by heart rate control with β-blockade. Fortunately, his previous presentation, during which he underwent cardiac catheterization, did not precipitate a crisis. This highlights the need for a high index of suspicion for this sometimes elusive tumor, particularly in patients who experience paroxysms of symptoms, in young patients with hypertension, or in patients with a suspicious family history. The coexisting medullary thyroid cancer and primary hyperparathyroidism were consistent with MEN 2a, and recognition of this enabled gene testing of the patient's family, ultimately resulting in the identification and prophylactic treatment of his affected daughter.

## Questions

1. Which is the most sensitive screening test for a patient with suspected pheochromocytoma?

   (a)  Urine norepinephrine and epinephrine
   (b)  Plasma metanephrines (total and fractionated)
   (c)  Plasma dopamine
   (d)  Urine metanephrines

2. A patient with an adrenal incidentaloma has elevated plasma metanephrine levels. Which is the best and first imaging procedure to be done?

   (a)  Abdominal ultrasound
   (b)  Magnetic resonance imaging
   (c)  Positron Emission (PET) scan
   (d)  123I-MIBG scan

3. A patient with pheochromocytoma is hypertensive with blood pressures in the range of 160–200/100–115 and intermittent headaches. Which is the best choice for initial blood pressure control?

   (a)  Intravenous enalapril
   (b)  Oral metoprolol
   (c)  Oral dibenzyline
   (d)  Intravenous furosemide

4. Which genetic syndrome is least likely to be associated with pheochromocytoma?

  (a) Neurofibromatosis
  (b) MEN-2
  (c) Adult polycystic kidney disease
  (d) Von Hippel–Lindau Syndrome

## Answers to Questions

1. (B)
2. (B)
3. (C)
3. (C)

## References

1. Manger WM. The protean manifestations of pheochromocytoma. Harm Metal Res. 2009; 41(9):658–63.
2. Zelinka T, Eisenhofer G, Pacek K. Pheochromocytoma as a catecholamine-producing tumor: implications for clinical practice. Stress. 2007;10(2):195–203.
3. Zuber AM, Kantorovich V, Pacek K. Hypertension in pheochromocytoma: characteristics and treatment. Endocrinol Metab Clin N Am. 2001;40(2):295–311.
4. O'Rourke MF, Staessen JA, Vlachopoulos C, et al. Clinical application of arterial stiffness; definitions and reference values. Am J Hypertens. 2002;15(5):426–44.
5. Manger W, Gifford RW. The clinical and experimental pheochromocytoma. 2nd ed. Malden, MA: Blackwell Science; 1996.
6. Sinclair AM, Isles CG, Brown I, Cameron H, Murray GD, Robertson JW. Secondary hypertension in a blood pressure clinic. Arch Intern Med. 1987;147(7):1289–93.
7. Anderson Jr GH, Blakeman N, Streeten DH. The effect of age on prevalence of secondary forms of hypertension in 4429 consecutively referred patients. J Hypertens. 1994;12(5): 609–15.
8. Omura M, Saito J, Yamaguchi K, Kakuta Y, Nishikawa T. Prospective study on the prevalence of secondary hypertension among hypertensive patients visiting a general outpatient clinic in Japan. Hypertens Res. 2004;27(3):193–202.
9. Schwartz GL. Screening for adrenal-endocrine hypertension: overview of accuracy and cost-effectiveness. Endocrinol Metab Clin N Am. 2011;40(2):279–94.
10. Young Jr WF. Endocrine hypertension. In: Melmed S, Polonsky KS, Larsen PR, Kronenberg HM, editors. Williams textbook of endocrinology. 12th ed. Philadelphia, PA: Elsevier; 2011.
11. Young Jr WF. Endocrine hypertension: then and now. Endocr Pract. 2010;16(5):888–902.
12. Mantero F, Terzolo M, Arnaldi G, Osella G, Masini AM, Alì A, Giovagnetti M, Opocher G, Angeli A. A survey on adrenal incidentaloma in Italy. Study Group on Adrenal Tumors of the Italian Society of Endocrinology. J Clin Endocrinol Metab. 2000;85(2):637–44.
13. Mansmann G, Lau J, Balk E, Rothberg M, Miyachi Y, Bornstein SR. The clinically inapparent adrenal mass: update in the diagnosis and management. Endocr Rev. 2004;25(2):309–40.
14. Neumann HP, Bausch B, McWhinney SR, Bender BU, Gimm O, Franke G, Schipper J, Klisch J, Altehoefer C, Zerres K, Januszewicz A, Eng C, Smith WM, Munk R, Manz T, Glaesker S, Apel TW, Treier M, Reineke M, Walz MK, Hoang-Vu C, Brauckhoff M, Klein-Franke A,

Klose P, Schmidt H, Maier-Woelfle M, Peçzkowska M, Szmigielski C, Eng C, Freiburg-Warsaw-Columbus Pheochromocytoma Study Group. Germ-line mutations in nonsyndromic pheochromocytoma. N Engl J Med. 2002;346(19):1459–66.

15. Pacek K, Eisenofer G, Ahlman H, Bornstein SR, Giminez-Roqueplo AP, Grossman AB, Kimura N, Mannelli M, McNichol AM, Tischler AS. Pheochromocytoma: recommendations for clinical practice from the First International Symposium. Nat Clin Pract Rev. 2007;3(2):92–102.

16. Eisenhofer G, Tischler AS, de Krijger RR. Diagnostic tests and biomarkers for pheochromocytoma and extra-adrenal paraganglioma: from routine laboratory methods to disease stratification. Endocr Pathol. 2012;23(1):4–14.

17. Eisenhofer G. Screening for pheochromocytomas and paragangliomas. Curr Hypertens Rep. 2012;14(2):130–7.

18. Eisenhofer G, Goldstein DS, Walther MM, Friberg P, Lenders JW, Keiser HR, Pacak K. Biochemical diagnosis of pheochromocytoma: how to distinguish true-from false-positive test results. J Clin Endocrinol Metab. 2003;88(6):2656–66.

19. Eisenhofer G, Huysmans F, Pacek K, Walther MM, Sweep FC, Lenders JW. Plasma metanephrines in renal failure. Kidney Int. 2005;67(2):668–77.

20. Peaston RT, Graham KS, Chambers E. Performance of plasma free metanephrines measured by liquid chromatography-tandem mass spectrometry in the diagnosis of pheochromocytoma. Clin Chim Acta. 2010;411(7–8):546–52.

21. Kölby L, Bernhardt P, Levin-Jakobson AM, Johanson V, Wängberg B, Ahlman H, Forssell-Aronsson E, Nilsson O. Uptake of meta-iodobenzylguanidine in neuroendocrine tumors is mediated by vesicular monoamine transporters. Br J Cancer. 2003;89(7):1383–8.

22. Lentschener C, Gaujoux S, Tesniere A, Dousset B. Point of controversy: perioperative care of patients undergoing pheochromocytoma removal—time for a reappraisal? Eur J Endocrinol. 2011;165(3):365–73.

23. Därr R, Lenders JWM, Hofbauer LC, Naumann B, Bornstein SR, Eisenhofer G. Pheochromocytoma-update on disease management. Ther Adv Endocrinol Metab. 2012; 3(1):11–26.

24. Phitayakorn R, McHenry CR. Perioperative considerations in patients with adrenal tumors. J Surg Oncol. 2012;106(5):604–10.

25. Bravo EL, Tagle R. Pheochromoocytoma: state-of-the-art and future prospects. Endocr Rev. 2003;24(4):539–53.

26. Prys-Roberts C. Phaeochromocytoma-recent progress and its management. Br J Anaesth. 2000;85(1):44–57.

27. Krakoff LR, Garbowit D. Adreno-medullary hypertension: a review of syndromes, pathophysiology, diagnosis, and treatment. Clin Chem. 1991;37(10 Pt 2):1849–53.

28. Kinney MA, Narr BJ, Warner MA. Perioperative management of pheochromocytoma. J Cardiothorac Vasc Anesth. 2012;16(3):359–69.

29. Chobanian AV, Bakris GL, Black HR, Cushman WC, Green LA, Izzo Jr JL, Jones DW, Materson BJ, Oparil S, Wright Jr JT, Roccella EJ, National Heart, Lung, and Blood Institute Joint National Committee on Prevention, Detection, Evaluation, and Treatment of High Blood Pressure, National High Blood Pressure Education Program Coordinating Committee. The seventh report of the Joint National Committee on prevention, detection, evaluation, and treatment of high blood pressure: the JNC 7 report. JAMA. 2003;289(19):2560–72.

30. Erlic Z, Rybicki L, Peczkowska M, Golcher H, Kann PH, Brauckhoff M, Müssig K, Muresan M, Schäffler A, Reisch N, Schott M, Fassnacht M, Opocher G, Klose S, Fottner C, Forrer F, Plöckinger U, Petersenn S, Zabolotny D, Kollukch O, Yaremchuk S, Januszewicz A, Walz MK, Eng C, Neumann HP, European-American Pheochromocytoma Study Group. Clinical predictors and algorithm for genetic diagnosis of pheochromocytoma patients. Clin Cancer Res. 2009;15(20):6378–85.

31. Jiménez C, Cote G, Arnold A, Gagel RF. Review: should patients with apparently sporadic pheochromocytomas or paragangliomas be screened for hereditary syndromes? J Clin Endocrinol Metab. 2006;91(8):2851–8.

# Part VI
# Hyperparathyroidism

# Chapter 24
# Introduction

Claudio Marcocci

## Calcium Homeostasis

The maintenance of calcium homeostasis within strict limits in humans is guaranteed by the actions of three hormones: parathyroid hormone (PTH), 1,25-dihydroxyvitamin D [1,25(OH$_2$)D], and fibroblast growth factors 23 (FGF 23) [1]. The large majority of calcium (more than 99 %) is stored in bone, predominantly as hydroxyapatite. Serum calcium concentrations ranges between 8.4 and 10.4 mg/dl (2.1–2.6 mmol/l); about half of it is in the form of ionized calcium (Ca$^{2+}$) and the remaining is either bound to protein (45 %, mostly albumin) or complexed with small organic ions (5–10 %, bicarbonate, citrate, and phosphate). The maintenance of adequate levels of plasma Ca$^{2+}$ is required for bone mineralization, neuromuscular function, and many other physiological functions.

Despite the Ca$^{2+}$ is the metabolically active form, the total calcium is commonly measured in clinical practice. Albumin concentration may affect serum calcium levels and therefore total serum calcium level should be corrected by means of the following formula:

$$\text{corrected total calcium} = \text{total calcium}\left(\text{mg}/\text{dl}\right) + 0.8 \times \left[4\text{-serum albumin}\left(\text{g}/\text{dl}\right)\right]$$

Thus, hypoalbuminemia observed in patients with several chronic illnesses, malnourished or hospitalized, may be responsible for a reduction in total serum calcium concentration.

Minimal changes of the plasma Ca$^{2+}$ concentrations are sensed by the parathyroid calcium sensing receptor (CaSR) and the PTH secretion is adjusted accordingly [2].

C. Marcocci, M.D. (✉)
Department of Clinical and Experimental Medicine, University of Pisa and Endocrine Unit 2, University of Pisa, Via Paradisa 2, 56124 Pisa, Italy
e-mail: claudio.marcocci@med.unipi.it

© Springer Science+Business Media New York 2015
T.F. Davies (ed.), *A Case-Based Guide to Clinical Endocrinology*,
DOI 10.1007/978-1-4939-2059-4_24

A short-term increase in extracellular $Ca^{2+}$ concentration results in an increased cleavage of PTH (1–84) and a decreased secretion of stored PTH from secretory vesicles; a suppression of the expression and transcription of the PTH gene also occurs when the increase of $Ca^{2+}$ is long lasting [3]. Opposite cellular responses are induced by a decrease of serum $Ca^{2+}$. Moreover, a long term decline in serum $Ca^{2+}$ is associated with an increased in the size and proliferation of parathyroid cells.

The compensatory response of PTH to a decreased of $Ca^{2+}$ is mediated by an increased release of calcium from the skeleton, an increased renal calcium reabsorption and phosphate excretion, and, indirectly, by enhancing intestinal calcium absorption by stimulation the renal production of $1,25(OH)_2D$.

The CaSR is expressed in several other tissues outside the parathyroid gland including the kidney, bone, cartilage, and many others. In the kidney activation of the receptor by $Ca^{2+}$ inhibits calcium reabsorption in the cortical thick ascending limb, thus allowing a regulation of renal calcium handling independently of PTH.

In addition to $Ca^{2+}$, PTH secretions is also regulated by $1,25[OH_2]D$ and serum phosphate. It is well known that vitamin D deficiency is associated with an increased PTH production, owing to a decreased suppression of PTH secretion by $1,25[OH_2]D$ and $Ca^{2+}$. A decreased rate of transcription of the PTH gene accounts for the suppression of PTH secretion induced by $1,25[OH_2]D$. Hyperphosphatemia (as in chronic kidney failure) stimulates PTH synthesis and secretion and parathyroid cell proliferation either directly or by lowering serum $Ca^{2+}$ due to its binding to phosphate. In addition, hyperphosphatemia stimulates the secretion of FGF23 by osteoblast/osteocytes. The main effect FGF23 is to increase phosphate excretion and suppress the renal $1\alpha$-hydroxylase enzyme. FGF23 also acts directly, in a Klotho-dependent fashion, on the parathyroid cell inhibiting PTH secretion.

# Primary Hyperparathyroidism

Hyperparathyroididm may occurs as a primary disorder of the parathyroid gland where PTH secretion is increased or abnormally elevated in the face of PTH-induced hypercalcemia [primary hyperparathyroidism, (PHPT)] or as a compensatory response to hypocalcemia or peripheral resistance to PTH (secondary hyperparathyroidism). Finally, HPT may occur in setting of previous SHPT, when PTH secretion continues despite the correction of the triggering cause (tertiary hyperparathyroidism), as in end-stage chronic kidney disease.

## Clinical Presentation

PHPT is the most common endocrine disorder after thyroid diseases and diabetes and is the most common cause of hypercalcemia [4]. The estimated prevalence ranges between 1 and 4 cases per 1,000 persons in different countries and may reach up 2.6 % in older women in Sweden. The incidence of PHPT peaks in the sixth-seventh decade and is most common in women (female/male ratio 3:1). PHPT is most often caused by a single adenoma (80–85 %) and less frequently by multiple gland disease (10–15 %) or carcinoma (less than 1 %). It mainly occurs as a sporadic disease (90–95 %), but may be part of hereditary disorders (multiple endocrine neoplasia types 1 and 2A or the hyperparathyroidism–jaw tumor syndrome).

In the Western Countries the clinical profile has shifted from a symptomatic disease (hypercalcemic symptoms, kidney stones, overt bone disease) to one with absent or nonspecific manifestations (asymptomatic PHPT).

The diagnosis is usually made by the finding of a mild increase of albumin-adjusted serum calcium on routine biochemistry or in evaluating women with postmenopausal osteoporosis.

Plasma PTH measurement is the next step in the differential diagnosis of hypercalcemia. The simultaneous elevation of serum calcium and PTH (or an inappropriately normal PTH level) indicates the diagnosis of PHPT. Exceptions to this rule are the use of lithium or thiazides, tertiary hyperparathyroidism of end-stage renal failure, and familial hypocalciuric hypercalcemia.

Patients may complain of weakness and easy fatigability, anxiety, and cognitive impairment. Abnormalities of glucose and lipid metabolism are seen. Low-bone mineral density (BMD), particularly at sites enriched in cortical bone (e.g., distal 1/3 radius), is found in most patients. Nephrolithiasis has been reported in up to 7 % of patients with asymptomatic PHPT undergoing renal ultrasonographic evaluation.

Recently, another phenotype of PHPT, with increased PTH concentration in the absence of hypercalcemia (normocalcemic PHPT), has been detected particularly in women evaluated for low BMD [5]. Normocalcemic PHPT should be diagnosed only after exclusion of all causes of secondary hyperparathyroidism.

The natural course of PHPT depends upon its severity. Worsening usually occurs in symptomatic patients not undergoing parathyroidectomy. Conversely, studies most patients with asymptomatic mild PHPT have shown stability of serum calcium, PTH, creatinine, urinary calcium, and BMD for up to 8 years. Progression of the disease occurs in about one-third of patients, particularly in those aged less than 50 years [6].

## Surgical Treatment

Parathyroidectomy, with removal of all hyperfunctioning parathyroid tissue, is indicated in all patients with symptomatic PHPT and should be recommended in those with asymptomatic disease who met the criteria for surgery established by international guidelines [7] (Table 24.1). In experienced hand parathyroidectomy is successful in up to 95–98 %, with a low rate (1–3 %) of complications (laryngeal nerve injury and less frequently permanent hypocalcemia). A minimally invasive approach can be offered to most patients. Intraoperative PTH monitoring may be helpful in this setting. A single, benign chief-cell adenoma is usually found at histology. When histology is equivocal or suggests a possible malignancy, molecular studies may help to define the diagnosis [8]. Successful surgery is followed by a prompt normalization of PTH and serum and urinary calcium. BMD increases, mostly during the first few postoperative years. Recurrence of nephrolithiasis is rare. Recurrence of

**Table 24.1** Guidelines for the management of patients with asymptomatic primary hyperparathyroidism

| Measurement | Criteria for parathyroidectomy[a] | Surveillance without surgery |
|---|---|---|
| Serum calcium | >1.0 mg/dl above upper limit of normal | Annually |
| Creatinine clearance (calculated)[b] | Reduced to <60 ml/min | Annually |
| | 24-h urinary calcium >400 mg (>10 mmol) and increased stone risk by biochemcial stone risk analisys | 24-h biochemical stone profile and renal imaging, if renal stones suspected |
| | Presence of nephrolithiasis or nephrocalcinosis | |
| BMD (by DXA) | T-score <−2.5 at any site[c] | Every 1–2 years (3 sites) |
| | Vertebral fracture | Vertebral fracture assessment if clinically suspected (eg. back pain, height loss) |
| Age | <50 years | Not applicable |

[a]Surgery should also be advised to patients in whom surveillance is not feasible
[b]The estimated glomerular filtration rate (ml/min per 1.73 $m^2$) should be evaluated from serum creatinine concentration, demographic characteristics (age, sex, and ethnicity), and other serum measurements [4]
[c]Z-scores instead of T-scores should be used in evaluating BMD in premenopausal women and men aged less than 50 years [4]

PHPT is rare in patients with sporadic PHPT, but it may occur in familial cases, unless total parathyroidectomy is performed.

## Surveillance

A normal calcium intake should be recommended in patients not undergoing parathyroidectomy. Vitamin D deficiency, which appears to be associated with a more severe disease, should be corrected. Monitoring of serum calcium and creatinine every year and measurement of BMD every 1–2 years should be recommended to patients not undergoing parathyroidectomy. Vertebral fracture assessment should be done is clincally indicated. If renal stones suspetced, 24-h biochemical stone profile and renal imaging should be performed.

## Medical Treatment

Medical therapy might be considered to reduce serum calcium or increase BMD in some of these patients. Beneficial effects of antiresorptive therapy have been shown in placebo-controlled clinical trials in postmenopausal women. In one trial of 2 years duration estrogen therapy (0.625 mg conjugated estrogen associated with 5 mg medroxyprogesterone daily) increased femoral neck and lumbar spine BMD

[9], but long-term treatment with estrogen is no longer used because of the increased cardiovascular and breast-cancer risks. In another trial alendronate (10 mg daily for 2 years) reduced bone turnover markers and increased BMD at the lumbar spine and hip, but not at the distal radius. Serum calcium and PTH did not change significantly [10]. The calcimimetic cinacalcet may be considered in patients in whom BMD is not low. It has been show to decrease and often normalize serum calcium levels across a broad range of disease severity [11, 12], including patients with parathyroid carcinoma [13]. PTH levels declined only modestly and generally remained elevated. BMD did not change in patients given cinacalcet for up to 5.5 years. Cinacalcet may be associated with antiresorptive therapy in patients with low BMD. It is worth noting that no single or combined medical therapy is associated with a complete cure of PHPT and therefore medical therapy should not be offered as an alternative to patients who met the criteria for parathyroidectomy.

## Hypoparathyrodism

Hypoparathyroidism (HPT) in an uncommon endocrine disorder characterized by the combination of symptoms and signs due to inadequate production of PTH (parathyroid insufficiency) [14, 15]. HPT rarely occurs as a spontaneous condition, and in this setting mostly occurs as a congenital disorder, either isolated or associated with other organ defects, which may be classified according to the genetic defect, including abnormalities of PTH biosynthesis and/or secretion, parathyroid gland development or destruction. Postoperative HPT, and less frequently autoimmune HPT, are the most common forms of acquired HPT. Magnesium deficiency or excess may also cause a functional HPT. Patients with HPT present with low serum calcium levels, elevated serum phosphorus levels, and undetectable or inappropriately low PTH concentration. The clinical presentation depends on the duration, severity, and rate of development of hypocalcaemia. Symptoms related to increased neuromuscular irritability are usually present and include paresthesia, cramps or tetany, bronchospasm, laryngospasm; seizures and cardiac arrhythmias may also be present. In chronic HPT patients may be asymptomatic even if serum calcium is extraordinarily low. Increased neuromuscular irritability may be demonstrated at the bedside by eliciting the Chvostek's and Trousseau's signs.

HPT should be considered in the differential diagnosis of hypocalcemia [14]. The first step should be to exclude "pseudohypocalcemia" by measuring serum albumin. Hypoalbuminemia may be observed in patients with several chronic illnesses, malnourished or hospitalized. HPT is diagnosed if a patient with subnormal albumin corrected total serum calcium also has intact PTH concentration either normal or inappropriately low, once hypomagnesemia has been ruled out. The finding of elevated serum PTH suggests a non-parathyroid cause of hypocalcemia (PTH resistance or secondary hyperparathyroidism).

A careful review of the patient's medical history may be helpful to further refine the diagnosis of HPT. A family history of hypocalcemia may indicate a genetic cause; a history of neck surgery may suggest a postoperative HPT. The coexistence of candidiasis or other autoimmune endocrine disease (i.e. adrenal insufficiency) prompts the diagnosis of type I polyglandular autoimmune syndrome.

## Postoperative HPT

Postoperative HPT in the majority of cases is due to unintentional damage or removal of parathyroid glands at the time of neck surgery (mainly thyroid and parathyroid surgery). Hypocalcemia usually manifests within a few days after surgery. Postoperative HPT can be transient or permanent. Transient HPT is usually due to reversible parathyroid ischemia and usually resolves within a few weeks, but may persist up to 6 months after surgery. Permanent HPT is diagnosed when insufficient PTH secretion to maintain normocalcemia persists 6 months after surgery [14, 15]. The rate of either transient or permanent postoperative HPT varies according to the experience of the surgeon and in tertiary referral centers it may be as low as 5.4–9.6 % and 0.5–1.7 %, respectively [16]. Transient HPT may be asymptomatic and its prevalence underestimated if serum calcium is not routinely assessed, but only measured in patients with hypocalcemic symptoms.

The risk for postoperative HPT is higher following thyroidectomy for retrosternal goiters, Graves' disease, thyroid cancer, and radical neck lymph node dissections. Other factors, such as low 25-hydroxyvitamin D levels, magnesium depletion, and high-bone turnover state, due to preoperative severe hyperthyroidism or hyperparathyroidism, may contribute to the development of postoperative symptomatic hypocalcemia.

The clinical manifestations of postoperative HPT are directly related to the severity and speed of onset of hypocalcemia. Postoperative hypocalcemia can range from asymptomatic, if the decrease in serum calcium is mild, to a severe, life-threatening condition that requires rapid and intensive treatment.

Postoperative HPT typically develops within few days after surgery. Usually, patients become hypocalcemic on the first postoperative day, but calcium levels may reach the lowest value even 3 days after surgery. Thus hypocalcemia can become clinically manifest even 3–4 days after the operation in patients almost asymptomatic before.

The measurement of albumin-corrected serum calcium or ionized calcium, where available, in the perioperative period is a reliable method to exclude or confirm postsurgical HPT. In the latter case serum phosphate is high or in the high normal range because of the lack of the phosphaturic action of PTH.

## Prevention

Prevention of postoperative HPT is important since hypocalcemia can delay the patient's discharge from the hospital and increase the morbidity after neck surgery.

In addition to preserve the parathyroid glands and maintain their blood supply during surgery, the preoperative assessment of other risk factors may help to prevent or limit the occurrence of postoperative hypocalcemia. In this regard it is important to check vitamin D status and serum magnesium concentration and start supplementation in deficient patients [16].

## *Management*

The goal of treatment is to maintain total serum calcium in the low-normal range, serum phosphate in the high–normal range, 24-h urinary calcium excretion below 300 mg (7.5 mmol) and the calcium-phosphate product below 55 $mg^2/dl^2$ (4.4 $mmol^2/l^2$) [15–17].

Patients with symptomatic severe hypocalcemia, as well as patients with mild symptoms but serum calcium lower than 7.6 mg/dl (1.9 mmol/l), require intravenous administration of calcium. Calcium gluconate is usually employed. One vial of 10 % calcium gluconate contains 93 mg of elemental calcium. One commonly employed protocol is to infuse 1–2 vials in 100 ml 5 % dextrose in 5–10 min and then start slow infusion of calcium gluconate in 1 liter of 5 % dextrose or 0.9 % saline, administered over several hours or a few days, at a rate of 1–3 mg of elemental calcium/kg of body weight/h. Meanwhile, oral supplementation of calcium and active vitamin D metabolites should be started (see below).

Chronic treatment of HPT requires oral calcium and active vitamin D metabolites.

Calcium carbonate and calcium citrate, containing 40 % and 21 % of elemental calcium, respectively, are commonly used. Calcium citrate should be used if proton pump inhibitors are taken or in the case of atrophic gastritis. The daily amount of calcium supplementation may range from 1 g to 6 g, but daily doses of 1–2 g are usually used.

Partially active vitamin D metabolites, which do not require the renal 1α hydroxylation, are preferably used, since this enzymatic activity is impaired in patients with HPT [16]. Calcitriol [1,25(OH)$_2$D$_3$] is the biologically active form of vitamin D. It promptly (with a maximum after 10 h) increases intestinal calcium and phosphate absorption, with a washout time of 2–3 days. Alfacalcidiol (1α-hydroxyvitamin D$_3$ or 1α-OHD$_3$) is rapidly converted to calcitriol by hepatic hydroxylation. The clinical effectiveness is comparable to that of calcitriol, but it has a longer half-life. The use of cholecalciferol, ergocalciferol, and calcifediol should be limited or avoided since they require the renal hydroxylation to be fully activated.

Treatment with active vitamin D analogs does not correct a poor vitamin D status, if present. Cholecalciferol or ergocalciferol administration, in addition to active vitamin D metabolites, might be advised in vitamin D-deficient patients.

In the author's experience some patients with chronic HPT may be kept eucalcemic by taking only vitamin D metabolites, provided that an adequate dietary calcium is guaranteed.

Serum calcium, phosphate, creatinine and urinary calcium should be checked periodically until a stable regimen is established. If urinary calcium is greater than 300 mg/24 h, a low salt diet and eventually a thiazide diuretic should be given in order to decrease hypercalciuria and maintain normocalcemia.

## PTH Replacement Therapy in Chronic HPT

Parathyroid insufficiency is only endocrinopathy for which the replacement of the missing hormone is not currently employed.

Treatment with calcium and vitamin D metabolites does not fully restore quality of life in patients with HPT [18]. The efficacy of an alternative approach using teriparatide (PTH 1–34) [19] and intact PTH (1–84) [20] administered subcutaneously has been tested in these patients and promising results have been generated, but no long-term efficacy and safety data are available at this time.

# References

1. Brown EM. Physiology of calcium homeostasis. In: Bilezikian JP, Marcus R, Levine MA, editors. The parathyroids: basic and clinical concepts. 2nd ed. San Diego, CA: Academic Press; 2001. p. 167–81.
2. Brown EM, MacLeod RJ. Extracellular calcium sensing and extracellular calcium signaling. Physiol Rev. 2001;81:239–97.
3. Nissenson RA, Jüppner H. Parathyroid hormone. In: Rosen CJ, Compston JE, Lian JB, editors. Primer on the metabolic bone diseases and disorders of mineral metabolism. 7th ed. Washington, DC: American Society of Bone and Mineral Research; 2008. p. 123–7.
4. Marcocci C, Cetani F. Clincial practice: primary hyperparathyroidism. N Engl J Med. 2011;36:2389–97.
5. Lowe H, McMahon DJ, Rubin MR, Bilezikian JP. Normocalcemic primary hyperparathyroidism: further characterization of a new clinical phenotype. J Clin Endocrinol Metab. 2007; 93:3001–5.
6. Rubin MR, Bilezikian JP, McMahon DJ, Jacobs T, Shane E, Siris E, Udesky J, Silverberg SJ. The natural history of primary hyperparathyroidism with or without parathyroid surgery after 15 years. J Clin Endocrinol Metab. 2008;93:3462–70.
7. Bilezikian JP, Brandi ML, Eastell R, Silverberg SJ, Udelsman R, Marcocci C, Potts Jr JT. Guidelines for the management of asymptomatic primary hyperparathyroidism: Summary statement from the Fourth International Workshop. J Clin Endocrinol Metab. 2014;99:3561–9.
8. Marcocci C, Cetani F, Rubin MR, Silverberg SJ, Pinchera A, Bilezikian JP. Parathyroid carcinoma. J Bone Min Res. 2008;23:1869–80.
9. Grey AB, Stapleton JP, Evans MC, Tatnell MA, Reid IR. Effect of hormone replacement therapy on bone mineral density in postmenopausal women with mild primary hyperparathyroidism: a randomized, controlled trial. Ann Intern Med. 1996;125:360–8.
10. Khan AA, Bilezikian JP, Kung AW, Ahmed MM, Dubois SJ, Ho AY, Schussheim D, Rubin MR, Shaikh AM, Silverberg SJ, Standish TI, Syed Z, Syed ZA. Alendronate in primary hyperparathyroidism: a double-blind, randomized, placebo-controlled trial. J Clin Endocrinol Metab. 2004;89:3319–25.

11. Marcocci C, Cetani F. Update on the use of cinacalcet in the management of primary hyperparathyroidism. J Endocrinol Invest. 2012;35:90–5.
12. Peacock M, Bolognese MA, Borofsky M, Scumpia S, Sterling LR, Cheng S, Shoback D. Cinacalcet treatment of primary hyperparathyroidism: biochemical and bone densitometric outcomes in a 5-year study. J Clin Endocrinol Metab. 2009;94:4860–7.
13. Silverberg SJ, Faiman C, Bilezikian JP, Peacock M, Shoback DM, Smallridge R, Schwanauer LE, Olson KA, Tuner SA, Bilezikian JP. Cinacalcet HCl effectively reduces serum calcium concentration in parathyroid carcinoma. J Clin Endocrinol Metab. 2007;93:3803–8.
14. Shoback D. Clinical practice: hypoparathyroidism. N Engl J Med. 2008;359:391–403.
15. Bilezikian JP, Khan A, Potts Jr JT, Brandi ML, Clarke BL, Shoback D, Jüppner H, D'Amour P, Fox J, Rejnmark L, Mosekilde L, Rubin MR, Dempster D, Gafni R, Collins MT, Sliney J, Sanders J. Hypoparathyroidism in the adult: epidemiology, diagnosis, pathophysiology, target-organ involvement, treatment, and challenges for future research. J Bone Miner Res. 2011; 26:2317–37.
16. Marcocci C, Cianferotti L. The Parathyroids. In: Miccoli P, Terris DJ, Minuto MN, Seybet MW, editors. Thyroid surgery. Preventing and managing complications. Oxford: Wiley-Blackwell; 2013. p. 227–36.
17. Cooper MS, Gittoes NJ. Diagnosis and management of hypocalcaemia. BMJ. 2008;336: 1298–302.
18. Arlt W, Fremerey C, Callies F, Reincke M, Schneider P, Timmermann W, Allolio B. Well-being, mood and calcium homeostasis in patients with HPT receiving standard treatment with calcium and vitamin D. Eur J Endocrinol. 2002;146:215–22.
19. Winer KK, Sinaii N, Reynolds J, Peterson D, Dowdy K, Cutler Jr GB. Long-term treatment of 12 children with chronic HPT: a randomized trial comparing synthetic human parathyroid hormone 1–34 versus calcitriol and calcium. J Clin Endocrinol Metab. 2010;95:2680–8.
20. Cusano NE, Rubin MR, McMahon DJ, Zhang C, Ives R, Tulley A, Sliney Jr J, Cremers SC, Bilezikian JP. Therapy of hypoparathyroidism with PTH(1–84): a prospective four-year investigation of efficacy and safety. J Clin Endocrinol Metab. 2013;98:137–44.

# Chapter 25
# Complex Primary Hyperparathyroidism

F. Cetani and F. Saponaro

## Objective

- Evaluation of a complex case of Primary Hyperparathyroidism
- Focus on a rare disease with a poor prognosis: parathyroid cancer
- Evaluation of clinical, biochemical, instrumental, and histopathological features suggesting malignancy
- Description of new genetic and immunohistochemical tools available

## Case Presentation

A 53-year-old man was evaluated for recurrent primary hyperparathyroidism (PHPT). The clinical history was notable for recurrent nephrolithiasis since the age of 20 years. At the age of 38 years, severe PHPT (calcium 15 mg/dl and PTH >1000 ng/l) with *osteitis fibrosa cystic* was diagnosed. He underwent neck exploration with excision of a markedly enlarged left parathyroid gland. Histology reported chief-cell parathyroid adenoma. Ten years later there was evidence of recurrent PHPT with progressive increase of serum calcium and PTH. Neck imaging studies were negative. A second neck operation was performed with excision of apparently slightly enlarged right parathyroid glands. The histology showed minimal chief cell hyperplasia. Postoperative serum calcium and PTH levels remained elevated. Treatment with cinacalcet 270 mg daily was started. There was no family history of PHPT. The physical examination was unremarkable except the neck scar.

F. Cetani, M.D., Ph.D. (✉) • F. Saponaro, M.D.
Endocrine Unit 2, University Hospital of Pisa, Pisa, Italy
e-mail: cetani@endoc.med.unipi.it

© Springer Science+Business Media New York 2015
T.F. Davies (ed.), *A Case-Based Guide to Clinical Endocrinology*,
DOI 10.1007/978-1-4939-2059-4_25

His laboratory data were as follows (reference ranges are reported in parentheses):

Total serum calcium = 11.4 mg/dl (8.4–10.2) while taking cinacalcet
Albumin = 4 g/l (3.4–5.0)
Ionized calcium = 6.4 mg/dl (4.52–5.28)
Serum creatinine = 1.3 mg/dl (0.4–1.25)
Intact PTH = 201 ng/l (10–75)
Serum bone alkaline phosphatase = 37.7 µg/l (2–15)
Serum C- telopeptide = 7,091 pmol/l (<5,100)
24-h urinary calcium = 560 mg (100–300)

Bilateral nephrocalcinosis was detected by ultrasound of the abdomen. [99mTc]-sestamibi scintigraphy and neck ultrasound did not show any residual parathyroid tissue. A chest CT, however, showed a 1.5 cm nodule in the inferior right pulmonary lobe. Orthopantography of the jaw was negative. Osteoporosis was detected by DXA. There was no evidence of other endocrinopathies. Upon revision by our pathologist of the original slides of the left parathyroid gland removed at the time of the initial surgery, oncocytic cells arranged in trabeculae, the presence of fibrous bands, and atypical frequent mitoses were observed (Fig. 25.1). These features were

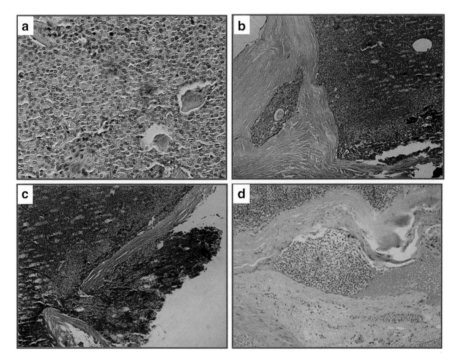

**Fig. 25.1** Pathology of the parathyroid tumor. Panel (**a**) Trabecular pattern of the tumor (hematoxylin and eosin, ×200). Panel (**b**) Capsular pseudoinvasion with trapping of tumor cells within the capsule. Panel (**c**) Capsular invasion with a "tongue like" protrusion through the collagenous fibers. Panel (**d**) Vascular invasion (**b**, **c** and **d** hematoxylin and eosin, ×100)

at least consistent with the diagnosis of atypical parathyroid adenoma or parathyroid carcinoma. Both parathyroid glands that were removed at the time of the second neck operation were read as normal. Because of the clinical suspicion of parathyroid carcinoma, further slides of the left parathyroid tumor were obtained and examined. In addition to the features already shown in the original slides minimal signs of capsular and vascular invasion were present, indicating the diagnosis of parathyroid carcinoma (Fig. 25.1). The lung lesion was excised and the histology showed a metastasis of parathyroid carcinoma. Following surgery, PTH becomes undetectable (<15 ng/l), hypocalcemia developed (1.75 mmol/l), and treatment with calcium and calcitriol was started with stable normocalcemia. Genetic analysis of *CDC73/HRPT2* gene was carried out since inactivating mutations of this gene are responsible for the hyperparathyroidism–jaw tumor syndrome (where a high prevalence of parathyroid cancer is present) and detected in up to 70 % parathyroid cancers. A heterozygous mutation (E115X) was detected in the left parathyroid tumor. The analysis of constitutional DNA showed that the mutation was germline. Loss of parafibromin (the protein encoded by *CDC73/HRPT2*) staining was evident at immunohistochemistry.

## Review of How the Diagnosis Was Made

The clinical features of parathyroid cancer are primarily due to hypercalcemia rather than to tumor mass or distant metastases, and therefore the challenge to the clinician is to distinguish this rare variant of PHPT from its much more common benign counterpart [1]. Several clinical manifestations may suggest a malignant lesion: male gender, young age, marked hypercalcemia, severe and concomitant bone disease, and renal involvement [2]. In addition, intraoperative findings can be helpful (large and stony-hard mass, adherence to the adjacent tissues, and most important, gross local infiltration), but they may be absent; frozen section is of little value. When considered together, the clinical features and the size of the parathyroid lesion at initial surgery raised the possibility of parathyroid carcinoma. The negative cervical exploration at the time of the second operation also raised doubts about the initial benign diagnosis.

As in many endocrine neoplasms, the histopathological distinction between benign and malignant parathyroid tumors is difficult and, in the absence of local invasion or metastases at initial surgery, a definite diagnosis cannot be established with certainty [3, 4]. Taken together, these considerations may account for diagnostic "underreading" in our patient of the initial parathyroid pathology. Misdiagnosis may have important psychological and clinical consequences. Indeed, the incorrect diagnosis of benign adenoma suggested a possible multiglandular disease at the time of recurrence, justifying a second neck operation, and delaying a more appropriate investigation and management. Several presenting features of our patient at initial evaluation might have suggested a malignant etiology of PHPT, but the course after surgery did not appear to counter the diagnosis of a benign parathyroid tumor. On the other hand, it is well known that parathyroid cancer is an indolent neoplasm with a relatively low malignant potential and both local recurrence and metastases may occur late in the course of the disease. Indeed our patient had a disease-free interval of 10 years between initial surgery and recurrence. This case illustrates the difficulty for an inexperienced endocrine pathologist to recognize a parathyroid carcinoma at initial surgery in the absence of local invasion or metastases. Moreover, when the clinical course of PHPT is at variance with the expected course, it may be valuable to have the slides reviewed again and eventually perform molecular analysis on pathologic tissue for *CDC73/HRPT2* mutations and immunohistochemistry for parafibromin. This combined diagnostic approach could be of great utility in parathyroid tumors with equivocal histological features, since both the *CDC73/HRPT2* gene inactivating mutation and loss of parafibromin immunostaining have been reported in up to 70 % of parathyroid cancers and in hyperparathyroidism–jaw tumor syndrome [5, 6].

Although there was no history of familial PHPT, the *CDC73/HRPT2* mutation in our patient was unexpectedly germline and this prompted us to perform genetic analyses in first-degree relatives. The *CDC73/HRPT2* mutation was detected in one of the two sons and in a liver specimen of the deceased father, who underwent partial hepatectomy for a benign nodule. The recognition of the carrier status in a kindred carrying a germline *CDC73/HRPT2* mutation enabled the early detection of a parathyroid cancer in an apparently healthy subject [7]. Thus, a regular surveillance of subjects carrying a germline *CDC73/HRPT2* mutation should be performed using serum calcium and PTH assays and neck ultrasound for early detection of affected individuals.

*Diagnosis*: Parathyroid carcinoma.

## Lesson Learned

- Male gender, relatively young age, markedly elevated serum calcium and PTH, bone and renal involvement, and a large size of the parathyroid lesion may suggest a malignant lesion
- The histopathological distinction between benign and malignant parathyroid tumors may be difficult
- In a patient with recurrent PHPT, the initial diagnosis of parathyroid adenoma may suggest a multiglandular disease with asynchronous parathyroid involvement. However, the severity of PHPT at initial diagnosis and at the time of recurrence, and the persistence of PHPT after the second operation, should raise the possibility of a malignant disease.
- Physician should be aware of the possibility that even endocrine pathologists inexperienced in parathyroid pathology may have some difficulties in distinguishing an atypical parathyroid adenoma from a parathyroid cancer.
- In selected patients with recurrent PHPT and clinical features suggestive of malignancy, it may be valuable to have the slides reviewed by an experience

parathyroid pathologist. Molecular analysis for *CDC73/HRPT2* and immunohistochemistry for parafibromin could also be helpful in selected cases
* Family screening is recommended and genetic testing of *CDC73/HRPT2* should
be offered when a germline mutation is detected.

## Questions

1. Parathyroid cancer may occur with higher prevalence in association with the
following conditions:

   a. Familial isolated hyperparathyroidism
   b. Multiple endocrine neoplasia type 1
   c. Multiple endocrine neoplasia type 2
   d. Hyperparathyroidism–jaw tumor syndrome
   e. Familial benign hypocalciuric hypercalcemia

2. Which of the following pathological features is diagnostic for parathyroid cancer?

   a. Fibrous band
   b. Trabecular growth
   c. Capsular invasion
   d. Vascular invasion
   e. C and D

3. The following features can be seen in parathyroid cancer:

   a. Male gender
   b. Markedly elevated serum calcium and PTH
   c. Bone and renal involvement
   d. Large size of the parathyroid lesion
   e. All

4. Medications useful in treating hypercalcemia include:

   a. Glucocorticoids
   b. Calcimimetic agents
   c. Loop diuretics
   d. Calcitonin
   e. All

## Answers to Questions

1. d. Hyperparathyroidism–jaw tumor syndrome
2. d. Vascular invasion
3. e. All
4. e. All

# References

1. Marcocci C, Cetani F. Clinical practice. Primary hyperparathyroidism. N Engl J Med. 2011;365:2389–97.
2. Marcocci C, Cetani F, Rubin MR, Silverberg SJ, Pinchera A, Bilezikian JP. J Bone Miner Res. 2008;23:1869–80.
3. De Lellis RA. Parathyroid carcinoma. An overview. Adv Anat Pathol. 2005;12:53–61.
4. Grimelius L, DeLellis RA, Bondenson L, et al. Parathyroid adenoma. In: DeLellis RA, Lloyd RV, Heitz PU, Eng C, editors. Pathology and genetics. Tumours of endocrine organs. WHO Classification of Tumour. Lyon: IARC; 2004. p. 128–32.
5. Cetani F, Pardi E, Borsari S, et al. Genetic analyses of the HRPT2 gene in primary hyperparathyroidism: germline and somatic mutations in familial and sporadic parathyroid tumors. J Clin Endocrinol Metab. 2004;89:5583–91.
6. Cetani F, Ambrogini E, Viacava P, et al. Should parafibromin staining replace HRPT2 gene analysis as an additional tool for histologic diagnosis of parathyroid carcinoma? Eur J Endocrinol. 2007;156:547–54.
7. Guarnieri V, Scillitani A, Muscarella LA, Battista C, Bonfitto N, Bisceglia M, Minisola S, Mascia ML, D'Agruma L, Cole DE. Diagnosis of parathyroid tumors in familial isolated hyperparathyroidism with HRPT2 mutation: implications for cancer surveillance. J Clin Endocrinol Metab. 2006;91:2827–32.

# Chapter 26
# Differential Diagnosis of Hypocalcemia

**E. Vignali and Antonella Meola**

## Objectives

– Overview of multiple causes of hypocalcemia
– Accurate assessment of serum calcium level
– Importance of monitoring magnesium level in clinical practice

## Case Presentation

A 53-year-old woman was referred to our outpatient clinic for episodes of tingling and muscle cramps which started 6 months before. Previous blood tests revealed moderate hypocalcemia associated with mild hypomagnesemia and low serum 25OHD levels. She was treated with cholecalciferol and oral calcium and magnesium supplements, with partial remission of the above symptoms. Her past medical history included bilateral congenital sensor neural hearing loss, a duplex kidney with a bifid renal pelvis and bifid uterus, right renal cell carcinoma treated with nephrectomy, and a hiatal hernia with reflux esophagitis treated with esomeprazole since 1 year. There was no family history of hypocalcemia or other autoimmune endocrinopathies. Bowel function was regular. The current treatment included cholecalciferol (800 IU daily), calcium carbonate (1 g daily), and esomeprazole (20 mg daily).

E. Vignali, M.D. (✉) • A. Meola, M.D.
Endcorine Unit 2, University Hospital of Pisa, Via Paradisa 2, 56124 Pisa, Italy
e-mail: edda.vignali@tin.it

© Springer Science+Business Media New York 2015
T.F. Davies (ed.), *A Case-Based Guide to Clinical Endocrinology*,
DOI 10.1007/978-1-4939-2059-4_26

Physical examination was normal with the exception of a right abdominal side scar. BMI was 30. Trousseau and Chvostek's signs were positive. The blood pressure was 120/75 mmHg.

The laboratory data were as follows (reference ranges are reported in parentheses):

Total serum calcium 7.6 mg/dl (8.4–10.2)
Serum albumin 4.2 g/dl (3.4–5.0)
Albumin-corrected total serum calcium = 7.4 mg/dl (8.4–10.2)
Serum ionized calcium = 4.1 mg/dl (4.5–5.3)
Serum phosphorus = 3.7 mg/dl (2.7–4.5)
Serum magnesium = 1.07 mg/dl (1.73–2.26)
Serum creatinine = 0.8 mg/dl (0.5–0.9)
Intact PTH = 34 pg/ml (10–75)
25OHD = 24 ng/ml (>30)

## Review of How the Diagnosis Was Made

The diagnostic testing in patients with hypocalcemia should include the determination of total serum calcium, magnesium, phosphorus, creatinine, intact PTH, and 25OHD. The correction of total serum calcium for albumin may help to exclude the so-called pseudohypocalcemia, a condition in which the decreased total serum calcium is due to a decrease of serum albumin [1].

The causes of hypocalcemia can be divided into those in which the secretion of parathyroid hormone (PTH) is impaired (PTH-dependent) and those in which the secretion of PTH is increased (reactive secondary hyperparathyroidism, or PTH-independent) (Table 26.1) [2, 3]. In the former the phosphorus concentration is increased or in the upper normal range, whereas in the latter decreased or in the low normal range.

In our patient, on the basis of serum phosphorus and intact PTH concentrations, all causes of hypocalcemia associated with reactive secondary hyperparathyroidism could be excluded. Therefore, we focused on PTH-dependent causes. The decreased levels of magnesium raised the possibility that this might be the cause. Hypomagnesemia may be due to gastrointestinal disorders, renal loss, endocrine and metabolic disorders (Table 26.2) [4].

A decreased of serum magnesium in the short term is associated with an increased PTH secretion, whereas when intracellular magnesium depletion develops, the PTH secretion is impaired, resulting in a decrease of serum PTH and hypocalcemia [5]. Primary renal hypomagnesemia could be excluded on the basis of normal urinary magnesium excretion. All other causes of hypomagnesemia could be excluded on the basis of the medical and pharmacological history.

Recently an association between hypomagnesemia and chronic treatment with proton-pump inhibitors (PPIs) has been described [6, 7].

**Table 26.1** Causes of hypocalcemia

| |
|---|
| **PTH-dependent**[a] |
| *Hypoparathyroidism* |
|   • Parathyroid agenesis |
|   • PTH gene mutations |
|   • Postoperative (transient or permanent) |
|   • Autoimmune |
| – Isolated |
| – Combined with multiple endocrine deficiencies |
|   • Activating mutations of the calcium sensing receptor |
|   • Developmental abnormalities of the parathyroids (Di George syndrome, etc.) |
|   • Neonatal hypocalcaemia |
|   • Infiltrative processes (iron overload, Wilson's disease, metastases) |
|   • Radiation therapy |
|   • Hypomagnesemia |
|   • Hypermagnesemia |
| **PTH-independent**[b] |
| *PTH resistance* |
|   • Pseudohypoparathyroidism (1a, 1b, 1c, 2) |
|   • Hypomagnesemia |
| *Alterations of vitamin D metabolism* |
|   • Acquired deficiency of vitamin D |
| – Lack of sunlight exposure |
| – Nutritional deficiency |
| – Malabsorption |
| – End-stage liver disease and cirrhosis |
| – Anticonvulsants |
|   • Hereditary disorders of Vitamin D metabolism |
| – $1\alpha$ hydroxylase deficiency |
| – Vitamin D-dependent rickets type 1 |
| – Vitamin D-dependent rickets type 2 |
| *Miscellaneous causes* |
|   • Increased osteoblastic activity |
| – Hungry bone syndrome (post-parathyroidectomy, post-thyroidectomy for Graves' disease) |
| – Osteoblastic metastases |
|   • Drugs reducing serum calcium levels |
| – Forcarnet |
| – Intravenous bisphosphonate therapy |
|   • Hyperphosphatemia |
|   • Large transfusions of citrate-containing blood |
|   • Acute pancreatitis |
|   • Rhabdomyolysis |
|   • Acute critical illness |

[a]Hypocalcemic conditions caused by impaired/absent PTH secretion
[b]Hypocalcemic conditions in which the secretion of PTH is increased

**Table 26.2** Causes of magnesium deficiency

| |
|---|
| *Gastrointestinal disorders* |
| • Prolonged nasogastric suction/vomiting |
| • Acute and chronic diarrhea |
| • Intestinal and biliary fistula |
| • Malabsorption syndromes |
| • Extensive bowel resection or bypass |
| • Acute hemorrhagic pancreatitis |
| • Protein-calorie malnutrition |
| • Primary intestinal hypomagnesemia |
| *Endocrine and metabolic disorders* |
| • Diabetes mellitus |
| • Phosphate depletion |
| • Primary hyperparathyroidism (hypercalcemia) |
| • Hypoparathyroidism (hypercalciuria, hypercalcemia caused by overtreatment with vitamin D) |
| • Primary aldosteronism |
| • Hungry bone syndrome |
| • Excessive lactation |
| *Renal loss* |
| • Primary renal hypomagnesemia (genetic defects in Mg transport) |
| • Chronic parenteral fluid therapy |
| • Osmotic diuresis (glucose, urea, mannitol) |
| • Hypercalcemia |
| • Alcohol |
| • Diuretics (e.g., furosemide) |
| • Cisplatin |
| • Amphotericin B |
| • Pentamidine |
| • Cyclosporin |
| • Tacrolimus |
| • Proton pump inhibitors |
| • Metabolic acidosis |
| • Chronic renal disorders with magnesium deficiency |
| • Mutation of mitochondrial RNA |

Magnesium is absorbed in the small intestine, through two different mechanisms: an active system, mediated by ion channels TRPM6 and TRPM7 (30 % of magnesium absorption), and a passive system (70 % of magnesium absorption) through enterocyte tight junction [5]. Experimental data indicate that the function of these ion channels is pH-sensitive. Thus, it might be possible that the function of TRPM6 and TRPM7 might be reduced by the lack of protons; alternatively, the patients might be carrying a heterozygous mutation of the TRPM6 gene [8].

We decided to discontinue omeprazole therapy and start magnesium supplementation. Serum magnesium and calcium returned normal levels after 4 weeks (magnesium 1.84 mg/dl; total calcium 9.7 mg/dl, PTH 64 pg/ml). Magnesium supplementation was withdrawn and normal serum magnesium and calcium concentrations were found thereafter.

*Diagnosis:* Hypomagnesemia and Hypocalcemia due to PPIs.

## Lessons Learned

- The total serum calcium level should be corrected for serum albumin
- The presence of normal serum phosphorus level and normal or low intact PTH concentration can exclude reactive secondary hyperparathyroidism
- In patients with hypocalcemia, it is important to measure serum magnesium
- The monitoring of serum magnesium levels should be considered in patients with chronic use of PPIs
- Mild hypomagnesemia is often asymptomatic and may be underdiagnosed because of the low frequency of monitoring magnesium levels in routine clinical practice

## Questions

1. The term "pseudohypocalcemia" refers to:

   a. Normal total serum calcium and reduced albumin-adjusted serum calcium
   b. Normal total serum calcium and decreased ionized calcium
   c. Decreased total serum calcium and normal albumin-adjusted total serum calcium
   d. Decreased total serum calcium and normal ionized serum calcium
   e. C and D

2. Which is the effect of chronic severe hypomagnesemia on PTH secretion?

   a. Secretion of PTH is not influenced by magnesium
   b. Increased
   c. Reduced
   d. It depends on serum calcium level

3. Which is the mechanism of intestinal magnesium absorption?

   a. Active mechanism
   b. Passive mechanism
   c. A and B
   d. It depends on calcium serum levels

4. Which is the correct therapy of hypomagnesemia?

   a. Calcitriol and magnesium
   b. Calcium alone
   c. Magnesium and cholecalciferol
   d. Magnesium alone

## Answers to Questions

1. e. C and D
2. c. Reduced
3. c. A and B
4. d. Magnesium alone

## References

1. Downs RW. Hypoparathyroidism in the differential diagnosis of hypocalcemia. In: Bileziakian JP, Marcus R, Levine MA, editors. The parathyroids: basic and clinical concepts. 2nd ed. San Diego, CA: Academic Press; 2001. p. 755–7.
2. Shoback D. Hypocalcemia: definition, etiology, pathogenesis, diagnosis, and management. In: Rosen CJ, Compston JE, Lian JB, editors. Primer on the metabolic bone diseases and disorders of mineral metabolism. 7th ed. Washington, DC: American Society of Bone and Mineral Research; 2008. p. 313–25.
3. Shoback D. Clinical practice. Hypoparathyroidism. N Engl J Med. 2008;359:391–403.
4. Rude RK. Magnesium deficiency. In: Bileziakian JP, Marcus R, Levine MA, editors. The parathyroids: basic and clinical concepts. 2nd ed. San Diego, CA: Academic Press; 2001. p. 763–77.
5. Rude RK. Magnesium depletion and hypermagnesemia. In: Rosen CJ, Compston JE, Lian JB, editors. Primer on the metabolic bone diseases and disorders of mineral metabolism. 7th ed. Washington, DC: American Society of Bone and Mineral Research; 2008. p. 325–35.
6. Matsuyama J, Tsuji K, Doyama H, Kim F, Takeda Y, Kito Y, Ito R, Nakanishi H, Hayashi T, Waseda Y, Tsuji S, Takemura K, Yamada S, Okada T, Kanaya H. Hypomagnesemia associated with a proton pump inhibitor. Intern Med. 2012;51:2231–4.
7. Cundy T, Dissanayake A. Severe hypomagnesaemia in long-term users of proton-pump inhibitors. Clin Endocrinol (Oxf). 2008;69:338–41.
8. Schlingmann KP, Weber S, Peters M, Niemann NE, Vitzthum H, Klingel K, Kratz K, Haddad E, Ristoff E, Dinour D, Syrrou M, Nielsen S, Sassen M, Waldegger S, Seyberth HW, Konrad M. Hypomagnesemia with secondary hypocalcemia is caused by mutations in TRPM6, a new member of the TRPM gene family. Nat Genet. 2002;31:166–70.

# Chapter 27
# Management of Hypoparathyroidism

C. Banti and G. Viccica

## Objective

- Diagnosis and differential diagnosis of hypoparathyroidism
- Therapy and management of hypoparathyroidism
- Side effects and risks of overtreatment

## Case Presentation

A 50-year-old woman was referred to our outpatient clinic for advice concerning management of postoperative hypocalcaemia.

Six months before she had undergone total thyroidectomy for multinodular goiter. Histology showed a colloid cystic goiter. One day after surgery she had acute hypocalcemia with tetany, which was treated with intravenous calcium gluconate.

At the time of hospital discharge, treatment with calcitriol (1 mcg/die) and calcium carbonate (2 g/die) was recommended. Monitoring of serum calcium was not satisfactory, despite several adjustments or treatment.

At the time of our evaluation, the patient was treated with levothyroxine 87.5 µg, 1 g calcium carbonate, and calcitriol 1.25 µg daily. The patient reported paresthesia and a positive Chvostek and Trousseau' signs were detected at physical examination. The past medical history was unremarkable, with the exception of cluster headache and constitutional slimness. Serum calcium and PTH were normal before surgery.

Her laboratory data were as follows. Normal values are reported in parenthesis. Total serum calcium 8.2 mg/dl (8.4–10.2)

C. Banti, M.D. (✉) • G. Viccica, M.D.
Endocrine Unit 2, University Hospital of Pisa, Pisa, Italy
e-mail: chiara_banti@virgilio.it

© Springer Science+Business Media New York 2015
T.F. Davies (ed.), *A Case-Based Guide to Clinical Endocrinology*,
DOI 10.1007/978-1-4939-2059-4_27

243

Serum albumin 4.5 g/dl (3.4–5.0)
Albumin-corrected total serum calcium (see below) 7.8 mg/dl
PTH < 10 ng/ml (10–75)
Serum phosphate 4.8 mg/dl (2.7–4.5)
24-h urinary calcium 416 mg (150–300)

## Diagnosis

Postoperative hypoparathyroidism with hypocalcemia partially controlled with calcium carbonate and calcitriol complicated by hypercalciuria.

## Review of How the Diagnosis Was Made

Postoperative hypoparathyroidism is the most likely diagnosis in a patient with hypocalcemia, previously submitted to total thyroidectomy. This might not be the case in the rare patient with primary hypoparathyroidism. Hypoparathyroidism is the most common complication of parathyroid or thyroid surgery and is generally caused by damage to the parathyroid gland and/or their blood supply or inadvertent/unavoidable removal [1].

Postoperative hypoparathyroidism can be transient or permanent; the transient variant is due to a reversible parathyroid damage and commonly resolve within a few weeks, but may persist up to 6 months after surgery. Permanent postoperative hypoparathyroidism is diagnosed when it persist for at least 6 months after surgery [2, 3].

The diagnosis of postoperative hypoparathyroidism is based upon the finding of hypocalcemia and undetectable or inappropriately low/normal intact PTH level [4]. The serum calcium levels should be corrected for serum albumin:

$$\text{Albumin}-\text{corrected total serum calcium}=\text{measured total calcium}\left(\text{mg}/\text{dl}\right)$$
$$+\left[0.8\times4.0-\text{patient s serum albumin concentration}\left(\text{g}/\text{dl}\right)\right].$$

The diagnosis of postoperative hypoparathyroidism can be confirmed by the finding of low-ionized calcium level and normal serum level of magnesium. Serum phosphorus levels are usually high or at the upper normal range. In a few patients with severe primary hyperparathyroidism, postoperative hypocalcemia may persist despite standard treatment, because of the uptake of calcium into the remineralizing bone ("hungry bone syndrome"). In this condition, hypocalcemia is with low phosphorus and appropriately elevated PTH levels.

The goal of therapy is to relieve symptoms of hypocalcemia and maintain serum calcium in the low–normal range and serum phosphorus in the high–normal range. The standard treatment includes oral calcium and vitamin D metabolites and analogs. Calcitriol [$1,25(OH)_2D_3$] is preferred (over vitamin $D_2$ or $D_3$) because of its potency and rapid onset and offset of action. The analogue alfacalcidol ($1\text{-}\alpha OHD_3$), which is converted to calcitriol, may also be used [1] (Table 27.1).

**Table 27.1** Orally active vitamin D analogs commonly used in the management of chronic hypoparathyroidism

| | $1,25(OH)_2D_3$, calcitriol | $1\alpha OHD_3$, alfacalcidiol | DHT, dihydrotachysterol |
|---|---|---|---|
| Dose | 0.5–2.0 μg once or twice daily | 0.5–3.0 μg once daily | 0.2–1.0 mg once daily |
| Time to onset of action | 1–2 days | 1–2 days | 4–7 days |
| Time of offset of action | 2–3 days | 5–7 days | 7–21 days |
| Pharmaceutical formulation | Capsules | Capsules/drops | Drops |

The potential side effects of overtreatment are hypercalcemia, hyperphosphatemia, and hypercalciuria; the latter can determine nephrocalcinosis and nephrolithiasis [5]. Hypercalciuria may develop before serum calcium increases, because of the lack of PTH-mediated calcium reabsorption in the renal distal tubule. A low-salt diet and eventually a thiazide diuretic may be helpful to reduce hypercalciuria and maintain normocalcemia.

In our patient, a low-salt diet (100 mEq of sodium per day) together with hydrochlorothiazide 25 mg daily restored normocalcemia (albumin-corrected total serum calcium 8.8 mg/dl) and reduced urinary calcium excretion (250 mg/24 h).

## Lessons Learned

- The total serum calcium level should be corrected for serum albumin.
- The diagnosis of postoperative hypoparathyroidism is based upon the finding of hypocalcemia and undetectable or inappropriately low/normal intact PTH level
- The goal of therapy is to relieve symptoms of hypocalcemia and maintain serum calcium in the low–normal range and serum phosphorus in the high–normal range.
- The potential side effects of hypoparathyroidism overtreatment are hypercalcemia, hyperphosphatemia, and hypercalciuria; the latter can determine nephrocalcinosis and nephrolithiasis
- When hypercalciuria occurs, a low-salt diet and eventually a thiazide diuretic may be helpful to reduce hypercalciuria and maintain normocalcemia.

## Questions

1. The most common cause of hypocalcemia:

    a. Parathyroid gland agenesis
    b. DiGeorge syndrome
    c. Vitamin D deficiency
    d. Hyperphosphatemia
    e. Postoperative hypoparathyroidism

2. The following symptoms can be seen in hypocalcemia

   a. Paresthesias
   b. Tetany
   c. Hypertension
   d. Stipsis
   e. A and B

3. Which of the following treatment options are commonly used in patients with postoperative hypoparathyroidism

   a. Calcium alone
   b. Calcitriol
   c. Vitamin $D_2$
   d. Calcium and calcitriol
   e. Vitamin $D_3$

4. Which of the following side effects may occur during therapy of hypoparathyroidism

   a. Hypercalciuria
   b. Hypophosphatemia
   c. Urinary infection
   d. Hyperphosphatemia
   e. A and D

## Answers to Questions

1. e. Postoperative hypoparathyroidism
2. e. A and B
3. d. Calcium and calcitriol
4. e. A and D

## References

1. Shoback D. Clinical practice: hypoparathyroidism. N Engl J Med. 2008;359:391–403.
2. Pattou F, Combemale F, Fabre S, Carnaille B, Decoulx M, Wemeau JL, Racadot A, Proye C. Hypocalcemia following thyroid surgery: incidence and prediction of outcome. World J Surg. 1998;22:718–24.
3. Page C, Strunski V. Parathyroid risk in total thyroidectomy for bilateral, benign, multinodular goitre: report of 351 surgical cases. J Laryngol Otol. 2007;121:237–41.
4. Cooper MS, Gittoes NJ. Diagnosis and management of hypocalcaemia. BMJ. 2008;336:1298–302.
5. Bilezikian JP, Khan A, Potts Jr JT, Brandi ML, Clarke BL, Shoback D, Jüppner H, D'Amour P, Fox J, Rejnmark L, Mosekilde L, Rubin MR, Dempster D, Gafni R, Collins MT, Sliney J, Sanders J. Hypoparathyroidism in the adult: Epidemiology, diagnosis, pathophysiology, target organ involvement, treatment, and challenges for future research. J Bone Miner Res. 2011;26:2317–37.

# Chapter 28
# Osteomalacia and Primary Hyperparathyroidism

**Antonella Meola and Silvia Chiavistelli**

## Objective

- Diagnosis of osteomalacia
- Diagnosis and natural history of normocalcemic primary hyperparathyroidism

## Case Presentation

A 60-year-old man was evaluated for severe vitamin D deficiency, associated with muscle weakness pain at the upper limbs and back lasting since 1 year.

His medical history included arterial hypertension, benign prostatic hyperplasia, bladder cancer treated with surgical intervention.

On examination, the patient appeared reasonably well. The BMI was 22, the blood pressure 140/80 mmHg, and the pulse rate 72 per minute. The neurologic examination revealed bilateral muscle weakness and hypotonia that affected the proximal shoulder and hip-girdle muscles.

His laboratory data were as follows (reference ranges are reported in parentheses):

Total albumin-corrected serum calcium = 8.2 mg/dl (8.4–10.2)
Serum ionized calcium = 1.05 mmol/l (1.13–1.32)
Phosphorus = 2.2 mg/dl (2.7–4.5)
Serum creatinine = 0.8 mg/dl (0.5–0.9)
eGFR = 108 ml/min × 1.73 m²

A. Meola, M.D. (✉) • S. Chiavistelli, M.D.
Endocrine Unit 2, University Hospital of Pisa, Via Paradisa 2, Pisa, Italy
e-mail: antonella.meola@hotmail.it

© Springer Science+Business Media New York 2015          247
T.F. Davies (ed.), *A Case-Based Guide to Clinical Endocrinology*,
DOI 10.1007/978-1-4939-2059-4_28

Intact PTH = 212 pg/ml (15–75)
25OHD = 8.5 ng/ml (>30)
Alkaline phosphatase = 280 U/l (40–129)
24-h urinary calcium = 100 mg (150–300)
Anti-transglutaminase antibody = <10 U/ml (<10)

Bone scintigraphy (TC99m HDP) showed an enhanced radioisotope uptake in the calvaria, ribs, clavicles, and spine suggestive of osteogenic process.

Bone mineral density (BMD) was decreased at the lumbar spine (T-score −1.6) and hip (T-score −2.4), and markedly reduced at the one-third distal radius (T-score −3.4).

## Review of How the Diagnosis Was Made

The medical history and biochemical examination were consistent with the diagnosis of secondary hyperparathyroidism due to severe vitamin D deficiency and osteomalacia [1]. Vitamin D deficiency is the most common cause of secondary hyperparathyroidism. Patients with low 25OHD should be replaced with vitamin D and reevaluated. Occasionally these patients will become hypercalcemic, thus unmasking the more typical hypercalcemic primary hyperparathyroidism (PHPT). Cholecalciferol treatment was started (25,000 IU weekly for 8 weeks and subsequently 50,000 IU monthly). Three months later the patient's general conditions and muscle function were improved and the bone pain decreased. Results of laboratory tests were as follows:

Total albumin-corrected serum calcium = 9.3 mg/dl
Serum phosphorous = 2.5 mg/dl
Intact PTH = 132 pg/ml
25OHD = 39 ng/ml
Alkaline phosphatase = 139 U/l
24-h urinary calcium = 180 mg

Neck ultrasound showed a right hypoechoic lump, posterior to the thyroid lobe, compatible with an enlarged parathyroid gland.

The finding of persistently elevated intact PTH despite normalization of serum calcium and 25OHD prompted us to further evaluate the patient. The normal urinary calcium excretion, and the negative history for liver and renal diseases, gastrointestinal diseases associated with malabsorption, other metabolic bone disease (e.g., Paget's disease), and use of drugs (loop diuretics, bisphosphonates, and anticonvulsants) that could affect PTH levels raised the question that the patients might have normocalcemic PHPT (NPHPT) [2]. This entity has been recently described in women evaluated in their early postmenopausal years for parameters of skeletal health, as well as a consequence of measuring PTH in all subject undergoing evaluation for low BMD [3].

Total albumin-corrected serum calcium and ionized calcium should be normal on several determinations, since occasional normal serum calcium levels may be present in patients with mild classical PHPT.

Measurement of total serum calcium weekly for 3 weeks confirmed normocalcemia. The patients underwent neck ultrasound evaluation which showed a nodule of 10 mm hypoechoic compatible with an enlarged parathyroid gland.

Measurements of serum calcium and intact PTH over a 18-month follow-up period confirmed normocalcemia associated with moderately increased PTH levels. No other manifestations related to PHPT developed.

It has been suggested that PHPT has a biphasic disease course: the first phase is characterized by elevated serum level of PTH, while hypercalcemia is not present yet. In the second phase hypercalcemia occurs. NPHPT could represent the first phase of PHPT [4, 5].

Limited data are available on the natural history of NPHPT, but observational studies provided evidence that some individuals may develop hypercalcemia or evidence of disease progression.

In the Columbia experience with a median follow-up of 3 years further signs of PHPT developed in about one-third of patients [hypercalcemia ($n=7$), kidney stone ($n=1$), fracture ($n=1$), osteoporosis ($n=4$), and hypercalciuria ($n=2$)] [6]. A parathyroid adenoma was shown by sestamibi scan in 8 of the 16 patients tested. Successful parathyroid surgery was performed in 7 patients. Because of hypercalcemia ($n=3$), osteoporosis ($n=3$), or patient choice ($n=1$), serum calcium normalized in hypercalcemic patients after surgery but did not change in normocalcemic patients, despite a significant fall in PTH levels.

In another series 32 patients with NPHPT were followed for a mean of 3.7 years [7]. Parathyroid surgery was performed in 12 patients with positive preoperative localization studies and a significant decline in PTH and serum calcium was observed. At variance with the Columbia experience none of the 20 patients followed without parathyroidectomy showed a progression of the disease.

The finding that disease progression is demonstrable in some but not all cases, even after a rather long follow-up, suggests that there is no uniform time course for the development of hypercalcemia in NPHPT and that some patients might never develop the hypercalcemic phenotype.

*Diagnosis*: Normocalcemic primary hyperparathyroidism.


# Lesson Learned

- Vitamin D deficiency is the most common cause of secondary hyperparathyroidism
- Bilateral muscle weakness and hypotonia at the hip-girdle muscles associated with vitamin D deficiency might suggest the diagnosis of osteomalacia
- The finding of elevated plasma PTH levels associated with consistently normal albumin-adjusted (or ionized) serum calcium concentration suggests NPHPT once all other causes of secondary hyperparathyroidism have been excluded
- NPHPT can be detected only if PTH is measured in normocalcemic individuals
- An enlarged parathyroid gland may be detected at imaging studies in individuals with NPHPT

- The course of NPHPT is not uniform: some patients may show disease progression with appearance of hypercalcemia and other disease manifestations, whereas others might never develop the hypercalcemic phenotype

## Questions

1. Which is the most common cause of secondary hyperparathyroidism?

   a. Vitamin D deficiency
   b. Gastrointestinal diseases associated with malabsorption
   c. Paget's disease
   d. Drugs (estrogens, loop diuretics, bisphosphonates, and anticonvulsants)

2. Which is the biochemical profile of patients with osteomalacia?

   a. Elevated PTH and elevated serum calcium levels
   b. Elevated PTH and normal serum calcium levels
   c. Elevated PTH and low or low/normal serum calcium levels
   d. Low PTH and low serum calcium levels.

3. Patients with NPHPT have:

   a. Intermittently normal total albumin-adjusted serum calcium and elevated PTH
   b. Consistently normal total albumin-adjusted serum calcium and intermittent elevation of PTH
   c. Consistently normal total albumin-adjusted serum calcium and elevated PTH
   d. Alternate finding of increased total albumin-adjusted serum calcium and normal ionized calcium in individuals with elevated PTH

4. Which is the natural history of patients with NPHPT:

   a. All patients become hypercalcemic within 3 years
   b. Some patients may develop hypercalcemia but other might never develop the hypercalcemic phenotype
   c. Serum calcium remains in the normal range and PTH normalized over time
   d. Hypercalcemia never occurs in the disease

## Answers to Questions

1. a. Vitamin D deficiency
2. c. Elevated PTH and low or low/normal serum calcium levels
3. c. Consistently normal total albumin-adjusted serum calcium and elevated PTH
4. b. Some patients may develop hypercalcemia but other might never develop the hypercalcemic phenotype

# References

1. Holick MF. Vitamin D deficiency. N Engl J Med. 2007;357:266–81.
2. Marcocci C, Cetani F. N Engl J Med. 2011;365:2389–97.
3. Bilezikian JP. Primary hyperparathyroidism. Updated 28 Feb 2012. http://www.endotext.org/parathyroid/parathyroid5/parathyroidframe5.htm.
4. Rao DS, Wilson RJ, Kleerekoper M, Parfitt AM. Lack of biochemical progression or continuation of accelerated bone loss in mild asymptomatic primary hyperparathyroidism: evidence for biphasic disease course. J Clin Endocrinol Metab. 1988;67:1294–8.
5. Silverberg SJ, Bilezikian JP. Incipient primary hyperparathyroidism: a "forme fruste" of an old disease. J Clin Endocrinol Metab. 2003;88:5348–52.
6. Lowe H, MacMahon DJ, Rubin MR, Bilezikian JP, Silverberg SJ. Normocalcemic primary hyperparathyroidism: further characterization of a new clinical phenotype. J Clin Endocrinol Metab. 2007;92(8):3001–5.
7. Tordjman KM, Greenman Y, Osher E, et al. Characterization of normocalcemic parimary hyperparathyroidism. Am J Med. 2004;117:861–3.

# Part VII
# Metabolic Bone Diseases

# Chapter 29
# Introduction

**Mone Zaidi, Se Min Kim, Tony Yuen, and Li Sun**

Over the past decade there has been a radical and rapid evolution not only in our understanding of the pathobiology of osteoporosis but also in our ability to diagnose skeletal fragility and effectively prevent and treat its consequences. This shift has resulted from the remarkable successes in our understanding, through the use of genetically modified mouse models, of how the skeleton is remodeled in time and space, as well as how the reparative process is modulated by hormonal, cytokine, and immune stimuli [1]. These insights have been buttressed by striking advances in technologies used to image the skeleton, resulting in ways by which microskeletal elements, which are responsible in maintaining bone strength and hence, its propensity to fracture, are now visualized by high resolution tomography and magnetic resonance imaging. There has also been a progression, *albeit* small, in the development and use of new therapies for osteoporosis, with new target-specific agents in development.

All of this has meant that we are able to expand the diagnosis of osteoporosis beyond the traditional realm of BMD-based methods alone. The WHO based the diagnosis of osteoporosis on T-scores that utilized epidemiologic criteria to label patients as osteopenic or osteoporotic. This method has stood the test of time and is currently being used most widely. However, T-scores are derived by comparing a patient's BMD, which is a measure of bone mineral content across a given area, against a database of ~30-year-old Caucasian women. Two sets of compelling evidence have nonetheless highlighted the need for a BMD-independent tool that can capture patients with fragile skeletons or those at a high risk of fracture. First, biomechanical studies show that the strength of bone is not derived solely from BMD, but that other elements, not yet measurable clinically, contribute to bone strength and fragility. Second, it is clear that patients that display normal BMDs do fracture and that increases in BMD with drug therapy do not necessarily correlate with reduced fracture risk.

M. Zaidi, M.D., Ph.D., F.R.C.P. (✉) • S.M. Kim, M.D. • T. Yuen, Ph.D. • L. Sun, M.D., Ph.D.
Mount Sinai Bone Program, Mount Sinai School of Medicine, New York, NY 10029, USA
e-mail: mone.zaidi@mssm.edu

© Springer Science+Business Media New York 2015
T.F. Davies (ed.), *A Case-Based Guide to Clinical Endocrinology*,
DOI 10.1007/978-1-4939-2059-4_29

In response to the clinical need for the identification of men and women at a high risk of fracture, the WHO developed a risk stratification tool, FRAX™, which allows us to estimate the 10-year absolute fracture risk in a given patient [2]. This tool allows a country-specific and cost-effective extension of therapeutic thresholds to include patients with a high fracture risk, who otherwise would not be candidates for therapy under BMD-only guidelines. While this is considered a positive step, FRAX™ is said to have its gaps. On its own, it purposefully excludes the perimenopausal or early postmenopausal woman, who is undergoing the most rapid bone loss, but has yet not attained as high an absolute fracture risk as an older postmenopausal woman. Toward this end, there have been attempts to rationalize the use of bone turnover markers, which, to us, provide a valuable point estimate for the rate of bone removal, and hence can predict bone loss [3]. A fear is that, by relying solely on BMD- or fracture risk-based treatment thresholds, health maintenance organizations and third-party payers are likely to shy away further from these young, fast bone losers. On the basis of current evidence for rapid bone loss during and efficacy of therapies across the menopausal transition, we suggest that early identification, follow-up, and treatment of progressive "bone loss" are prudent approaches that will likely prevent a skeleton characterized by "lost bone" and a high fracture risk [3]. These diagnostic challenges have been highlighted in Chap. 29.

With our increased awareness of osteoporosis as a crippling disease, and an understanding of the molecular cross-talk between the skeleton and distant organs, such as the brain, pancreas, pituitary, and kidney, among others, there has been the realization that certain drugs (and diseases) have off-target effects on skeletal integrity and bone mass. Glucocorticoids constitute the most well-characterized example in this regard, but new evidence suggests that proton pump inhibitors, selective serotonin uptake inhibitors, tricyclic antidepressants, and certain antidiabetic agents, prominently thiazolidinediones, affect the formation and/or resorption of bone.

Evidence from observational studies, including case–control and cohort studies, has established important associations between the aforementioned drugs and fracture risk, thus offering new hypotheses amenable to testing. Biological testing of chemicals, such as thiazolidinediones, has shown that the drugs not only divert mesenchymal stem cells away from the bone-forming osteoblast to the adipocyte lineage, but that the agents can also increase bone resorption [4]. Furthermore, and complicating issues even further, is the realization that underlying diseases, such as type-2 diabetes and depression, can themselves cause bone loss and a high fracture risk through yet unclear mechanisms. However, clinically, it is clear that, the greater the number of risk factors, the higher is the risk of fracture [5], an idea that has been elaborated in Chap. 28.

In as much as certain drugs used for other diseases can impair skeletal integrity, there have been suggestions that bisphosphonates, the mainstay for osteoporosis therapy now for nearly two decades, can cause a rare, low-trauma fracture of the femur that displays certain atypical features [6]. This question has prompted a broader examination of the long-term effects of bisphosphonate use. Although certain case control and cohort studies show that there are a greater number of long-term bisphosphonate users have fractures with atypical radiologic features, the studies equally importantly reveal that non-bisphosphonate users also have fractures with this specific appearance. Furthermore, there are likely more atypical fracture patients on bisphosphonates because of their underlying high fracture risk, which is suggestive of indication bias within at least certain studies.

Some of the largest fracture trials conducted, namely the FIT, the FIT Long-Term Extension (FLEX) trial, and the HORIZON-PFT, have been reanalyzed to explore any association between bisphosphonates and subtrochanteric or femoral diaphyseal fractures. Compared with placebo, there was no significant increase in fracture risk associated with bisphosphonate use [7]. Furthermore, while oversuppression of bone remodeling by bisphosphonates has been implicated in the genesis of these fractures, there is no biologic plausibility that establishes a cause–effect relationship between bisphosphonate use and atypical femur fracture. In fact, questions arise as to how a drug that prevents fractures can be the cause of fractures, and more specifically, how a drug that prevents fractures at the femoral neck is the cause of a fracture just a few centimeters below. It is our opinion that the continued press on this issue, and the resulting fears in the minds of some patients and physicians, has significantly (and unfortunately) reduced the use of these and other medications that prevent osteoporosis-related fractures. This places the average postmenopausal woman at a high risk of debilitating osteoporosis-related fractures. Chapter 30 focuses on a fracture that was misdiagnosed as atypical femoral fracture.

# References

1. Zaidi M. Skeletal remodeling in health and disease. Nat Med. 2007;13:791–801.
2. Cauley JA, et al. FRAX®: Position Conference Members. Official Positions for FRAX® clinical regarding international differences from Joint Official Positions Development Conference of the International Society for Clinical Densitometry and International Osteoporosis Foundation on FRAX®. J Clin Densitom. 2011;14:240–62.
3. Zaidi M, et al. Bone loss or lost bone: rationale and recommendations for the diagnosis and treatment of early postmenopausal bone loss. Curr Osteoporos Rep. 2009;4:118–26.
4. Wan Y, et al. PPAR-$\gamma$ regulates osteoclastogenesis in mice. Nat Med. 2007;12:1496–503.
5. Cummings SR, et al. Risk factors for hip fracture in white women. N Engl J Med. 1995;332:767–72.
6. Shane E, et al. American Society for Bone and Mineral Research. Atypical subtrochanteric and diaphyseal femoral fractures: report of a task force of the American Society for Bone and Mineral Research. J Bone Miner Res. 2010;25:2267–94.
7. Whitaker M, Guo J, Kehoe T, Benson G. Bisphosphonates for osteoporosis–where do we go from here? N Engl J Med. 2012;366:2048–51.

# Chapter 30
# Multiple Risk Factors for Osteoporosis and Fracture

**Mone Zaidi and Li Sun**

## Objective

1. Understand that fracture risk can be increased in the presence of a near-normal BMD
2. Recognize that multiple risk factors can compound to increase the risk of an individual's fracture

## Case Presentation

The patient is a 75-year-old housewife, who underwent menopause about 20 years ago. She has a long-standing history of back and leg pain for over two decades. She was an avid treadmill user and undertook low impact exercises. There was no family history of osteoporosis or fracture. She had no prior fractures. She denies a history of smoking and reports minimal alcohol use during social occasions. She has been taking 1,200 mg calcium carbonate and a multivitamin daily as supplements. Her medications have also included hydrochlorothiazide for hypertension, crestor for hypercholesterolemia, Elavil (a tricyclic antidepressant, TCA), and Prozac (a selective serotonin reuptake inhibitor, SSRI) for chronic pain symptoms. She was also on prempro over the past 10 years initially at 0.625/2.5 mg/day, but this was later reduced to 0.3/2.5 mg/day and stopped 3 years ago. The patient underwent a bone mineral density measurement around 10 years ago with T-scores (and BMD) of −0.60 (1.032 g/cm$^2$) at the lumbar spine and −2.6 (0.701 g/cm$^2$) at the femoral neck. Lateral thoracolumbar spine X-rays revealed diffuse degenerative joint disease, but

M. Zaidi, M.D., Ph.D., F.R.C.P. (✉) • L. Sun, M.D., Ph.D.
Mount Sinai Bone Program, Mount Sinai School of Medicine, New York, NY 10029, USA
e-mail: mone.zaidi@mssm.edu; Li.Sun@mssm.edu

© Springer Science+Business Media New York 2015
T.F. Davies (ed.), *A Case-Based Guide to Clinical Endocrinology*,
DOI 10.1007/978-1-4939-2059-4_30

**Table 30.1** Renal Function
of the Patient in this Study

| Cr | BUN | eGFR |
|----|-----|------|
| 1.5 | 30 | 50 |
| 1.5 | 35 | 40 |
| 1.4 | 30 | 51 |
| 1.8 | 36 | 30 |
| 1.4 | 20 | 41 |
| 1.3 | 25 | 37 |

no evidence of compression deformity. Her FRAX™ score was 20 % and 9.5 % for all osteoporosis-related and hip, respectively. As the patient had osteoporosis and a high risk of fracture per FRAX™, she was treated with Actonel (35 mg once a week), and while BMDs remained stable over the next 3 years, the patient fractured her right hip when she slipped and fell in her bathroom. The fracture was treated surgically by an intramedullary nail and healed normally.

Around 2 years prior to fracture, the patient began developing renal insufficiency. Her BUN, creatinine, and eGFR are shown in Table 30.1 (weight ~125 lb).

## How the Diagnosis Was Made

The patient had osteoporosis and a high fracture risk, and despite stable BMDs on Actonel, sustained a hip fracture. She had several risk factors for a fracture, which included being female, her Caucasian descent, age, menopausal status, history of withdrawal of hormone replacement therapy, and the use of SSRIs and TCA. *Per* the Kidney Disease Outcomes Quality Initiative (KDOQI) of the National Kidney Foundation, the patient also had stage 3 (moderate) chronic kidney disease (eGFR = 30–59), likely due to her hypertension.

## Lessons Learned

1. This is a classic case in which a patient suffering from osteoporosis and being effectively treated with an antiresorptive medication, such as a bisphosphonate, sustains a hip fracture. Of note is that bisphosphonates and other skeletal osteoprotective therapies reduce, but do not eliminate fracture risk. Certain therapies have been shown to reduce hip fracture by ~40 %. The fracture in the patient should therefore not be seen as failure of therapy, as patients on statins are not exempt from heart attacks.
2. Figure 30.1 shows that no matter what a patient's BMD is, three or four risk factors increase the risk of fracture [1]. This was noted even in patients within the highest tertile of BMD values, which included those with normal BMDs. This was evident on the patient FRAX™ calculations (20 % and 9 % for all

**Fig. 30.1** Effect of the number of risk factors and bone mineral density on hip fracture risk. Redrawn from [1]

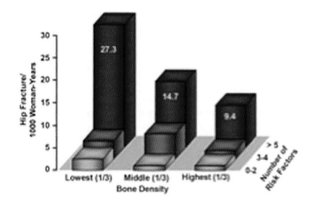

**Table 30.2** Changes in structural and material properties of bone with age leading to reduced bone strength

| *Structural properties* |
| --- |
| Thinning of cortical bone |
| Thinning and loss of trabecular structures |
| Increased cortical porosity |
| *Material properties* |
| Reduced bone mineral density |
| Altered collagen crosslinks and phosphorylation pattern |
| Increased crystal size |
| Changes in mineral-to-matrix ratio |
| Microcrack accumulation in cortical bone |

osteoporosis-related and hip fractures, respectively). However, FRAX™ may have in fact underestimated the patient's fracture risk, particularly as she had three further risk factors for a fracture, namely acute withdrawal of hormone replacement therapy, chronic kidney disease, PPI use, and TCA/SSRI use. Therefore, aggressive therapy was mandated.

3. No matter what one's BMD is, the older one gets, the higher the risk of fracture is at all sites. This effect of age is in part due to an increased propensity to fall in older individuals. However, there occur changes in structural and material properties of bone as one gets older (Table 30.2). These changes alter bone strength and increase its propensity to fracture. The implication of this is that if there is a T-score of −2.6 in a patient aged 80 years, his/her fracture risk is considerably higher than a patient who is 55 years of age with the same T-score. In other words, while a 14.1 % absolute fracture risk over 10 years, per FRAX™, requires a T-score of −3.0 at age 50 years, about the same fracture risk (14.6 %) at age 70 years just requires a T-score of −1.5. Therefore, the requirement of a low T-score to produce a given risk of fracture diminishes as one gets older, so that older patients, both men and women, fracture at considerably conserved T-scores.

4. While 0.625 mg/day estrogen is known to have a bone protective effect and can reduce fracture risk according to data from the Women's Health Initiative, in clinical practice, not all women show an equally robust BMD response to estrogen therapy. Women can continue to lose bone despite being on hormone replacement therapy.

5. It has been shown that withdrawal of hormone replacement therapy is followed by an increased annual rate of bone loss (−0.7 % to −1.6 %). This is accompanied by a marked increase of bone turnover markers after 6 months [2]. This rate of bone loss was found to be higher than in women who never received estrogen [2, 3]. Thus, upon withdrawal of estrogen replacement therapy, other follow-up therapies are mandated, as was the case with this patient.

6. End-stage renal disease is well known to be associated with a high fracture risk. However, there is considerable accruing evidence showing that moderate CKD, i.e., Stage 3 CKD, is also associated with a high fracture risk, particularly at the hip [4, 5]. A number of studies now show very clearly a significant association between hip fracture and moderate CKD, independently of age, BMI, and BMD. Very relevant to the patient, the analysis of the Women's Health Initiative database provided evidence for an increased risk of hip fracture in women with moderate CKD who were on hormone therapy.

7. The patient had a consistent pattern of antidepressant use for over a decade. The interaction between antidepressant drugs and fracture risk is considered complex mechanistically, in part because depression itself can lead to bone loss. A comprehensive meta-analysis found that the relative risk for fracture among antidepressant users do persist when the analysis is confined to studies that adjust for depression. The patient did not have depression; instead she used these agents for pain relief. Therefore, in her case, depression per se cannot be regarded as a contributor to her bone loss. There is good consensus from case control studies, cohort studies, and more recent meta-analyses that hip fracture risk is increased by as much as twofold in TCA and SSRI users compared to nonusers [6]. However, while SSRIs show evidence of dose dependence, the effect of dose is not a feature seen across all studies or among all classes. The effect on fracture risk is rapid, beginning within few months of initiation, continues to remain high, and declines considerably after cessation of therapy [7].

8. Whereas there is some consistency that SSRIs reduce BMD, this is not seen with TCAs. For TCAs, the data indicates that fracture risk is increased in the absence of BMD.

## Questions

1. True or False: The effect of age in increasing fracture risk is:

    1. Seen clinically in that older patients fracture at higher (less negative) T-scores than younger patients
    2. Results, in part from, microcrack accumulation in aging bone

   3. Not due to an increased propensity to fall in older patients

   4. A key determinant of FRAX™

2. True or False: For a patient who is on a PPI for recurrent GERD:

   1. One should always use the citrate form of calcium as a supplement

   2. There should be no concern of an increased risk of fracture

   3. Calcium should not be used as supplement

3. True or False: Chronic renal failure:

   1. Is always associated with hyperparathyroidism

   2. Can cause a high fracture risk

   3. Rarely presents with hypercalcemia

   4. Initially elevates serum phosphorous to change the $Ca \times P$ product

4. True or False:

   1. There is evidence that both SSRIs and TCAs reduce BMD

   2. There is evidence that both SSRIs and TCAs elevate fracture risk

   3. The mechanism of action of TCAs on the skeleton is unclear and may be related to increase in falls

   4. TCAs increase fracture risk earlier than SSRIs

   5. There is evidence that the effect of TCAs and SSRIs on the skeleton is synergistic

## Answers to Questions

1. 1: True; 2: True; 3: False; 4: True
2. 1: True; 2: False; 3: False
3. 1: False; 2: True; 3: True; 4: True
4. 1: False; 2: True; 3: True; 4: True; 5: False

## References

1. Cummings SR, Nevitt MC, Browner WS, Stone K, Fox KM, Ensrud KE, et al. Risk factors for hip fracture in white women. Study of Osteoporotic Fractures Research Group. N Engl J Med. 1995;332(12):767–73.
2. Sornay-Rendu E, Garnero P, Munoz F, Duboeuf F, Delmas PD. Effect of withdrawal of hormone replacement therapy on bone mass and bone turnover: the OFELY study. Bone. 2003;33(1):159–66.
3. Epstein S, Inzerillo AM, Caminis J, Zaidi M. Disorders associated with acute rapid and severe bone loss. J Bone Miner Res. 2003;18(12):2083–94.

4. Nickolas TL, McMahon DJ, Shane E. Relationship between moderate to severe kidney disease and hip fracture in the United States. J Am Soc Nephrol. 2006;17(11):3223–32.
5. Miller PD. Diagnosis and treatment of osteoporosis in chronic renal disease. Semin Nephrol. 2009;29(2):144–55.
6. Rabenda V, Nicolet D, Beaudart C, Bruyere O, Reginster JY. Relationship between use of antidepressants and risk of fractures: a meta-analysis. Osteoporos Int. 2013;24(1):121–37.
7. Rizzoli R, Cooper C, Reginster JY, Abrahamsen B, Adachi JD, Brandi ML, et al. Antidepressant medications and osteoporosis. Bone. 2012;51(3):606–13.

# Chapter 31
# Delayed Diagnosis of Osteoporosis

**Mone Zaidi and Tony Yuen**

## Objective

- Emphasize the importance of using "osteoporosis" as a diagnosis when there is a fragility fracture, even in the absence of a low T-score.
- Appreciate that bone loss begins during the late perimenopause, and that the most rapid rates of bone loss occur during this transition.
- Recognize the importance of intervention during early menopausal bone loss.

## Case Presentation

A 65-year-old Caucasian woman, otherwise healthy, underwent menopause at 53 years of age. Since then, she has been on hormone replacement therapy (0.62 mg/2.5 mg) for hot flashes. However, over a year ago, she discontinued HRT upon reading about the risks of breast cancer and heart disease. She has not taken any vitamin D or calcium on a regular basis, but does use a multivitamin tablet occasionally. She was diagnosed with gastro-esophageal reflux (GERD), for which she has been on pantoprazol over the past 6 years. She is also lactose intolerant. She indicates that she has lost 2 in. in height. Approximately 10 years ago, the patient fell on a sidewalk and broke her forearm, which was managed by her orthopedic surgeon. There is no history of osteoporosis. The patient has never smoked and drinks wine socially. Her mother had a hip fracture at age 68 years.

She came in for a consultation asking whether she needed additional therapy to treat or prevent her osteoporosis. Examination on presentation was unremarkable,

M. Zaidi, M.D., Ph.D., F.R.C.P. (✉) • T. Yuen, Ph.D.
Mount Sinai Bone Program, Mount Sinai School of Medicine, New York, NY 10029, USA
e-mail: mone.zaidi@mssm.edu; tony.yuen@mssm.edu

© Springer Science+Business Media New York 2015                                                    265
T.F. Davies (ed.), *A Case-Based Guide to Clinical Endocrinology*,
DOI 10.1007/978-1-4939-2059-4_31

specifically with no thyromegaly or spinal tenderness. Her height was 5 ft 4 in. and weight was 125 lbs. Her most recent bone densitometry (DXA) showed the following T-scores (and BMD values): −2.2 of the AP lumbar spine (0.825 g/cm$^2$); −2.0 at the total hip (0.640 g/cm$^2$); and −2.2 at the femoral neck (0.629 g/cm$^2$). Her basic metabolic profile was normal, but her 25-OH vitamin D was 31 ng/mL. PTH levels were normal, as was her urine calcium. The physician labeled her with a diagnosis of osteopenia, prescribed 50,000 IU vitamin D (ergocalciferol) per week for 12 weeks followed by 50,000 IU per month continuing indefinitely, and counseled her on an appropriate exercise regimen.

Notably, the patient was not prescribed anti-osteoporosis drug therapy and was advised to repeat her BMD in 1 year at the time of her mammogram. The patient missed her mammography appointment, and had a repeat BMD at 18 months. The following T-scores were noted: −2.6 of the AP lumbar spine (0.744 g/cm$^2$) and −2.3 at the total hip (0.60 g/cm$^2$). This represented a 5.2 % drop in BMD (0.04 g/cm$^2$) at the spine and a 4 % drop (0.04 g/cm$^2$) at the total hip. These represented clinically significant changes, considering the least significant change for the spine and total hip to be 0.03 and 0.035 g/cm$^2$, respectively. FRAX™ assessment using BMD values obtained at her initial presentation indicated a fracture risk of 28 % for all osteoporosis-related fractures, and 3.6 % for a hip fracture. In hindsight, this exceeded the 20 % and 3 % triggers for all osteoporosis-related and hip fracture risk, respectively. Urine N-telopeptide level at the second visit was 69 nmol/mmol Cr. The upper end of the premenopausal range is 38 nmol/mmol Cr, above which increased levels predict a decline in BMD.

## How the Diagnosis Was Made

The patient was mislabeled as osteopenia based on her T-scores, without consideration of her wrist fracture history and loss of height. Further evaluation by lateral X-ray of thoracolumbar spine revealed two compression deformities at T12 and L2. This, together with her prior history of wrist fractures would have placed her in the severe osteoporosis category. A FRAX™ score was not calculated despite her history of a wrist fracture. Because of this misdiagnosis and the absence of remodeling marker measurements, the patient was left untreated for over 18 months, at which time bone remodeling continued to be high, as evidenced by an elevated N-telopeptide level, and the patient consequently suffered a further decline in her BMD, putting her at an even higher risk of fracture.

## Lessons Learned

1. At the outset, the patient should have not been labeled as osteopenic, but should have undergone a lateral X-ray of the spine, which would have likely revealed vertebral compression fractures. A FRAX calculation would have shown a high

fracture risk, essentially mandating therapy before her condition worsened. The diagnosis and therapy of osteoporosis has traditionally been based heavily on T-scores [1]. Basic and clinical research over the past decade has revealed that the strength of bone, which determines its propensity to fracture, is not derived solely from BMD. Patients with normal BMDs do fracture. In response to the clinical need for the early identification of women at a high risk of fracture, the World Health Organization (WHO) developed a risk stratification tool, FRAX™, which allows us to estimate the 10-year absolute fracture risk in a given patient.

2. If there is a fragility fracture, as was the case in the patient, the diagnosis converts to osteoporosis, no matter what the BMD is. Unfortunately only 3 % of patients with wrist fracture—wrist fracture being the commonest fracture in the early post-menopausal years—ever receive a BMD test. A fracture also begets a future fracture. A wrist fracture not only increases the risk of a future wrist fracture by three-fold, but also dramatically increases the risk of vertebral and hip fractures, respectively, by 70 and 90 %. Importantly, known therapies reduce the risk of future fractures, *albeit* not eliminating them. Furthermore, vertebral fractures, as were diagnosed late in this patient despite her complaint of height loss, can cause as much morbidity and mortality as hip fractures.

3. FRAX™ will not capture a perimenopausal or early postmenopausal woman, aged 48 years, who has no fractures or loss of height and has a T-score of −1.8 at the lumbar spine and −1.5 at the total hip. Understand that the most rapid resorption, architectural deterioration, and bone loss occurs during this period. FRAX™ excludes healthy, late perimenopausal or early postmenopausal women, who are losing bone rapidly, but display a low absolute risk of fracture.

4. A substantial body of new evidence supports the premise that bone loss starts as early as the late perimenopause, even when estrogen levels are normal, and continues for 10–15 years at a rapid pace. Multiple studies document reductions in BMD and high resorption levels starting as early as 2–3 years before the last menstrual period. The Study of Women's Health Across the Nations (SWAN) presents both cross-sectional and 4-year longitudinal analyses of high-turnover bone loss in relatively eugonadal perimenopausal women, aged between 42 and 52 years. Despite this severe perimenopausal and early postmenopausal bone loss, T-scores were mostly within the normal limits. In these women, bone markers often rise even before the onset of irregular menstrual cycles, and a notable acceleration of activation frequency, a histomorphometric measure of bone resorption, is noted at 1 year of the menopause. SWAN further shows that changes in remodeling markers and BMD do not correlate with changes in serum estradiol, but instead display a strong negative correlation with changes in serum FSH, a marker of the menopause (Fig. 31.1).

5. Concordant with the rapidity of the bone loss across the menopausal transition, histology and high resolution μCT of bone biopsies show evidence of trabecular perforation and loss. Perforation is far more detrimental to bone strength than thinning. Perforation reduces strength by two- to fivefold more than does thinning. Consequently, a woman undergoing rapid bone loss may also be losing bone strength due to trabecular perforation, even if her BMD has not decreased substantially. Of particular importance is the irreversibility of this process.

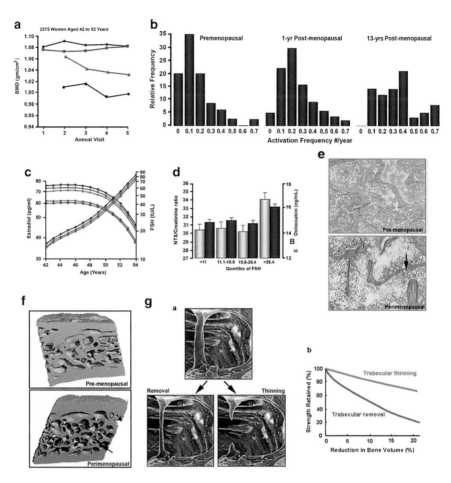

**Fig. 31.1** (**A**) Bone loss at the lumbar spine in enrollees of the Study of Women's Health Across the Nations over 4 years of follow-up. Upon entry into the trial, these women were classified as premenopausal (*purple*), early perimenopausal (*green*), late perimenopausal (*red*) and early post-menopausal (*blue*). Drawn from data in [2]. (**B**) Activation frequency in iliac crest bone biopsy specimens from women premenopausal women and women at 1 and 13 years postmenopause. Redrawn from [3]. (**C**) Estradiol and FSH levels in women of different races (*blue*: Hispanics; *red*: Caucasians; *dark green*: African Americans; *pink*: Japanese; *light green*: Chinese) across the menopausal transition. Of note is that estrogen levels can be normal during the late perimenopause, while FSH levels have risen by about threefold. Redrawn from [4]. (**D**) Urinary N-telopeptide/ creatinine ratio (*grey*) and serum osteocalcein (*black*) in enrollees of the Study of Women Across Nations (SWAN) plotted as a function of quartiles of serum FSH, a marker of the menopause. Redrawn from [5]. (**E**) Representative iliac crest bone biopsy of a woman taken before and after menopause subject to 2D histomorphometry. From [6]. (**F**) Iliac crest bone biopsy of a woman taken before and after menopause subject to 3-D μ-CT. This sensitive technology yielded significant decrements in structural parameters, such as bone volume and trabecular thickness and number, across the menopausal transition. From [6]. (**G**) Simulated loss of bone from a trabeculum. (a) Mild bone loss might result in trabecular thinning (*left panel*), whereas more aggressive bone loss associated with high remodeling results in complete removal of the trabeculum (*right panel*). (b) The latter severely decreases bone strength. Trabecular thinning will cause a 17 % loss in strength if 10 % of the bone tissue is lost. The same loss in bone tissue will result in a 50 % loss in bone strength if the trabeculae are removed. From [7], adapted with permission

**Table 31.1** Bone remodeling markers

| |
|---|
| *Bone formation markers* |
| Serum osteocalcin |
| Serum bone-specific alkaline phosphatase |
| Serum intact N-terminal propeptide of type 1 procollagen (PINP) |
| Serum intact C-terminal propeptide of type 1 procollagen (PICP) |
| Fragments of osteocalcin (experimental) |
| *Bone resorption markers* |
| Urinary hydroxyproline (now obsolete) |
| Urinary N-telopeptide (cross-links of N-terminal telopeptide of type 1 collagen) |
| Urinary hydroxypridinium crosslinks of type 1collagen |
|    Urinary pridinoline |
|    Urinary deoxypridinoline (DpD) |
| Serum C-telopeptide (crosslinks of C-terminal telopeptide of type 1 collagen) |
| Serum α and β C-telopeptides |
| Serum tartrate-resistant acid phosphatase 5B (experimental) |

Once lost, trabeculae are not rebuilt, so the lost bone strength occurring across menopausal transition is most likely permanent.

6. BMD measurements cannot quantify the *rate* of bone loss. Neither can they capture trabecular perforation and thinning. Bone turnover markers can be valuable point estimates of the rate of loss [8]. Unlike two BMD determinations, which provide an interval estimate of "lost bone," the single measurement of a remodeling marker will positively predict the risk of ongoing "bone loss." [9] Hence, elevated marker levels can be clinically useful during early menopause. Studies show strikingly positive correlations of bone loss and urinary N-telopeptide levels. Urinary N-telopeptide levels are 19 % higher in perimenopausal than postmenopausal women. An increase of 1 SD in N-telopeptide and osteocalcin levels increased the odds of losing spinal BMD, the most affected site during the early menopause, by 2.1 % and 1.6 %, respectively. SWAN showed cross-sectional correlations between urinary N-telopeptide and serum FSH levels; the latter, in turn, predicted bone loss over 4 years. With further validation, bone remodeling markers will likely be utilized increasingly to predict early bone loss across the menopausal transition (Table 31.1). Our patient's elevated N-telopeptide level was consistent with the decline in BMD noted during her treatment-free interval.

7. Estrogen, when used for osteoporosis prevention, has been shown to enhance BMD. Likewise, raloxifene displays positive effects on BMD associated with bone marker suppression in young osteopenic women. When taken off either therapy, in the case of our patient being taken off hormone replacement therapy, there is acute rapid and severe bone loss with a high fracture risk due to accelerated bone resorption [10].

8. In the EPIC (Early Postmenopausal Intervention Cohort) trial, the bisphosphonate alendronate increased BMD over 2 and 5 years. Likewise, young postmenopausal women showed a conserved BMD with risedronate (daily regimen), ibandronate (monthly regimen), and zoledronic acid (once every 1 or 2 years).

9. In a patient, such as the one described, we suggest yearly instead of biennial BMD measurements to examine for least significant change. Bone remodeling markers should be measured every 3–6 months, particularly, if these are outside of the premenopausal range. If there is a history of fracture as was the case in this patient, treatment should be initiated irrespective of BMD considerations. If there is no history of documented fracture, and should BMD show a significant drop, or resorption markers rise into the postmenopausal range, active pharmacological intervention should be considered, again irrespective of basal BMD. Treatment should be continued until BMD and bone turnover markers are within the normal range, after which both parameters should be monitored yearly, and treatment reinitiated if necessary. If the BMD remains within the low bone mass or osteoporotic range, treatment should be continued.

## Questions

1. An initial and repeat (after 2 years) bone mineral density (BMD) measurement at the lumbar spine (L1–L4) in a 56-year-old otherwise healthy patient on adequate calcium and vitamin D supplementation showed the following:

   - Initial: 0.650 g/cm$^2$
   - 2 years later: 0.620 g/cm$^2$
   - The least significant change (LSC) of the machine is 0.02 g/cm$^2$

True or False:

   1. There has been a significant decline as the change in BMD in g/cm$^2$ is greater than the LSC
   2. The BMD does not show a significant decline as it is not greater than 10 % over 2 years
   3. More information, including a change in T-scores, is required before a judgment can be made

2. The following are risk factors included in FRAX™:

True or False:

   1. Age
   2. Prior history of fracture
   3. Bone turnover markers
   4. Bone mineral density at femoral neck (T-score)
   5. Recurrent falls

3. An 80-year-old woman with a perception of height loss was noted to have a compression fracture at T12 on lateral X-ray of the thoracolumbar spine. The lumbar spine T-score was −2.3, and her hip T-score was −1.7.

True or False:

1. The patient should be diagnosed as having osteopenia
2. The patient should be diagnosed as having osteoporosis
3. The compression is normal at the patients age and no diagnosis of osteoporosis is required
4. A compression fracture at the vertebral column begets a future fracture at all sites

4. Bone turnover markers:

True or False:

1. Are valuable in monitoring changes in fracture risk
2. Are commonly used to assess compliance and persistence on anti-resorptive therapy
3. If high, can predict a fall in BMD
4. Rise early during menopause
5. Are only measured in spot urine samples

## Answers to Questions

1. 1: True; 2: False; 3: False
2. 1: True; 2: True; 3: False; 4: True; 5: False
3. 1: False; 2: True; 3: False; 4: True
4. 1: False; 2: True; 3: True; 4: True; 5: False

## References

1. Miller PD. Guidelines for the diagnosis of osteoporosis: T-scores vs fractures. Rev Endocr Metab Disord. 2006;7(1-2):75–89.
2. Sowers MR, Jannausch M, McConnell D, Little R, Greendale GA, Finkelstein JS, et al. Hormone predictors of bone mineral density changes during the menopausal transition. J Clin Endocrinol Metab. 2006;91(4):1261–7.
3. Recker R, Lappe J, Davies KM, Heaney R. Bone remodeling increases substantially in the years after menopause and remains increased in older osteoporosis patients. J Bone Miner Res. 2004;19(10):1628–33.
4. Randolph JF, Jr., Sowers M, Bondarenko IV, Harlow SD, Luborsky JL, Little RJ. Change in estradiol and follicle-stimulating hormone across the early menopausal transition: effects of ethnicity and age. J Clin Endocrinol Metab. 2004;89(4):1555–61.
5. Sowers MR, Greendale GA, Bondarenko I, Finkelstein JS, Cauley JA, Neer RM, et al. Endogenous hormones and bone turnover markers in pre- and perimenopausal women: SWAN. Osteoporos Int. 2003;14(3):191–7.

6. Akhter MP, Lappe JM, Davies KM, Recker RR. Transmenopausal changes in the trabecular bone structure. Bone. 2007;41(1):111–6.
7. Guo XE, Kim CH. Mechanical consequence of trabecular bone loss and its treatment: a three-dimensional model simulation. Bone. 2002;30(2):404–11.
8. Rosen CJ, Chesnut CH 3rd, Mallinak NJ. The predictive value of biochemical markers of bone turnover for bone mineral density in early postmenopausal women treated with hormone replacement or calcium supplementation. J Clin Endocrinol Metab. 1997;82(6):1904–10.
9. Zaidi M, Turner CH, Canalis E, Pacifici R, Sun L, Iqbal J, et al. Bone loss or lost bone: rationale and recommendations for the diagnosis and treatment of early postmenopausal bone loss. Curr Osteoporos Rep. 2009;7(4):118–26.
10. Epstein S, Inzerillo AM, Caminis J, Zaidi M. Disorders associated with acute rapid and severe bone loss. J Bone Miner Res. 2003;18(12):2083–94.

# Chapter 32
# Misdiagnosis of Atypical Femur Fractures

**Mone Zaidi and Semin Kim**

## Objective

1. Recognize a true atypical fracture of the femur.
2. Evaluate critically the literature that links long-term bisphosphonate usage to the risk of atypical fracture.

## Case Presentation

A 60-year-old Caucasian female was brought to the Emergency Room with a fracture of the right femur and severe leg pain. *Per* first responder reports, the patient fell in her patio, but she was unclear of the precise circumstances relating to the fall. Until the day of the fracture, the patient was in her usual state of good health. X-ray on the day of admission reported fracture of the proximal femoral diaphysis, with comminution. Her vitals were normal on admission. The patient was admitted for surgical repair by open reduction and intramedullary rodding. Her postoperative course was complicated with anemia due to blood loss. Acute physical and occupational rehabilitation enhanced her capacity to ambulate. While her pain improved, she continued to complain of leg spasms for which she received Percocet. Discharged with a wheelchair and walker, the patient underwent 6 further months of strength training. Repeat X-rays showed good alignment of the fragments.

Prior to this injury, she was an avid runner. She had no fractures in the past, was not diabetic, and used intranasal steroids for her allergies. There was no history of

**Disclosure** M.Z. consults for Merck and Roche Pharmaceuticals.

M. Zaidi, M.D., Ph.D., F.R.C.P. (✉) • S. Kim, M.D.
Mount Sinai Bone Program, Mount Sinai School of Medicine, New York, NY 10029, USA
e-mail: mone.zaidi@mssm.edu; ksm8099@gmail.com

© Springer Science+Business Media New York 2015                                          273
T.F. Davies (ed.), *A Case-Based Guide to Clinical Endocrinology*,
DOI 10.1007/978-1-4939-2059-4_32

kidney stones. She became perimenopausal 10 years prior to her fracture. For ~3 years, she was on hormone replacement therapy (Prempro 0.625 mg/2.5 mg). Other medical history included diffuse degenerative disc disease and hypercholesterolemia for which she was on crestor (10 mg qd). She had a 30-pack-year history of smoking, but had stopped 5 years ago. Her mother and older sister both suffered from vertebral compression fractures.

The patient underwent a bone density (DXA) scan at age 52 at the recommendation of her primary care physician. Her T-scores were: −0.6 in the lumbar spine AP view; −2.2 in the lumbar spine lateral view; −1.9 at the femoral neck; and −1.3 at the total hip. In view of her osteopenia and the high risk of developing osteoporosis because of her maternal history and smoking history, the patient was started on alendronate (10 mg qd) by her primary care physician. Therapy was continued over the following 8 years. A repeat DXA measurement 4 years later showed the following T-scores: +0.5 at the lumbar spine AP view, −1.8 at the lumbar spine lateral view, −1.7 at the femoral neck; and −1.3 at the total hip. Her alendronate was stopped following her fracture, which was suggested as being "atypical" and caused as a result of long-term alendronate therapy (see below).

Blood chemistries were unremarkable, except for notable abnormalities in serum calcium and PTH. Her serum calcium levels were noted as high or high–normal on several occasions, notably 10.5 mg/dL, 10.3 mg/dL, 10.8 mg/dL, 10 mg/dL, 10.7 mg/dL (around the time of her fracture), 10.8 mg/dL, 10.6 mg/dL, and 10.5 mg/dL. Phosphorous levels were in the low to low–normal range. Corresponding to a calcium of 10.7 mg/dL, her PTH was 40 pg/mL. While in the normal range (12–68 pg/mL), this represents inappropriate elevation with respect to serum calcium. A repeat blood level 5 days later again showed an inappropriately elevated PTH (33 pg/mL) *versus* her serum calcium (10.5 mg/dL). Her serum ionized calcium was high at 6.0 mg/dL (4.5–5.4 mg/dL) with high urine calcium of 269 mg/day (<250 mg/day). These findings are consistent with primary hyperparathyroidism. Vitamin D levels remained largely normal.

## How the Diagnosis Was Made

The question is whether the patient had an atypical fracture. Atypical femur fractures (AFFs) are a rare type of low trauma femur fracture occurring below the greater trochanter. Between 2007 and 2008, three case series described femur fractures that displayed features that were inconsistent with typical osteoporosis-related fractures. A proportion of the patients reported in these studies had been on alendronate therapy for periods close to or over 5 years. The authors suggested that "long-term" alendronate use may in fact be the culprit underlying these unusual insufficiency fractures, although none of these case series could prove anything more than temporal association, much less cause and effect.

The phenotypic features of these fractures included cortical thickening in the lateral aspect of the subtrochanteric region; transverse fracture; medial cortical spiking; bilateral findings of stress reactions or fractures; and prodromal pain. These features ultimately became the basis of a formal definition enacted by the American Society for Bone and Mineral Research (ASBMR) Task Force in 2010 [1]. The Task Force stated that, in order for a fracture to be designated as "atypical," it must include all the following radiographic features classified as *major criteria:* Notably the fracture must be:

1. Located in the subtrochanteric or femoral shaft region of the femur
2. Associated with minimal or no trauma
3. Transverse or short oblique in orientation
4. Complete or incomplete (complete fractures may have a medial spike and incomplete fractures must involve the lateral cortex),
5. Without comminution

Minor criteria included cortical thickening, a periosteal reaction of the lateral cortex, bilaterality, prodromal pain, and delayed fracture healing, together with the presence of comorbid conditions and concomitant drug exposure. The European Society on Clinical and Economic Aspects of Osteoporosis and Osteoarthritis (ESCEO), and the International Osteoporosis Foundation (IOF) Working Group essentially endorsed that definition, as did the Food and Drug Administration (FDA).

In 2013, the ASBMR produced a revised case definition for AFFs. The only mandated criterion relates to the location of the fracture, which must occur along the femoral diaphysis from just distal to the lesser trochanter to just proximal to the supracondylar flare. Additionally, four out of five features must be present for it to qualify as an AFF, namely:

• Associated with minimal or no trauma
• Substantially transverse or short oblique in orientation ('substantially' has been added)
• Complete or incomplete (complete fractures may have a medial spike and incomplete fractures must involve the lateral cortex),
• Noncomminuted or minimally comminuted ("minimally" added, but extent not qualified)
• Periosteal reaction of the lateral cortex (prior minor feature)

Several issues arise from these new criteria. First, there is still little consensus on how precisely to define an AFF, elements of which continue to evolve. Second, while qualifiers such as "substantially" and "minimally" have been added, there is no mention as to their precise extent. Third, the idea that a fracture is designated as an atypical femoral fracture if it meets four out of five criteria, although providing flexibility, is an essentially difficult concept. For example, consider a fracture that meets four out of five criteria, but is spiral in configuration. Under the revised criteria, that fracture could be classified erroneously as an atypical femur fracture. Finally, considering that AFFs occur in bisphosphonate naive individuals, as well as in patients on other anti-resorptives, such as raloxifene and denosumab, the ASBMR Task Force removed the use of any drug as even a minor criterion for diagnosis. In clinical practice, the incidence of such fractures is extraordinarily low.

The patient's fracture was diagnosed as being atypical, but it did not meet all of the major criteria as required by the ASBMR Task Force at the time. It did meet two major criteria, namely location in the mid-disphyseal region and completeness of the fracture. However, the fracture was objectively comminuted and spiral in orientation. It was also unclear, as is often the case, how precisely the fracture occurred and the extent of trauma that caused it. With our patient, a fall from standing height appeared certainly not atraumatic as it was associated with enough force to fragment the bone. Thus, while it is tempting to make a diagnosis of atypical femur fracture in a patient on long-term bisphosphonates, this is an example of a patient whose fracture could not be classified as being atypical using the ASBMR's Task Force Guidelines.

## Lessons Learned

1. As the patient had degenerative disc disease, it was highly likely that her AP spine T-score (−0.6) was a gross overestimate. DXAs do not differentiate between normal bone tissue and calcified arthritic tissue. Specifically, the presence of osteophytes increases bone density falsely and results in an artificially raised T-score. Other artifacts that falsely elevate T-scores include fractured vertebrae, underlying calcified aorta, and external objects. In contrast, a lateral lumbar spine was performed prudently in this patient that showed a low T-score of −2.2.
2. The diagnosis of osteoporosis or osteopenia (now termed low bone mass) continues to come from the lowest T-score at any given site. One cannot have osteopenia/low bone mass at one site and osteoporosis or a normal bone density at the other.
3. Initial treatment was based on the patient's low bone mass on DXA, and at least two additional risk factors for osteoporosis, namely a maternal history of osteoporosis and fracture and a history of smoking. The judgement to start a bisphosphonate also fell in line with published treatment guidelines available at the time.
4. In relation to the patient's smoking history, several cohort studies have reported that ex-smokers have intermediate BMD values between those of current and nonsmokers. The MINOS study demonstrated almost no differences in BMD between current and former smokers except in forearm bones. Furthermore, a difference was reported in BMD between former smokers and those who had never smoked at most skeletal sites, which was further augmented in subjects of the lowest tertile in weight (<75 kg). Hence, this study suggested that smoking cessation does not result in BMD recovery and reinforces the notion of a smoking history, even remote, as a risk factor.
5. The patient was mislabeled as a case of atypical femoral fracture. Her fracture was traumatic due to a trip and twisting action and does not meet criteria of the ASBMR Task Force for classification.
6. Most studies have shown conclusively in randomized blinded interventional trials with bisphosphonates that increments in bone density translate into fracture risk reduction [2]. In contrast, only nonrandomized, nonblinded observational, case–control studies evaluating the odds of a particular fracture pattern being associated with bisphosphonate users point to an association between the atypical pattern and long-term bisphosphonate use [3].

7. It has been suggested that long-term therapy with bisphosphonates can reduce bone remodeling and impair the repair of microcracks, thereby contributing to atypical femur fractures [4]. Although bisphosphonates have been associated with the accumulation of microcracks by lowering turnover of bone in beagle dogs (generally at doses much higher than those used clinically for osteoporosis), this is not seen in humans. Even in beagle dogs, any microcrack accumulation is balanced by therapeutic hypermineralization, which strengthens rather than weakens bone. There is also no evidence that the decreased bone heterogeneity observed in patients on bisphosphonates translates into an increased propensity to fracture.

8. High serum calcium levels suppress PTH levels by negative feedback. An inappropriately suppressed PTH means clinically that the high serum calcium is arising from excessive PTH production which it can barely suppress—evidence for the diagnosis of hyperparathyroidism. A SPECT scan was equivocal and showed asymmetric uptake, whereas ultrasonography showed bilateral superior midlevel echoes, suspicious of parathyroid adenoma. The fact that the patient had hyperparathyroidism meant that she could not conceivably have grossly suppressed bone turnover, which has been purported as being a theoretical risk for atypical fracture.

9. Bisphosphonates and other antiresorptives reduce bone turnover from a postmenopausal high level to a premenopausal normal level. Osteoclastic bone resorption is reduced, which is followed by some reduction of bone formation, as the two processes are coupled [5]. Bisphosphonates can only reduce resorption so much—there is a floor beyond which resorption and formation cannot be lowered due to the fact that the skeleton is vast and the supply of osteoclasts and osteoblasts is unlimited.

## Questions

1. True or False: Atypical femoral fractures

   1. Do not occur in bisphosphonate naive individuals
   2. Must occur with minimal trauma
   3. Only occur when the cortices are thickened
   4. Are a rare form of femoral fractures with specific radiological features

2. True or False: The following lower bone turnover

   1. Bisphosphonates
   2. Human recombinant parathyroid hormone
   3. Osteopetrosis
   4. Infusion of calcium
   5. Hyperthyroidism

3. True or False: Primary hyperparathyroidism

    1. Is always associated with a serum calcium level above the normal range
    2. Is always associated with inappropriately suppressed PTH
    3. Occurs most commonly due to vitamin D deficiency
    4. May counteract the therapeutic suppression of bone remodeling by antiresorptive agents
    5. Will cure postmenopausal osteoporosis

4. True or False: Bone density measurements are most reliable when:

    1. Made at the lumbar spine particularly if the patient has degenerative disc disease
    2. Performed on the same machine with a high precision
    3. Conducted using a heel ultrasound device
    4. Performed on male subjects

## Answers to Questions

1. 1: False; 2: True; 3: False; 4: True
2. 1: True; 2: False; 3: True; 4: True; 5: False
3. 1: False; 2: True; 3: False; 4: True; 5: False
4. 1: False; 2: True; 3: False; 4: False

## References

1. Shane E, Burr D, Ebeling PR, Abrahamsen B, Adler RA, Brown TD, et al. Atypical subtrochanteric and diaphyseal femoral fractures: report of a task force of the American Society for Bone and Mineral Research. J Bone Miner Res. 2010;25(11):2267–94.
2. Pazianas M, Epstein S, Zaidi M. Evaluating the antifracture efficacy of bisphosphonates. Rev Rec Clin Trials. 2009;4(2):122–30.
3. Whitaker M, Guo J, Kehoe T, Benson G. Bisphosphonates for osteoporosis–where do we go from here? N Engl J Med. 2012;366(22):2048–51.
4. Chapurlat RD, Arlot M, Burt-Pichat B, Chavassieux P, Roux JP, Portero-Muzy N, et al. Microcrack frequency and bone remodeling in postmenopausal osteoporotic women on long-term bisphosphonates: a bone biopsy study. J Bone Miner Res. 2007;22(10):1502–9.
5. Zaidi M. Skeletal remodeling in health and disease. Nat Med. 2007;13(7):791–801.

# Part VIII
# Endocrine Disorders of Men

# Chapter 33
# Introduction

**Stephen J. Winters and Sathya Krishnasamy**

## Introduction

Testicular function is under the control of gonadotropin-releasing hormone (GnRH) produced by neurons in the anterior hypothalamus. GnRH stimulates the synthesis and secretion of the pituitary gonadotropic hormones, luteinizing hormone (LH), and follicle-stimulating hormone (FSH), which are composed of a common alpha subunit, shared with TSH and hCG, and a specific β-subunit (LH-β or FSH-β). LH and FSH are released into the circulation in pulses and activate G-protein-coupled receptors on Leydig and Sertoli cells, respectively, in order to stimulate testosterone production and spermatogenesis.

Normal testicular function is also maintained by an elaborate negative feedback mechanism controlling GnRH and gonadotropin synthesis and secretion. Sex steroids inhibit GnRH production by affecting neurons that produce Kisspeptin-1, which in turn, stimulate GnRH secretion. While androgens suppress GnRH, estrogen negative feedback plays an important role in males to suppress GnRH and directly inhibit pituitary responsiveness to GnRH perhaps by regulating proteins involved in hormone exocytosis (SNARE proteins). The testicular peptide inhibin-B is a selective regulator of FSH. This dimeric glycoprotein member of the TGF-β family competes with activin for binding to its receptor on gonadotrophs but fails to initiate activin signaling, thereby blocking activin stimulation of FSH and GnRH-receptor synthesis. When the testes are damaged, inhibin-B production and circulating levels fall, and unopposed activin causes FSH secretion to increase. These control mechanisms are summarized in Fig. 33.1.

S.J. Winters, M.D. (✉) • S. Krishnasamy, M.D.
Division of Endocrinology, Metabolism and Diabetes, University of Louisville,
ACB-A3G11, 550 Jackson Street, Louisville, KY 40202, USA
e-mail: sjwint01@louisville.edu

© Springer Science+Business Media New York 2015
T.F. Davies (ed.), *A Case-Based Guide to Clinical Endocrinology*,
DOI 10.1007/978-1-4939-2059-4_33

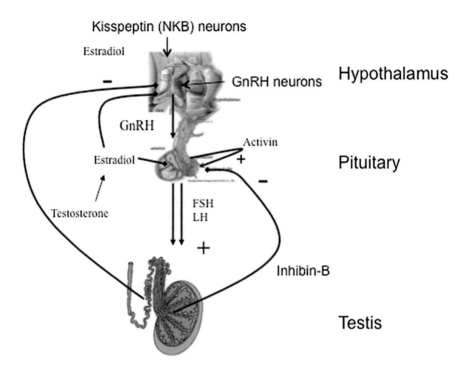

**Fig. 33.1** Diagram showing feedforward and feedback mechanisms governing hypothalamic–pituitary–testicular function

The willingness of men to discuss the symptoms of hypogonadism, and the availability of new, effective, and safe treatment approaches have increased substantially the number of men being evaluated and treated for hypogonadism. Men with hypogonadism present with symptoms and signs of androgen deficiency or with infertility. The symptoms are nonspecific, however, and the signs may be subtle. Other than azoospermia, the semen parameters that distinguish fertile from infertile men are indistinct. A careful medical history and physical examination to include measurement of testicular size is essential. Most often the total testosterone level is sufficient to confirm the clinical diagnosis of hypogonadism, with most reference ranges approximating 300–1,000 ng/dL. The level of sex-hormone-binding globulin (SHBG) is an important determinant of total testosterone, and increases or decreases in SHBG produce parallel changes in total testosterone. When total testosterone levels are borderline, or the total testosterone level is not consistent with the clinical findings, free testosterone or non-SHBG (bioavailable) testosterone levels should be measured. Direct analog assays for testosterone are inaccurate and should not be used to assess free testosterone.

Disorders that affect the testis are classically divided into those in which the gonadotropin drive to the testes is reduced (hypogonadotropic hypogonadism) or disorders that damage the testes directly (primary testicular failure). Systemic illnesses may affect both the production of GnRH and damage the testes. Three common illustrative cases are presented and discussed.

# Chapter 34
# Congenital Hypogonadotropic Hypogonadism

Stephen J. Winters

## Objectives

1. Review the variable clinical presentation of men with CHH
2. Summarize what is known about the gene defects causing CHH
3. Understand treatment options for gonadotropin-deficient men

## Case Presentation

A 20-year-old college student was referred because of hypogonadism. He was otherwise healthy, with a normal sense of smell, and there was no family history of hypogonadism or consanguinity, although both parents were from Beirut, Lebanon. On physical examination, he was healthy and well appearing. His height was 71 in., and his arm span was 72 in. His blood pressure was 120/76. He was hypogonadal in appearance with reduced muscle mass and little body hair, looking much younger than his stated age. There was no gynecomastia. The testes were each quite small, measuring about 1.5 cm in length (3 ml in volume).

Laboratory data: Serum testosterone 10 ng/dl, LH 0.5 U/l, FSH 1.1 U/l, Free T4 1.3 ng/dl, PRL 5 ng/ml, IGF-1 254 ng/ml (normal 114–492), AM cortisol 12 mcg/dl. DEXA scan: BMD of the lumbar spine T score was −2.4 and hip −1.5 S.D. Pituitary MRI was normal.

He was treated with increasing doses of testosterone enanthate and subsequently with transdermal testosterone. He married at age 31, and 1 year later treatment was changed to hCG 750 U three times a week. His testes increased in size to 5 ml over

S.J. Winters, M.D. (✉)
Division of Endocrinology, Metabolism and Diabetes, University of Louisville,
ACB-A3G11, 550 Jackson Street, Louisville, KY 40202, USA
e-mail: sjwint01@louisville.edu

© Springer Science+Business Media New York 2015

T.F. Davies (ed.), *A Case-Based Guide to Clinical Endocrinology*,
DOI 10.1007/978-1-4939-2059-4_34

6 months and the total testosterone level was 375 ng/dl. He remained azoospermic, however, and 75 IU rhFSH sc three times a week was added. Three months later his sperm count rose to 18 million/ml with normal sperm motility (40 %) and morphology, and 4 months later his wife became pregnant and subsequently delivered a healthy full-term female infant. He chose to continue hCG injections since they were planning for a second child.

## Review of How the Diagnosis Was Made

This young adult man presented with delayed puberty and clinical hypogonadism, but was otherwise healthy. His height was normal, and there was no clinical or biochemical evidence for hypothyroidism or cortisol deficiency. The PRL level was not increased. The testosterone level was typical for a prepubertal boy, and the serum levels of LH and FSH were in the low–normal range. There was no clinical evidence for a tumor or other pathological condition affecting the pituitary or suprasellar region, and mass lesions were excluded by the normal MRI. Thus the presumptive diagnosis was congenital isolated hypogonadotropic hypogonadism (CHH). The patient was not anosmic, and no congenital abnormalities were found. The family history was negative for hypogonadism and developmental defects.

A sporadic case with no family history suggested an autosomal recessive disorder or a spontaneous mutation. Patients with CHH are classically divided into those with anosmia or hyposmia (Kallmann syndrome) or those with normal olfaction [1]. He is in the latter subgroup. He wished to better understand the cause of his disease, and genetic testing was done which revealed compound heterozygous mutations in the GnRH-receptor gene (GNRHR, gln106 to arg (Q106R; 138850.0001) and arg262 to gln (R262Q; 138850.0002) [2].

## Lessons Learned

HH results from an inability to stimulate the secretion of the gonadotropic hormones from the pituitary with resultant testosterone deficiency. It can be acquired, e.g., pituitary tumor, or congenital, and CHH has various causes and a variable clinical presentation [1]. The prevalence of CHH is estimated at 1:10,000 males and 1:50,000 females. Men may present with sexual infantilism as newborns with a microphallus, with failure to enter puberty, or with infertility or osteoporosis as nearly sexually mature adults. The testes can be similar in size to those of a prepubertal child (<3 ml in volume) but are sometimes of normal adult size (20–25 ml). These latter patients were historically termed "Fertile Eunuchs" because they were clinically hypogonadal with soft smooth skin and reduced body hair, but the testes were not small. Affected females generally present with primary amenorrhea and minimal breast development.

The endocrine findings in CHH are also variable. The circulating testosterone level can range from <30 to 200–300 ng/dl; LH may be undetectable, or LH pulse amplitude or frequency may be reduced. Studies of the inheritance of CHH have been limited because infertility is a component of the syndrome, and there is incomplete penetrance of the clinical characteristics. However, inheritance can be X-linked, autosomal dominant, or autosomal recessive. This clinical, laboratory, and genetic variability implied that CHH is a syndrome with multiple etiologies.

## CHH and Anosmia

CHH is now known to result from at least 13 separate gene mutations (Table 34.1), and while CHH is a rare disorder, the identification of these genes has provided major insight into the pathways that are essential for the hypothalamic–pituitary control of reproduction. Recognition that some patients have digenic inheritance helps explain the variable reproductive and extragonadal phenotypic features within families with non-Mendelian inheritance patterns. The availability of commercial tests to detect these mutations can be found at the NIH-supported web site genet-ests.org. Mutations in genes known to cause CHH are identified in only 30 % of patients, indicating that other disease-causing genes remain to be discovered.

**Table 34.1** Causes of congenital isolated hypogonadotropic hypogonadism

| Gene | Inheritance | Phenotype | % of patients |
|------|-------------|-----------|---------------|
| *With development defects* | | | |
| KAL-1 | X linked recessive | Anosmia, ichthyosis, synkinesias, renal agenesis | 8–10 |
| FGF-R1 | Autosomal dominant | Anosmia | 10 |
| | | Craniofacial abnormalities | |
| | | Severe to mild hypogonadism | |
| FGF8 | Autosomal dominant | Anosmia | 1 |
| | | Craniofacial abnormalities | |
| ProK2 | Recessive, often heterozygotes—digenic | Anosmia | 2–3 |
| ProkR2 | Recessive, often heterozygotes—digenic | Anosmia, septo-optic dysplasia | 8–10 |
| *Without developmental defects* | | | |
| GnRH | Recessive | HH | |
| GnRH-R | Recessive | HH, partial or complete | 5–15 |
| Kisspeptin-R | Recessive | HH | |
| Kisspeptin | | HH | |
| Tach3 | Recessive | Microphallus | |
| | | HH with reversal in adults | |
| NK3R | Recessive | HH | 5 |

In 1944 Kallmann et al. reported several families in which men had CHH and anosmia, suggesting an X-linked trait. The discovery that CHH can be due to mutations of the KAL-1 gene, and its localization to the short arm of the X chromosome, provided an explanation for the male predominance of this disorder, and initiated extensive investigation into how GnRH secretion is linked to olfaction, a critical sense for reproductive success among lower animals. KAL-1 encodes a protein, anosmin, which shares homology with other proteins involved in axon path-finding and neuron migration. It is now known that GnRH neurons, uniquely among hypophysiotropic neurons, originate with olfactory epithelium outside of the brain, and migrate to arrive to their hypothalamic location during fetal development, and that this process fails to occur normally in Kalmann syndrome patients. Anosmin is thought to play a role in neuronal migration and in the development of the olfactory structures; hence the connection between anosmia and CHH. Many mutations of KALl-1 have been identified, with most mutations in exons 5–14 which encode four fibronectin III domains. These regions of the molecule have heparin sulfate (HS)-binding affinity and are present in a number of adhesion proteins that are involved in cell–cell or cell–matrix interaction. KAL-1 transcripts are found not only in the developing olfactory bulb together with GnRH mRNA but also in the retina, spinal column, and developing kidney. The latter location may explain the renal agenesis and horseshoe kidney that sometimes occur in affected patients, while involuntary movements, known as mirror movements, in some patients, are thought to result from disorganization of the pyramidal tracts of the spinal column. Men with KAL-1 mutation present with the most severe form of CHH with lack of LH pulsatile secretion, prepubertal testosterone levels, and sometimes with microphallus and/or cryptorchidism. Eight to ten percent of males with CHH have mutations in KAL-1 in most series.

Genetic studies in individuals with contiguous gene syndromes lead to the finding of FGFR-1 (fibroblast growth factor receptor) mutations in males and females with sporadic or autosomal dominant familial CHH [3]. In addition to hypogonadism, some CHH patients have cleft lip, cleft palate, dental agenesis, and other skeletal anomalies, as well as anosmia, and the disorder is therefore designated KAL-2. There are four functional FGF-receptors, and more than 20 FGFs that are paracrine stimulators of these receptors. At least 22 different mutations have been reported accounting for about 10 % of patients with CHH. FGF receptors are transmembrane receptor tyrosine kinases that activate phosphatidyl inositol and other signaling pathways by forming a dimer when stimulated by FGF and require a heparan sulfate glycosaminoglycans. FGF signaling is involved in the development and growth of a variety of tissues. Mutation of FGFR-1 in mice causes early embryonic death. Facial clefting and hypogonadotropic hypogonadism are also associated with mutation of FGF8. KAL-2 and KAL-1 may be functionally inter-related in that the KAL-1 gene product anosmin may function as a coreceptor for FGF signaling.

Mutations in the genes *PROK2* and *PROKR2* which encode prokineticin and its G-protein-coupled prokineticin receptor-2 have been found in approximately 10 % of Kallmann syndrome patients. Prokineticins are widely expressed and have diverse biological functions. PROKR2 is expressed in the olfactory bulb, and mice deficient in PROKR2 have hypoplasia of the olfactory bulbs and hypogonadotropic hypogonadism. Most CHH patients with mutations in these genes are heterozygotes, but the same mutations have also been found in apparently unaffected individuals. Among those heterozygotes with hypogonadism, a digenic disorder has been found in a few patients with mutations in other genes implicated in KS (KAL1, FGFR1 *PROKR2*, or *PROK2*), or in genes causing CHH without developmental defects (see below). The absence of mutations in other genes known to cause CHH implies that those hypogonadotropic patients with heterozygous mutation solely of *PROK2* or *PROKR2* must have mutations in other disease-causing genes that remain to be identified.

Semaphorins are proteins secreted by target tissues that repel or attract a wide range of neuronal and non-neuronal cells depending on the cellular targets and the expression of different subunits of its receptor complexes. Mice with deletion of the SEMA3A receptor have altered migration of GnRH neurons into the brain, and a few CHH patients heterozygous for mutations which disrupt secretion of SEMA-3A in vitro have been reported.

Less common causes of CHH with developmental defects are mutations in CHD7, *WDR11*, and *HS6S*. CHARGE syndrome, with ocular *coloboma*, congenital *heart* defects, choanal *atresia*, *retardation* of *growth* and development, *genital* hypoplasia, and *ear* anomalies and deafness, results from mutation of CHD7. WDR11 interacts with EMX1, a homeodomain transcription factor involved in the development of olfactory neurons. Like Kal-1, HS6ST, FGF17, IL17RD, DUSP6, SPRY4, and FLRT3 are genes involved in FGF receptor signaling and have been found to be mutated in a few CHH patients [3].

## *CHH Without Developmental Defects*

Normosmic CHH patients may have mutations in various genes including GnRH1, GnRHR, KISS, KISS-1R, TAC3, and TACR3. The protein products of these genes do not seem to play a role in the embryonic migration of GnRH neurons. Instead, the mutations disrupt GnRH synthesis and secretion or prevent the normal GnRH activation of gonadotrophs. GnRH activates a G-protein-coupled seven transmembrane receptor that signals primarily through the inositol phosphate–protein kinase C pathway to stimulate α-subunit, LH-β, and FSH-β gene transcription, as well as LH and FSH release from the pituitary. In each of these conditions, other than GnRH-R mutation, the pulsatile administration of GnRH will stimulate gonadal function.

The finding that LH secretion in some patients with CHH responds poorly or not at all to GnRH stimulation focused interest on the GnRH receptor gene on chromosome 4q13.1. At least 16 different mutations in 5–15 % of CHH patients have been associated with partial or complete GnRH resistance and hypogonadism. In these patients with autosomal recessive inheritance patterns, inactivating mutations are most often double heterozygotes but homozygotes are also found especially in inbred communities. Heterozygote carriers appear to be normal. The most common mutations are $Gln^{106}$ to $Arg^{106}$ and $Arg^{262}$ to $Gln^{262}$. These mutations result in loss of ligand binding or defective intracellular signaling, respectively. Males and females are affected, and predictably affected patients have no midline defects.

Perhaps the most significant advance in the neuroendocrinology of reproduction in the past decade was the identification of kisspeptin as a key upstream regulator of GnRH secretion for CNS sexual differentiation, the onset of sexual maturation, seasonal breeding, and the feedback control of GnRH by gonadal hormones and metabolic and environmental factors. This major breakthrough began with the identification of a few patients with normosmic CHH who were found to have loss of function mutations of a G-protein-coupled receptor, with homology to the galanin receptor, encoded by a gene on chromosome 19p13 (formerly called GPR54, but now termed the kisspeptin receptor KISS-1R). The disorder is rare with about 30 cases reported worldwide with a variety of homozygous or compound heterozygous mutations. The hypogonadism is generally severe, and some men have microphallus and/or cryptorchidism. Female siblings present with primary amenorrhea. The gene KISS1, encoding the peptide kisspeptin, is expressed in the arcuate and the anteroventricular periventricular nucleus of the hypothalamus in neurons that make direct synapses witih GnRH neurons. A large consanguineous family with four female siblings with CHH (and two unaffected males) associated with a loss-of-function mutation of *KISS1* was also recently described.

Some neurons in the arcuate nucleus that express kisspeptin coexpress the neuropeptides neurokinin B (NKB) and dynorphin, and mutations in *TAC3* and *TACR3* (encoding neurokinin B and its receptor, respectively) were shown to result in the hypogonadotropic phenotype, accounting for about 5 % of cases. NKB is a member of the substance P-related tachykinin family, and its receptor is expressed both on kisspeptin and GnRH neurons. Experiments in monkeys treated with kisspeptin and senktide, a synthetic NKB analogue, reveal that the NKB stimulation of GnRH release is upstream from KISS-1R.

While mutation of the GnRH gene was an obvious candidate for CHH, and a mouse with a large deletion within the GNRH1 gene (hpg) causing autosomal recessive hypogonadism in both sexes was discovered in 1977, it was not until 2009 that one female and two male subjects with homozygous inactivating mutations in the GNRH1 gene were reported. These patients provided definitive proof for the pivotal role of GnRH in human pubertal development and reproduction.

Several patients with inactivating mutations of the LH-$\beta$ gene have been reported with a variety of genotypic abnormalities. They have presented as phenotypic males with absent or impaired pubertal development, a low testosterone level, small testes, and hypospermatogenesis. Treatment with hCG markedly increased testosterone levels and produced virilization. While most mutations have resulted in LH deficiency due to abnormal LH-$\beta$ processing or inability to bind to the $\alpha$-subunit, one man with a high LH level due to a point mutation producing an immunoreactive LH molecule that was unable activate the LH-receptor has also been reported. FSH levels are normal or elevated. Affected men have a masculine phenotype because fetal testosterone production is governed by hCG, and only the postnatal production of testosterone under LH control is disrupted.

Mutations of the FSH-β gene causing FSH deficiency result in lack of sexual development and elevated serum LH levels in women. Affected male relatives were discovered to have small testes and azoospermia with variable but impaired Leydig cell function causing LH levels to increase. The abnormal FSH-β protein is unable to associate with the common α-subunit to form the active dimer. A polymorphism in the FSH-β gene promoter is also associated with lower levels of FSH and lower sperm counts in otherwise normal men.

Adrenal hypoplasia congenital (AHC) is a disorder characterized by primary adrenal failure in infancy or childhood, and CHH. Mutations in the *DAX1* gene (Dosage-sensitive sex reversal-Adrenal hypoplasia congenita (AHC) critical region on the X chromosome gene) cause X-linked AHC. More than 60 mutations have been reported. Frame-shift or missense mutations produce a truncated protein with limited function. DAX1 is a repressor of steroidogenic factor 1 (SF1)-mediated gene transcription with targets including the α-subunit, LH-β and GnRH-receptor genes accounting for the CHH.

Constitutional delay of puberty is a transient state of HH associated with prolongation of the physiological GnRH deficiency of childhood, and endocrinologists are often asked to distinguish healthy prepubertal teenage boys with CDP from those with CHH. In the absence of a positive family history or developmental defects such as anosmia, CHH in sporadic cases remains a consideration until there is spontaneous and complete pubertal development, otherwise extensive genetic testing for candidate genes is needed. The presence of developmental defects allows the clinician to favor the diagnosis of CHH, and certain phenotypic features such as synkinesia and renal anomalies (KAL1) or cleft lip and palate (FGFR1 or FGF8) can be useful for directing genetic screening.

Interestingly, a few patients with CHH with established genetic abnormalities appear to recover GnRH secretion in early adulthood [4] implying that a holiday from hormone replacement in early adulthood is worthwhile.

## Treatment Strategies

All forms of testosterone treatment (e.g., intramuscular injection or transdermal application) will stimulate secondary sex characteristics and increase male sexual behaviors. Testosterone will not appreciably activate spermatogenesis, however. The testes of men with CHH are variably immature and lacking in LH/FSH activation, but most men with CHH can produce sperm with diligent treatment. Coexistent cryptorchidism portends a poorer prognosis, however. To stimulate spermatogenesis, treatment of our patient was first changed to human chorionic gonadotropin (hCG). hCG purified from the urine of pregnant women, and a recombinant product from Chinese Ovary Hamster cells, is available as a therapeutic analog for LH to stimulate Leydig cell function. Recombinant hCG, while purer and with little batch-to-batch variation, is marketed as a 0.5 ml vial containing 250 µg hCG (equivalent to about 10,000 IU) for use in ovulation induction. Purified hCG is available in 10,000 IU vials as brand name and generic products that can be reconstituted in 10 ml of normal saline to deliver 1,000 IU/ml. A dose of 750–1,000 IU intramuscularly or subcutaneously three times weekly is generally sufficient; larger doses may increase estradiol production and produce gynecomastia. All products occasionally produce a rash and rarely a more serious allergic reaction.

hCG alone usually stimulates spermatogenesis in men with acquired HH due to pituitary tumors, and is sometimes effective as a sole agent in CHH, especially in men with partial gonadotropin deficiency (testes ≥5 ml prior to treatment) [5]. In this case, the testes were smaller in size, and although hCG treatment normalized testosterone levels and increased the size of the testes, the patient remained azoospermic after 6 months of treatment. Therefore, FSH was added [6]. Recombinant hFSH is available in vials containing 75 IU, and the usual dose is 75–150 IU three times weekly. Most men with partial CHH and more than 50 % of men with more severe CHH will produce sperm with this regimen, although pregnancy may take several years, and in vitro fertilization is sometimes performed for oligospermia. FSH is costly, and is often discontinued after pregnancy since hCG alone can maintain spermatogenesis even for extended periods although sperm counts gradually decrease.

GnRH can be administered using a pulsatile infusion pump to stimulate spermatogenesis in men with GnRH deficiency and normal pituitary function. GnRH administered continuously, however, will downregulate testicular function because GnRH receptors are depleted and GnRH receptor signaling is disrupted. The dose of GnRH that effectively increases adult testosterone levels and stimulates spermatogenesis has ranged from 5 to 20 μg/pulse.

There is a progressive increase in bone density throughout childhood, with a marked increase in bone mineralization during puberty. Testosterone and estradiol are important regulators of bone metabolism, and osteoporosis is a well-established complication of CHH [7]. Testosterone replacement increases bone density in young, previously untreated men with CHH but is less effective in older men. Bisphosphonates are also generally recommended.

## Questions

1. A 27-year-old man presents with delayed pubertal development. The family history is negative. He is otherwise healthy and has a normal sense of smell. He looks hypogonadal with sparse beard and body hair and lack of musculature. His height is 65 in. and his arm span is 68 in. His testes are each 4.0×2 cm. There are no other positive findings. Which of the following mutations might explain his condition?

   a. Kal-1
   b. FGF-R1
   c. GnRH-R
   d. IGF-1
   e. Prop-1

2. Your clinical diagnosis of hypogonadotropic hypogonadism is confirmed with a testosterone level of 35 ng/dl, LH 1.2, and FSH 2.5 U/l. Each of the following should be assessed at this time, except:

   a. PRL level
   b. MRI pituitary
   c. Iron and iron-binding capacity
   d. Peripheral blood karyotype
   e. Free thyroxine

3. Other than hypogonadotropic hypogonadism, his endocrine function is normal, the percent iron saturation is 35 %, and there is no mass on the MRI. Which additional tests are needed at this time?

   a. DEXA scan
   b. Inhibin-B
   c. GnRH stimulation test
   d. Estradiol
   e. hCG stimulation test

4. The patient and his wife would like to have children. After obtaining a baseline semen analysis, you recommend which of the following treatments:

   a. hFSH
   b. Testosterone gel
   c. hCG
   d. hGH
   e. Clomiphene

## Answers to Questions

1. c. Missense mutations in the GnRH-receptor gene result in a variable defect in GnRH signaling and a range of phenotypes. Parents of affected individuals are asymptomatic carriers, and there is no abnormality of neuronal migration or associated abnormalities.

2. d. The karyotype is invariably normal 46,XY in men with CHH. While hemochromatosis is a very rare cause of hypogonadism in adolescents, it can be fatal and screening is advised.

3. a. Men with congenital hypogonadotropic hypogonadism are deficient in testosterone and estradiol, have reduced peak bone mass in early adulthood, and are at increased risk for osteoporosis.

4. c. While parenteral testosterone will produce virilization in men with CHH, it has little effect on spermatogenesis. Some men with CHH will produce sperm with hCG alone, and although coadministration of hFSH may ultimately be needed, the drug is very costly, and treatment is generally begun after 6 months of hCG if the patient remains azoospermic. hFSH is ineffective without cotreatment with hCG.

# References

1. Balasubramanian R, Crowley Jr WF. Isolated GnRH deficiency: a disease model serving as a unique prism into the systems biology of the GnRH neuronal network. Mol Cell Endocrinol. 2011;346(1–2):4–12.
2. Chevrier L, Guimiot F, de Roux N. GnRH receptor mutations in isolated gonadotropic deficiency. Mol Cell Endocrinol. 2011;346(1–2):21–8.
3. Miraoui H, Dwyer AA, Sykiotis GP, Plummer L, Chung W, Feng B, Beenken A, Clarke J, Pers TH, Dworzynski P, Keefe K, Niedziela M, Raivio T, Crowley Jr WF, Seminara SB, Quinton R, Hughes VA, Kumanov P, Young J, Yialamas MA, Hall JE, Van Vliet G, Chanoine JP, Rubenstein J, Mohammadi M, Tsai PS, Sidis Y, Lage K, Pitteloud N. Mutations in FGF17, IL17RD, DUSP6, SPRY4, and FLRT3 are identified in individuals with congenital hypogonadotropic hypogonadism. Am J Hum Genet. 2013;92:725–43.
4. Laitinen EM, Tommiska J, Sane T, Vaaralahti K, Toppari J, Raivio T. Reversible congenital hypogonadotropic hypogonadism in patients with CHD7, FGFR1 or GNRHR mutations. PLoS One. 2012;7:e39450.
5. Burris AS, Rodbard HW, Winters SJ, Sherins RJ. Gonadotropin therapy in men with isolated hypogonadotropic hypogonadism: the response to human chorionic gonadotropin is predicted by initial testicular size. J Clin Endocrinol Metab. 1988;66(6):1144–51.
6. Matsumoto AM, Snyder PJ, Bhasin S, Martin K, Weber T, Winters S, Spratt D, Brentzel J, O'Dea L. Stimulation of spermatogenesis with recombinant human follicle-stimulating hormone (follitropin alfa; GONAL-f): long-term treatment in azoospermic men with hypogonadotropic hypogonadism. Fertil Steril. 2009;92:979–90.
7. Laitinen EM, Hero M, Vaaralahti K, Tommiska J, Raivio T. Bone mineral density, body composition and bone turnover in patients with congenital hypogonadotropic hypogonadism. Int J Androl. 2012;35:534–40.

# Chapter 35
# Klinefelter Syndrome

**Stephen J. Winters and Sathya Krishnasamy**

## Objectives

1. Recognize the clinical presentation of men with Klinefelter Syndrome
2. Review the pathophysiology and genetics of Klinefelter syndrome
3. Discuss the clinical implications of undiagnosed primary testicular failure
4. Review management options for men with testicular failure

## Case Presentation

A 20-year-old man was referred by his pediatrician because of small testes. He had a patent ductus arteriosus that was repaired at age 9 months and is followed with yearly echocardiograms for partial anomalous pulmonary venous return. He is otherwise healthy. He began shaving his beard at age 14 and now shaves every 2–3 days. He has some chest hair, but much less than his father and brother. He seems shy and reserved. He is 6′1″ tall and is the tallest member in his family; his father is 5′10″, mother is 5′6″, and a brother is 5′9″. He is tall and thin, with an unusually long face. There is no thyromegaly. He has bilateral gynecomastia. The testes were each 2.3 cm in length (3 mL L, 4 ml R). The phallus was 6 cm long and had two meatal openings: the dorsal opening was a shallow blind pit, and an opening on the ventral surface of the glans was the urinary channel. The testosterone level was 316 ng/dL, LH 36.9, and FSH 66.3 U/L. The SHBG was 45 nmol/L, and the non-SHBG testosterone was 81.6 ng/dL (normal > 110). The peripheral blood karyotype was 47,XXY.

S.J. Winters, M.D. (✉) • S. Krishnasamy, M.D.
Division of Endocrinology, Metabolism and Diabetes, University of Louisville,
ACB-A3G11, 550 Jackson Street, Louisville, KY 40202, USA
e-mail: sjwint01@louisville.edu

© Springer Science+Business Media New York 2015
T.F. Davies (ed.), *A Case-Based Guide to Clinical Endocrinology*,
DOI 10.1007/978-1-4939-2059-4_35

**Table 35.1** Causes of primary testicular failure

| Congenital | Acquired |
| --- | --- |
| Klinefelter syndrome | Trauma |
| Cryptorchidism | Orchitis |
| Immune polyglandular failure | Spinal cord injury |
| Congenital anorchia | Medications: ketoconazole, cancer chemotherapy |
| Noonan's syndrome | X-irradiation |
| Lawrence–Moon–Bardet–Biedl syndrome | Retroperitoneal fibrosis |
| Myotonic dystrophy | Amyloidosis |
| Sickle cell disease | AIDS |
| Noonan syndrome | Alcoholic liver disease |
| | Chronic kidney disease |

# Review of How the Diagnosis Was Made

The very small testes, gynecomastia, and signs of moderate androgen deficiency suggested primary testicular failure, and the elevated serum LH and FSH levels confirmed the clinical diagnosis. There was no history of head trauma or headaches, no evidence for dysfunction of other endocrine systems, and no visual disturbance to suggest hypogonadotropic hypogonadism. Of the causes of testicular failure (Table 35.1), many were readily excluded by the medical history and physical examination. The phenotype, urogenital abnormality and congenital heart disease suggested a sex chromosome aneuploidy. 50 cells were analyzed to exclude a mosaic karyotype. Klinefelter syndrome (KS) is a relatively common disorder affecting about 1 in 500–1,000 men. Tall stature due to long legs, delayed puberty, clinical androgen deficiency, gynecomastia, small firm testes and infertility, and psychosocial disorders are common in KS patients [1, 2], and that diagnosis was confirmed by the 47,XXY karyotype.

# Lessons Learned

In 1942 Klinefelter et al. described nine unrelated adult men with gynecomastia, small firm testes, scant body hair, and elevated FSH levels (a bioassay for FSH in urine based on the development of the reproductive tract in mice was performed at that time). While the authors wrote that "nothing has been found in these patients to explain the testicular lesion", after an inactivated X-chromosome was identified in normal women (Barr body) in 1949, the 47,XXY chromosomal basis of the disorder was described in 1959. It is now known that KS syndrome is the most common form of congenital male hypogonadism and X and Y chromosome variation, and accounts for approximately 11 % of azoospermic men. The prevalence in the general population is 0.1–0.2 %. Intrauterine mortality does not appear to be a feature of Klinefelter syndrome (KS). The diagnosis is made in the course of prenatal screening, in newborns with cryptorchidism or microphallus, in boys with language delay, learning disabilities, or behavioral problems, as teenagers with delayed or incomplete pubertal development or gynecomastia, or in adults with hypogonadism or infertility. Bojesen et al. [3] estimated that only one fourth of adult men in Denmark with KS are ever diagnosed.

## Genetics/Etiology

In individuals with more than one X chromosome, all in excess of one condense to form Barr bodies, a darkly staining mass of chromatin at the cell's nuclear rim. A karyotype is performed using rapidly dividing T-lymphocytes in peripheral blood that are chemically arrested in metaphase and stained to establish the diagnosis. The extra X chromosome in KS results from nondisjunction during meiotic division in germ-cell development, or in less than 5 %, during early embryonic mitotic division. About half of the cases are paternally derived and result from the formation of an XY sperm in meiosis-1, whereas maternal XX oocytes can result from errors in either meiosis-1 or meiosis-11. The risk of KS appears to increase in mothers older than age 40.

About 10 % of men with KS have a mosaic peripheral blood karyotype, usually 47,XXY/46,XY, and have a milder phenotype. The karyotype may occasionally be normal, especially if only 20 cells are counted, and a karyotype of skin fibroblasts or testicular biopsy specimen may be needed to confirm the mosaic diagnosis. Higher grade chromosome aneuploidies (48,XXXY; 48,XXYY; 49,XXXXY) also produce the Klinefelter phenotype, but are rare, and cause psychomotor retardation.

When two X chromosomes are present, most genes on one X are silenced as a result of the X-chromosome inactivation. Some genes escape X-inactivation, however, and are expressed from both the active and inactive X chromosome. About 15 % of X-chromosome genes, especially genes in the pseudoautosomal region, escape X-inactivation in KS, and thus have a higher level of expression than in normal men. The overexpression of these genes in various tissues of the body, together with the hypogonadism, produce the Klinefelter phenotype.

Some men with primary testicular failure have a 46,XX karyotype. This condition generally results from the translocation during paternal meiosis of the distal end of the short arm of the Y chromosome, containing the testis determining gene (SRY), to the X chromosome, or sometimes to an autosome.

## Phenotypic Manifestations

The major manifestations of KS are listed in Table 35.2 [4]. In general, the greater the number of X chromosomes, the more marked are the phenotypic consequences. While stature and body hair are variable polygenic traits, all men with classical 47,XXY KS can be readily diagnosed because they have small firm testes.

**Table 35.2** Clinical features of Klinefelter syndrome (adapted from [2])

| Feature | Frequency % | Feature | Frequency % |
|---|---|---|---|
| Infertility | 91–99 | Cryptorchidism | 27–37 |
| Small testes (bitesticular size <6 ml) | >95 | Learning disabilities (children) | >75 |
| Increased gonadotropins | >95 | Delay of speech development (children) | 40 |
| Azoospermia | >95 | Psychiatric disturbances | 25 |
| Decreased testosterone | 63–85 | Increased height (prepubertal, adults) | 30 |
| Decreased facial hair | 60–80 | Abdominal adiposity (adults) | ~50 |
| Decreased pubic hair | 30–60 | Metabolic syndrome (adults) | 46 |
| Gynecomastia | 38–75 | Osteopenia (adults) | 5–40 |
| Breast cancer | 30× incr | Type 2 diabetes (adults) | 10–39 |
| Mediastinal cancers | 50× incr | Decreased penile size (children) | 10–25 |

Klinefelter patients are often tall, but rather than classic eunuchoidal skeletal proportions (arm span at least 6 cm >height), they have exaggerated pubis-floor growth. Even prepubertal boys with KS may have long legs, implying that this abnormality may not be from a sex hormone disturbance. Long legs are instead thought to be due to overexpression of short stature homeobox (SHOX) gene, on pseudoautosomal region1 of the X chromosome that plays a major role in growth [5].

*Gynecomastia* While breast enlargement was the essential finding in the cases reported by Klinefelter et al., not all men with KS have gynecomastia. Early studies found elevated circulating estradiol levels whereas more recent studies report normal estradiol levels in KS men. However, all cases have low testosterone in relation to estradiol levels. It is also possible that gynecomastia is due partly to effects on the breast of X-linked genes that escape silencing. Breast pain may occur, and gynecomastia can be psychologically disturbing, especially to adolescents. Long-standing gynecomastia generally contains extensive fibrous stroma as well as glandular tissue, and may be irreversible, and claims that antiestrogens or aromatase inhibitors substantially decrease breast tissue mass have come from open labeled uncontrolled trials with self-reported outcomes. These drugs are unapproved for this purpose and cannot be recommended at this time. Plastic surgery techniques restore the breast contour with minimal scarring and protect areolar anatomy and sensation. Subcutaneous mastectomy with liposuction through a circum-areolar approach is most often used. Corrective surgery will often favorably impact the emotional disturbance and academic difficulties that these boys endure.

*Bone mineral density* is reduced, and osteoporosis occurs more often in men with KS than in normal men, and the age-related decrease in bone mass is thought to be more pronounced [6]. Free testosterone levels are inversely correlated with bone mineral density in some studies; however, testosterone deficiency alone does not appear to explain the low bone mass in KS. BMD may increase after the initiation of testosterone replacement especially in younger men.

*Language-based learning disabilities*, reading disorders, developmental dyspraxia with neuromotor dysfunction, speech and language abnormalities, and social dysfunction are common in KS. 47,XXY individuals have lower verbal IQ than performance IQ with normal full-scale IQ whereas patients with higher grade aneuploidies tend to be mentally retarded. Babies with KS tend to have expressive language delay, while school-age boys demonstrate a verbal cognitive deficit with significant underachievement in reading, spelling, and writing. Some also have reduced mathematical ability. These learning disabilities lead to poor school performance and to less skilled occupations in adulthood. Behavioral problems and difficulty with social relationships may accompany academic underachievement. Many patients are quiet, sensitive and insecure, with lack of insight and poor judgment. On the other hand, some men with KS are intelligent, and professionally and financially successful. Between- subject variability in the overexpression of X-chromosome genes, and variable CAG repeat length in the androgen receptor promoter are thought to account for the inconstant phenotype. It is often written that quality of life would be considerably more favorable if the diagnosis were made in childhood, and information, counseling, support, and hormone treatment were given beginning at an early age; but this is unproven.

## Laboratory Findings

Serum LH and FSH levels are almost always elevated in adults with KS and indicate lack of negative feedback signals due to Leydig cell and seminiferous tubule dysfunction. Rare exceptions are men with coexistent gonadotropin deficiency due to pituitary tumor, acute or chronic illnesses, or morbid obesity. Mean total testosterone levels are lower than those of normal men, but many KS men have total testosterone levels in the low normal range although non-SHBG (bioavailable) testosterone levels are more often subnormal. Hormone values in prepubertal boys with KS are generally within the normal range although the neonatal increase in FSH may be slightly greater and the rise in testosterone slightly less than in normal boys [7]. Inhibin-B levels decline to barely detectable values during mid-late puberty rather than increase as in normal adolescents because germ cells and Sertoli cells die and are replaced by fibrosis.

## Histopathology of Testis

Nearly all men with KS are azoospermic, and microscopic examination of testicular tissue generally reveals absent spermatogenesis with hyalinizing fibrosis of the seminiferous tubules (Fig. 35.1). In some individuals, however, there are tubules with Sertoli cells but no germ cells, and there may be focal areas of spermatogenesis [8]. Although the peripheral blood cells in these men may be 47,XXY, there may be

**Fig. 35.1** Testicular biopsy from a man with Klinefelter syndrome. Note the hyalinized seminiferous tubules (T) that are devoid of germ cells and Sertoli cells and the hyperplastic Leydig cells (LC). Photograph courtesy of Dr. C. Alvin Paulsen

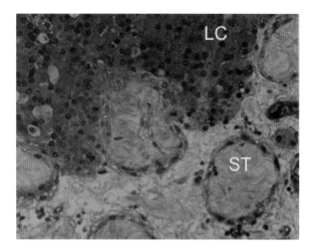

undiscovered 46,XY cell lines in testis. In spite of defective testosterone production, the number of Leydig cells is maintained or increased producing the histological picture of Leydig cell hyperplasia. Increased LH drive or disruption of the endocrine communication between Sertoli cells, germ cells, and Leydig cells may explain the abnormalities in Leydig cell structure and function.

The degenerative process may start during fetal life as testicular tissue from XXY fetuses have a fewer germ cells although tubules are nonsclerotic and Sertoli cells appear normal. In the first few years of life, the number of spermatogonia decreases, and their depletion accelerates as puberty begins. Germ cell differentiation is arrested at the spermatogonia or early primary spermatocyte stage, and rather than meiosis there is germ cell apoptosis. The testis of affected early teenage boys reveals hyalinization and hyperplastic Leydig cells. 10 % of the 1,000+ genes on the X-chromosome are expressed in testis, and the overexpression of these genes is presumably the proximate cause of the compromise in testicular function.

## Comorbid Conditions

Epidemiology studies indicate that KS is associated with a loss of 2.1 years in lifespan (3). Furthermore, there is increased risk for hospitalization (about 70 %) from infection, endocrine disorders, neurological and psychiatric conditions, circulatory, pulmonary, and gastrointestinal disorders. The comorbid conditions associated with KS are listed in Table 35.3.

Abdominal adiposity is common in KS men, and truncal fat is increased even before puberty, suggesting that factors beyond adult testosterone deficiency are important [9]. In one study of KS men age 19–66, 19 % had diabetes or impaired fasting glucose, and nearly 50 % met the criteria for metabolic syndrome, compared to 4 % and 10 % of controls, respectively. In another study of KS men compared to

**Table 35.3** Comorbid
conditions associated with
Klinefelter syndrome

| Glucose intolerance | Osteopenia |
|---|---|
| Dyslipidemia | Breast carcinoma |
| Chronic leg ulcerations | Germ cell cancers |
| Deep vein thrombosis and pulmonary embolism | Taurodontism |

men with obstructive azoospermia, fasting and glucose-stimulated insulin secretion were increased indicating insulin resistance. LDL and triglyceride levels are increased, and HDL cholesterol is reduced, and the risk for nonalcoholic fatty liver disease is increased in KS patients. Prospective randomized trials are needed to understand whether and how androgen replacement affects these metabolic conditions.

Varicose veins and leg ulcers are far more common in men with KS than in normal men and are thought to result from deep vein thrombosis. The risk for pulmonary embolism is also increased. Platelet hyperaggregation, factor V Leiden mutation, deficient fibrinolysis, and increased activity of factor VIII coagulant have all been proposed to explain DVTs and chronic leg ulcers.

Our patient had partial anomalous pulmonary venous return, and a variety of cardiovascular abnormalities have been reported as case reports, especially in higher grade chromosome aneuploidies, including aortic and mitral valve disease, atrial septal defect, pulmonary stenosis, Ebstein's anomaly, and tetrology of Fallot. Pulmonary diseases such as chronic bronchitis, bronchiectasis, and emphysema are also more common in KS than expected, and pneumonia was noted to occur more often than expected in the Danish registry study.

Men with KS are at increased risk for certain malignancies, including breast cancer, germ cell tumors, particularly extragonadal germ cell tumors involving the mediastinum, nonlymphocytic leukemia, non-Hodgkin lymphoma, and marrow dysplastic syndrome. For breast cancer, the data seem to support a risk about 20- to 30-fold higher than expected, although <1 % of KS patients will develop breast cancer. The risk for mediastinal germ cell tumors is more than 50-fold increased, and roughly 8 % of patients with mediastinal germ cell tumors have KS. Occasionally, mediastinal germ cell tumors produce hCG and may cause precocious puberty. A chest X-ray should be performed when KS men have progressive dyspnea. Several case reports also associate intra-abdominal and intracranial germ cell tumors with KS but it is not known how X-chromosome genes and/or the hormone disturbance contribute to these associations. Testicular failure predisposes to gonadotroph hyperplasia, and PRL levels may be slightly elevated, but pituitary tumors do not appear to occur more often in KS than expected.

Sex hormones and gender are important determinants in many autoimmune diseases. One study of 75 men found a slight decrease in free thyroxine levels but normal TSH levels and a normal prevalence of autoimmune thyroid disease among KS men. On the basis of case reports, the prevalence of systemic lupus and systemic sclerosis may be elevated, and there are case reports of KS patients with lupus treated with testosterone whose hematologic and serologic abnormalities, including elevated levels of anti-DNA antibodies and depressed complement levels, returned to normal.

## Treatment Strategies

Testosterone replacement corrects the classic features of hypogonadism including sexual infantilism, reduced muscle size and strength, osteopenia, anemia, and fatigue, and sexual interest and function improve. Some authors have suggested a low total testosterone level as the criteria for treatment of KS patients; however, non-SHBG testosterone is thought to be a more accurate and sensitive measure of testosterone deficiency, and is more often abnormal than is total testosterone in KS. Furthermore, the high level of LH reflects testosterone deficiency in the CNS. Thus, it is perhaps intuitive that androgen replacement should be begun in all patients with KS at midpuberty, but there are no placebo-controlled trials documenting the benefits of testosterone substitution, especially regarding the effects on cognitive and behavioral endpoints.

To avert mood changes, priapism, and acne, a tempered dose-escalation is suggested. This can be accomplished using intramuscular testosterone injections or with metered pumps that deliver testosterone in a gel. High levels of circulating testosterone are needed to suppress LH into the normal range in testicular failure perhaps because of increased GnRH receptor expression due to inhibin deficiency. Therefore, the level of non-SHBG testosterone, rather than the level of LH, should be used to guide the treatment dose.

Men with 47,XXY KS are usually azoospermic, whereas those with mosaic 46,XY/47,XXY karyotypes occasionally produce sperm and can be fertile, especially early in adulthood.

Reports of paternity and a few sperm in the ejaculate of 47,XXY men lead to the development of testicular sperm extraction (TESE) coupled with intracytoplasmic sperm injection as a method to help KS men be biological fathers. At surgery, the testis is widely opened and microdissected with examination of the morphology of seminiferous tubules using an operating microscope. Enlarged seminiferous tubules are removed, and the presence of sperm is evaluated in the operating room by an embryologist. The chance of finding sperm in the testis of KS patients is about 50 %, with successful pregnancy by ICSI in about 50 % of those men. So far, there are no useful preoperative predictors of successful sperm recovery. While there is concern for increased risk for producing sex chromosome or other aneuploidy in KS ICSI offspring, at least 149 healthy live born babies without anomalies have been conceived after TESE/ICSI from couples with an 47,XXY father worldwide. Even though conception in these men appears to be safe, preimplantation genetic diagnosis is generally offered in which one or two blastomeres are biopsied from embryos at the 8-cell stage.

Advancing age and testosterone treatment may reduce the fertility potential, and some authors recommend TESE in adolescents with cryopreservation of sperm for future ICSI, but the success of this approach remains to be demonstrated. Some authors have suggested that lowering LH and FSH with androgen replacement may reduce the likelihood that sperm will be found by TESE and may therefore negatively impact fertility. Further, they propose that if fertility is desired and the TESE/ICSI approach will be used, androgen treatment should be withheld and hCG, clomiphene, or an aromatase inhibitor should added. While thoughtful ideas, they are unproven, and they need to weighed against the consequences of eliminating androgen replacement.

## Questions

1. You are asked to evaluate a 13-year-old boy who has no palpable testes. He is otherwise healthy. He has soft smooth skin and little body hair. The phallus is 5 cm stretched and normally formed. Which of the following diagnostic tests should be performed at this time?
   a. Pituitary MRI
   b. Peripheral blood karyotype
   c. LH/FSH
   d. Free testosterone
   e. Inhibin-B

2. Which of the following statements with respect to testosterone replacement therapy is not correct:
   a. Erythrocytosis is more likely with transdermal testosterone than with long acting injectable testosterone preparations.
   b. Peliosis hepatis, hepatoma, and cholestatic jaundice are common side effects of 17-alkylated testosterone preparations
   c. Patients should be referred for prostate biopsy if a prostate nodule is palpated at any time or if the serum PSA concentration, confirmed by a repeat value, is >4.0 ng/mL initially or increases by 1.4 ng/mL in any 1 year period
   d. Overzealous treatment in adolescent male with open epiphyses can cause early fusion and limit linear growth.
   e. Testosterone treatment may be associated with fluid retention.

3. A 25-year-old man presents with gynecomastia and small testes but a normal phallus. The LH is 35 IU/L and the FSH is 46 U/L. While of the following is not in the differential diagnosis?
   a. XX Male
   b. Klinefelter syndrome
   c. 5-alpha reductase deficiency
   d. Mumps orchitis
   e. Congenital androgen insensitivity

4. Plasma levels of inhibin-B can be used to determine which men with Klinefelter syndrome will have testicular sperm for in vitro fertilization.
   a. true
   b. false

# Answers to Questions

1. c. From an endocrine perspective, the first step to establish the diagnosis in this patient is to determine if he has hypogonadotropic hypogonadism or primary testicular failure. The other tests may be indicted depending on these results.
2. a. Polycythemia occurs more often in men treated with testosterone esters intramuscularly than with topical application because of the high values that often occur on days 1–3 following injection.
3. c. 5-alpha reductase deficiency leads to ambiguous genitalia but estradiol levels are not elevated, and gynecomastia does not occur.
4. b. So far there is no reliable marker for sperm positive Klinefelter syndrome patients.

# References

1. Wikström AM, Dunkel L. Klinefelter syndrome. Best Pract Res Clin Endocrinol Metab. 2011;25:239–50.
2. Groth KA, Skakkebæk A, Høst C, Gravholt CH, Bojesen A. Clinical review: Klinefelter syndrome–a clinical update. J Clin Endocrinol Metab. 2013;98:20–30.
3. Bojesen A, Juul S, Birkebaek NH, Gravholt CH. Morbidity in Klinefelter syndrome: a Danish register study based on hospital discharge diagnoses. J Clin Endocrinol Metab. 2006;91:1254–60.
4. Aksglaede L, Skakkebaek NE, Almstrup K, Juul A. Clinical and biological parameters in 166 boys, adolescents and adults with nonmosaic Klinefelter syndrome: a Copenhagen experience. Acta Paediatr. 2011;100:793–806.
5. Ottesen AM, Aksglaede L, Garn I, Tartaglia N, Tassone F, Gravholt CH, Bojesen A, Sørensen K, Jørgensen N, Rajpert-De Meyts E, Gerdes T, Lind AM, Kjaergaard S, Juul A. Increased number of sex chromosomes affects height in a nonlinear fashion: a study of 305 patients with sex chromosome aneuploidy. Am J Med Genet A. 2010;152A:1206–12.
6. Ferlin A, Schipilliti M, Foresta C. Bone density and risk of osteoporosis in Klinefelter syndrome. Acta Paediatr. 2011;100(6):878–84.
7. Lahlou N, Fennoy I, Ross JL, Bouvattier C, Roger M. Clinical and hormonal status of infants with nonmosaic XXY karyotype. Acta Paediatr. 2011;100(6):824–9.
8. Aksglaede L, Juul A. Therapy of endocrine disease: testicular function and fertility in men with Klinefelter syndrome: a review. Eur J Endocrinol. 2013;168(4):R67–76.
9. Bojesen A, Kristensen K, Birkeback NH. The metabolic Syndrome is frequent in Klinefelter's syndrome and is associated with abdominal obesity and Hypogonadism. Diabetes Care. 2006;29:1591–8.

# Chapter 36
# Low Testosterone and the Metabolic Syndrome

Stephen J. Winters

## Objectives

1. Understand how obesity affects testicular function
2. Understand some pitfalls in the diagnosis of low testosterone in obese men
3. Summarize the benefits and risks of testosterone treatment for men with late onset hypogonadism

## Case Presentation

A 38-year-old man presented with his wife because of infertility. The couple had been married for 3 years. Prior to the marriage, he experienced low energy, low libido, a sleep disturbance, and mood swings. He weighed 350 lbs. The total testosterone level at 9 AM was 194 ng/dL (325–1,125) and the free testosterone level by direct analog assay was 7.0 pg/mL (8.7–25). PRL was 9.9 ng/mL, LH 3.8 mIU/mL (1.5–12), and FSH 6.3 mIU/mL (1.8–8.6) He was diagnosed with hypogonadism and treated with a testosterone gel. His symptoms improved, and he dieted and his weight fell to 306 lbs. The couple remained infertile and consulted with a specialist in Reproductive Endocrinology and Infertility who found the patient to be azoospermic. The testes measured $4.5 \times 2.5$ cm on the right and $4.0 \times 2.3$ cm on the left. He was advised that testosterone treatment might explain his infertility, and treatment was discontinued. Ten months later his wife conceived. The total testosterone level was 236 ng/dL and the non-SHBG (bioavailable) testosterone level was 128 ng/dL (normal >110).

S.J. Winters, M.D. (✉)
Division of Endocrinology, Metabolism and Diabetes, University of Louisville,
ACB-A3G11, 550 Jackson Street, Louisville, KY 40202, USA
e-mail: sjwint01@louisville.edu

© Springer Science+Business Media New York 2015
T.F. Davies (ed.), *A Case-Based Guide to Clinical Endocrinology*,
DOI 10.1007/978-1-4939-2059-4_36

# Review of How the Diagnosis Was Made

Obesity, sleep apnea, T2DM, and Metabolic Syndrome (MetS) are associated with low testosterone levels. This patient's low free testosterone and normal LH levels were thought to signify hypogonadotropic hypogonadism, perhaps due to a pituitary tumor, but no tumor was found on MRI. While testosterone deficiency is generally diagnosed by finding a morning total testosterone level below the reference range, the level of sex hormone-binding globulin (SHBG) is an important determinant of total testosterone, and men who have diabetes or MetS or are obese tend to have low levels of SHBG, and thereby low total testosterone levels. In these men, further testing, by measuring the free or non-SHBG (bioavailable) testosterone level, is essential to establish a correct diagnosis [1]. The direct free testosterone analog assay is a single-step, nonextraction method in which a $^{125}$I-labeled testosterone analog competes with free testosterone in plasma for binding to a testosterone-specific antiserum that has been immobilized on a polypropylene assay tube. The basis for the test is that the analog has a low affinity for SHBG and albumin. Studies have shown, however, that the result with this assay is related to the level of SHBG, much like the total testosterone level, and that free testosterone is undetectable using an analog assays in a dialysate of normal adult male serum where testosterone should be present. Thus, the free testosterone level determined with analog assays is inaccurate, provides essentially the same information as the total testosterone level, is not recommended. The result was misleading in this case, and when the pretreatment non-SHBG (bioavailable) testosterone level was calculated (www.issam.ch/freetesto.htm) from the levels of total testosterone (194 ng/dL) and SHBG (12 nmol), the result (136 ng/dL) was within the normal range (>110 ng/dL). If this information had been known, the MRI was probably unnecessary since the patient had no clinical features of hypogonadism, no headache or abnormality of vision, and his serum free thyroxine and PRL levels were normal. After stopping testosterone treatment, the AM non-SHBG testosterone level was within the reference range.

# Lessons Learned

Endocrinologists are often asked to evaluate men for low testosterone who have asthenia and erectile dysfunction and who are obese or have type 2 diabetes or dyslipidemia since these clinical findings may occur with hypogonadism [2]. This condition has been termed "late onset hypogonadism," although the term is also applied to the testosterone deficiency that occurs with aging. There is a well-established inverse relationship between total testosterone levels and BMI in adult men; however, much of the decrease is due to low SHBG. While hyperinsulinemia was thought to explain the low SHBG level in obesity, a mechanism related to hepatic fat signaling to the SHBG gene may be more important. Hypogonadism together with the metabolic syndrome may occur in Cushing's syndrome, acromegaly, or hemochromatosis, so these conditions should be considered.

Extreme obesity is associated with low free testosterone levels implying a decline in testosterone production. Mean LH levels in these men are generally within the reference range although values are slightly lower than in normal controls. Occasionally, high LH and/or FSH levels are found. Thus low testosterone in extreme obesity is most often associated with a disturbance in GnRH-LH secretion. Some pulsatility studies have found reduced LH pulse amplitude with normal pulse frequency, although other studies did not confirm this finding. Low LH pulse amplitude could be due to a reduction in GnRH production or to a decrease in responsiveness of gonadotrophs to GnRH activation because of changes in GnH receptor number or signaling. There is also some evidence that obesity impairs Leydig cell function directly.

The aromatase enzyme that converts androgens to estrogens is expressed in adipose tissue, and plasma estrone and estradiol levels are increased in most studies of obese men, and may cause the testosterone deficiency. Estrogens decrease LH secretion in men by slowing the GnRH pulse generator and by inhibiting the gonadotroph response to GnRH stimulation. Estrogen negative feedback effects on GnRH secretion are mediated by receptors on kisspeptin neurons while the mechanism for the inhibitory effects on the pituitary remains uncertain.

Men with Metabolic Syndrome also have increased levels of cytokines and adipokines. The cytokine interleukin-1β and its receptor are expressed in the hypothalamus of rats and humans and is the most potent inhibitor of GnRH secretion identified so far. TNFα, leukemia inhibitory factor, and ciliary neurotrophic factor have also been proposed to directly regulate the function of GnRH neurons. Obese individuals are believed to develop a functional leptin resistance which may also contribute to hypogonadism since leptin treatment not only reverses excessive food intake and body weight gain but also restores testosterone and fertility of genetically obese *ob/ob*$^{(-/-)}$ mice. While leptin levels predict low testosterone even after controlling for SHBG, LH, and estradiol in men, the impact of leptin treatment on testosterone in obese men remains to be determined.

Testosterone levels are low in men with obstructive sleep apnea although much of the effect is due to coexistent obesity [3]. Some studies have shown that continuous positive airway pressure (CPAP) treatment increases testosterone levels, but this is an inconstant finding, and might relate to changes in body weight and composition since SHBG may increase. U.S. Food and Drug Administration labeling of testosterone products states that "the treatment of hypogonadal men with testosterone may potentiate sleep apnea in some patients, especially those with risk factors such as obesity or chronic lung diseases."

With gradual weight loss, especially following bariatric surgery, SHBG and total testosterone levels rise substantially (Table 36.1). Estradiol levels tend to decrease and LH levels tend to rise. Likewise, metabolic parameters, and quality of life, including subjective and objective measures of sexual function, improve. Extreme low calorie diets, on the other hand, may lower testosterone levels because calorie restriction and energy deprivation suppress GnRH production.

**Table 36.1** Hormone levels in obese men before and 1–2 years following bariatric surgery

| Ref | Testosterone, ng/dL (nmol/L) | | SHBG (nmol/L) | | LH (mIU/mL) | | Estradiol, pg/mL (pmol/L) | |
|---|---|---|---|---|---|---|---|---|
| | Baseline | Post | Baseline | Post | Baseline | Post | Baseline | Post |
| 1 | 13.4±1.8 | +58 %* | | | 4.9±0.8 | +8 % | | |
| 2 | 340±21 | +100 %* | | | | | 39±3 | −21 %* |
| 3 | 340±130 | +106 %* | | | 4.8±1.7 | +21 % | 48±15 | −28 % |
| 4 | 256±120 | +100 %* | 25±12 | +92 %* | 3.69±1.87 | +5 % | 28±22 | +21 % |
| 5 | 8.75 | +58 % | 19.2 | +100 % | 2.31 | +53 % | 139.5 | −14 % |

* $p < 0.05$
1. Globerman H et al., Endocr Res 2005
2. Hammoud A et al., J Clin Endocrinol Metab 2009
3. Reis LO et al., Int J Androl 2010
4. Mora M et al., Surgical Endoscopy 2013
5. Luconi M et al., Fertil Steril 2012

There is some evidence that obesity disrupts spermatogenesis and predisposes to infertility [4]. A survey of American couples in Iowa and North Carolina revealed a twofold increase in infertility among men with BMI > 32 kg/m² after adjusting for age and female BMI. In another study, BMI was lower in a cohort of fathers than in men attending an infertility clinic, but fathers were also slightly older. There are reports of an inverse association between BMI and sperm concentration, motility and/or morphology, but other studies have not confirmed these findings. Several studies have found lower inhibin-B levels among obese men, and one idea is that reduced proliferation of Sertoli cells in obese adolescents results in lower sperm counts in adulthood [5]. Fertility may also be influenced by decreased libido and erectile dysfunction. Obese men are usually fertile, however, so obesity may be an additive factor when other causes of infertility are present.

## Treatment Strategies

Testosterone is often prescribed for men with symptomatic late onset hypogonadism because treatment usually increases mood and other quality-of-life measures [6]. Testosterone deficiency produced by GnRH analogs leads to a decrease in muscle mass and an increase in body fat. Thus testosterone deficiency may also be both a cause and a consequence of obesity and metabolic syndrome. Testosterone treatment tends to restore or to prevent the age-related decline in fat-free mass, reduces visceral adipose tissue, and improve insulin sensitivity. However, the changes are relative small in magnitude [7]. Testosterone treatment also tends to decrease both high-density lipoprotein and low-density lipoprotein cholesterol levels, but changes are again small and dose-dependent. Large doses of testosterone given to elderly men may cause edema and even contribute to congestive heart failure [8]. Testosterone stimulates erythropoiesis, and polycythemia, with its increased risk for stroke, may occur, especially in men with chronic lung disease treated with parenteral testosterone preparations.

Saad et al. [9] published a meta-analysis of the metabolic effects of various testosterone treatments on body composition in men with T2DM. They included 10 placebo-controlled studies of at least 6 months duration in which the increase in lean body mass was $2.49 \pm 1.64$ kg (range 0.8–6.2 kg) and the decrease in total fat mass was $-1.47 \pm 1.55$ kg (range −0.6 to 4.8 kg). Thus the results show a consistent benefit, and interestingly a reanalysis of their data reveals a strong correlation between the changes in these two variables among the studies, with men receiving testosterone by the parenteral route experiencing the greatest change implying a dose effect (Fig. 36.1). Insulin resistance may improve, and there are small reductions in HbA1C in some but not all studies. Thus the current evidence indicates that testosterone treatment positively affects some metabolic parameters in men with metabolic syndrome or type 2 diabetes but how these changes influence clinical cardiovascular disease remains controversial.

Several recent studies have shown that men treated with testosterone are at increased risk for CVD. The first was a retrospective analysis of older men who had undergone coronary angiography at several Veterans Administration medical centers. Men subsequently prescribed testosterone (14 % of the total) had a 30 % greater likelihood of death, compared to untreated men. A second report was a respective analysis of a U.S. commercial and Medicare insurance database in which the authors assessed the diagnosis of acute MI within 90 days of filling a first prescription for a testosterone product ($n = 55,593$) or a phosphodiesterase type 5 inhibitor ($n = 167,279$). Although the number of events was small, testosterone-treated men > 65 years, and those below age 65 with a history of heart disease, had double the risk of heart attack within the 90 day window. These findings, although inconclusive, mandate the correct diagnosis of testosterone deficiency before recommending testosterone treatment.

The potential impact of testosterone treatment on benign prostate hyperplasia and prostate cancer has also been a major concern. Prostate is an androgen target tissue, and prostate epithelium is stimulated by, and PSA levels will increase in proportion to the testosterone dose. Most studies using replacement doses of testosterone show no adverse effect on lower urinary tract symptoms, and some studies have shown unexpected improvement. The increase in PSA (average about 0.3 ng/mL) usually stabilizes over time, and it is uncommon for the PSA to exceed 4.0 ng/mL, but if so, referral to a Urologist for prostate biopsy is recommended. Both the prostate and cardiovascular effects of testosterone treatment continue to be actively investigated in randomized clinical trials.

While receiving testosterone treatment, our patient was found to be azoospermic, and when treatment was stopped, his wife conceived. Although a repeat semen analysis was not performed, testosterone administration will decrease circulating LH and FSH levels, and thereby reduce the level of intratesticular testosterone and other factors to suppress spermatogenesis, and recovery to pretreatment values generally

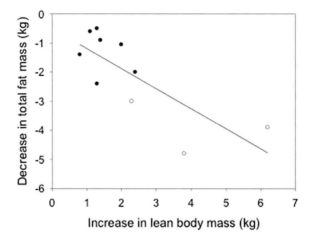

**Fig. 36.1** Relationship between the increase in lean body mass and the decrease in total body fat observed in 10 studies of hypogonadal men with T2DM treated with a variety of testosterone preparations for at least 6 months. *Open circles* are from studies in which men received testosterone enanthate, mixed esters, or injected testosterone undecanoate; the *closed circles* are from studies in which men were treated with a transdermal testosterone patch ($n=3$), a testosterone gel ($n=2$), or oral testosterone undecanoate ($n=2$). Data from Saad et al. [9]

occurs over 12–24 weeks [12]. When testosterone is given in slightly higher than replacement doses, approximately 70 % of volunteers develop azoospermia and the remaining men develop oligozoospermia.

Specific estrogen receptor response modifiers (SERMs), such as clomiphene or tamoxifen, that function as estrogen receptor antagonists in the hypothalamic–pituitary unit, or aromatase inhibitors that reduce estrogen production, increase LH and testosterone levels in men with late-onset hyponadism as in normal men because they interrupt estrogen negative feedback regulation of GnRH and LH secretion. These drugs therefore represent an alternate treatment approach for late onset hypogonadism since they increase testosterone levels without the suppression of spermatogenesis that occurs with testosterone treatment. No major safety concerns have been noted, but these drugs are not FDA approved for this purpose at this.

## Questions

1. A 42-year-old man presents with erectile dysfunction. He was married for 11 years and had two children, but divorced 2 years ago. He is otherwise healthy and takes no medications. His libido is strong. His maternal and paternal grandmothers each had type 2 diabetes. On physical examination, he is healthy and well-appearing. His height is 6′ and his weight is 190 lbs (BMI 26 kg/m²). There

is no goiter or gynecomastia. Both testes are 4.6×2.8 cm and 20–25 mL in volume. His total testosterone level was 236 ng/dL. Each of the following tests is useful at this time, except:

a. Lipid profile
b. Fasting blood sugar
c. Free testosterone
d. PRL
e. TSH

2. A 30-year-old man presents with bilateral breast enlargement. He was previously healthy and is the father of two children. Hypertension was diagnosed 2 years ago, and he is treated with lisinopril. He lost 10 lbs in weight during the past year. On physical examination, the pulse is 100. There is a small goiter. He has prominent breasts that are tender to palpation. The testes are each 4.8×2.7 cm. The serum testosterone level is 988 ng/dL. Each of the following tests is useful at this time except:

a. TSH
b. hCG
c. Mammogram
d. SHBG
e. LH/FSH

3. A 60-year-old African American man with a nonfunctional pituitary tumor is referred to you for treatment including testosterone replacement. His free T4 level is low at 0.7 ng/dL (normal 0.8–1.7) as is his total testosterone of 60 ng/dL. PRL is normal at 8.6 ng/mL and he responds normally to cortrosyn with a rise in cortisol from 8 to 21 μg/dL. He is a nonsmoker but the screening PSA is 3.8 ng/mL (normal <4). At this point which of the following would you recommend:

a. Insulin tolerance testing
b. Referral to a Urologist
c. Repeat PRL
d. hCG stimulation test
e. treatment with clomiphene

4. A 20-year-old man with cystic fibrosis is taking megestrol 400 mg daily to increase his appetite. Which of the following complications of therapy are likely to occur?

a. Hyperprolactinemia
b. Hypothyroidism
c. Hypogonadism
d. Osteoporosis
e. C & D

# Answers to Questions

1. d. The likely diagnosis is metabolic syndrome with low SHBG to explain the low total testosterone level. ED is a predictor of cardiovascular disease, and hypothyroidism results in a low SHBG level and may reduce sexual function. Hyperprolactinemia is a rare occurrence in men with ED whose libido is preserved, but should be measured if free testosterone proves to be low.
2. c. Gynecomastia is common in men with hyperthyroidism and may be the presenting complaint. One hypothesis is that the primary event is the potent increase in SHBG. hCG-producing tumors should always be excluded with gynecomastia whereas tender bilateral gynecomastia is hormonally stimulated, and a mammogram is almost always uninformative.
3. b. PSA levels are generally very low in men with hypopituitarism. Current guidelines suggest a urological consultation when the verified serum PSA concentration exceeds 3.0 ng/mL in men with increased risk for prostate cancer, e.g., Blacks.
4. e. Megestrol is a progestin and glucorticoid. It suppresses LH and thereby testosterone levels, and its glucocorticoid action adds to its effect to decrease bone mass.

# References

1. Elin RJ, Winters SJ. Current controversies in testosterone testing: aging and obesity. Clin Lab Med. 2004;24(1):119–39.
2. Dandona P, Dhindsa S. Update: hypogonadotropic hypogonadism in type 2 diabetes and obesity. J Clin Endocrinol Metab. 2011;96(9):2643–51.
3. Hoyos CM, Killick R, Yee BJ, Grunstein RR, Liu PY. Effects of testosterone therapy on sleep and breathing in obese men with severe obstructive sleep apnoea: a randomized placebo-controlled trial. Clin Endocrinol (Oxf). 2012;77(4):599–607.
4. Teerds KJ, de Rooij DG, Keijer J. Functional relationship between obesity and male reproduction: from humans to animal models. Hum Reprod Update. 2011;17(5):667–83.
5. Winters SJ, Wang C, Abdelrahaman E, Hadeed V, Dyky MA, Brufsky A. Inhibin-B levels in healthy young adult men and prepubertal boys: is obesity the cause for the contemporary decline in sperm count because of fewer Sertoli cells? J Androl. 2006;27(4):560–4.
6. Spitzer M, Huang G, Basaria S, Travison TG, Bhasin S. Risks and benefits of testosterone therapy in older men. Nat Rev Endocrinol. 2013;9(7):414–24.
7. Allan CA, Strauss BJ, Burger HG, Forbes EA, McLachlan RI. Testosterone therapy prevents gain in visceral adipose tissue and loss of skeletal muscle in nonobese aging men. J Clin Endocrinol Metab. 2008;93(1):139–46.
8. Basaria S, Coviello AD, Travison TG, Storer TW, Farwell WR, Jette AM, Eder R, Tennstedt S, Ulloor J, Zhang A, Choong K, Lakshman KM, Mazer NA, Miciek R, Krasnoff J, Elmi A, Knapp PE, Brooks B, Appleman E, Aggarwal S, Bhasin G, Hede-Brierley L, Bhatia A, Collins L, LeBrasseur N, Fiore LD, Bhasin S. Adverse events associated with testosterone administration. N Engl J Med. 2010;363(2):109–22.

9. Saad F, Aversa A, Isidori AM, Gooren LJ. Testosterone as potential effective therapy in treatment of obesity in men with testosterone deficiency: a review. Curr Diabetes Rev. 2012;8: 131–43.
10. Vigen R, O'Donnell CI, Baron AE, Grunwald GK, Maddox TM, et al. Association of testosterone therapy with mortality, myocardial infarction, and stroke in men with low testosterone levels. JAMA. 2013;310:1829–36.
11. Finkle WD, Greenland S, Ridgeway GK, Adams JL, Frasco MA, et al. Increased risk of non-fatal myocardial infarction following testosterone therapy prescription in men. PloS one. 2014;9:e85805.
12. Page ST, Amory JK, Bremner WJ. Advances in male contraception. Endocr Rev. 2008;29: 465–93.

# Part IX
# Pregnancy

# Chapter 37
# Introduction

Alex Stagnaro-Green

## Introduction

Pregnancy is a time of marked hormonal and immunological changes. Not only is there a disruption of the monthly alterations of FSH, LH, estrogen, and progesterone that accompany the menstrual cycle, but new hormonal and immune homeostasis is achieved. Simultaneously, new hormones are produced which have important metabolic impacts. Specifically, the placenta produces human chorionic gonadotropin (hCG) and human placental lactogen (HPL), both of which are critical to the progression of a normal pregnancy. However, both have unintended metabolic consequences. Human chorionic gonadotropin and thyrotropin-stimulating hormone (TSH) are composed of an alpha and beta subunit. The alpha subunit is identical in hCG and TSH, while the beta subunit in the two hormones shares approximately 85 % homology. Consequently, as hCG rises in the first trimester, it crossreacts with the TSH receptor resulting in a decrease in TSH levels and a constriction of the normal TSH range to 0.1–2.5 mIU/ml. Human placental lactogen peaks later in pregnancy and has the unintended impact of increasing insulin resistance. The selective immunosuppression which accompanies pregnancy has a direct impact on autoimmune diseases by impacting the titer of the etiological antibody. The present chapter discusses three common endocrinological abnormalities that are related to the hormonal and immunological perturbations of pregnancy. Specifically, this chapter will focus on a metabolic disorder which impedes a woman's ability to become pregnant (polycystic ovarian syndrome), impacts the natural course of the disease (Graves' disease), or results in the new onset of a disease state (gestational diabetes mellitus).

A. Stagnaro-Green, M.D., M.H.P.E. (✉)
Professor of Medicine, Obstetrics & Gynecology and Medical Education,
University of Illinois College of Medicine at Rockford,
1601 Parkview Avenue, Rockford, IL 61107, USA
e-mail: asg@uic.edu

© Springer Science+Business Media New York 2015
T.F. Davies (ed.), *A Case-Based Guide to Clinical Endocrinology*,
DOI 10.1007/978-1-4939-2059-4_37

Dr. Frankfurter presents a case of polycystic ovarian syndrome (PCOS) in which the patient presents with abnormal menses and infertility. Interestingly, despite decades of research the etiology of PCOS is still unknown and there is no single pathognomonic diagnostic test. Nevertheless, the treatment of infertility in PCOS is extremely effective with the vast majority of women able to conceive with appropriate management. Dr. Pearce discusses a case of thyrotoxicosis in the first trimester of pregnancy and presents a methodology by which the physician can differentiate gestational thyrotoxicosis (caused by the first trimester elevation of serum hCG) from Graves' hyperthyroidism (caused by a TSH receptor antibody). Specific focus is placed on utilizing the optimal antithyroid drug with propylthiouracil the agent of choice in the first trimester followed by methimazole in the second and third trimesters. Finally, Dr. Levy describes the diagnosis and management of gestational diabetes mellitus, a disease diagnosed de novo during pregnancy and caused by the insulin resistance that increases as a normal pregnancy progresses. Controversies remain regarding the criteria for diagnosis of gestational diabetes mellitus but consensus regarding the need for aggressive treatment to achieve euglycemia is universal.

The three cases presented provide a glimpse into the fascinating world of the impact of pregnancy on normal and abnormal endocrine function and disease. It is difficult to think of an endocrine system that is not impacted by pregnancy, through either an alteration in the normal range, direct impact on disease course, onset of new disease entities, or through an impact on the optimal management. Perhaps the most important lesson learned is that during pregnancy the endocrine system is in a state of flux.

# Chapter 38
# Getting Pregnant with PCOS

David Frankfurter

## Objectives

1. To describe the diagnostic features of polycystic ovarian syndrome.
2. To apply current therapies in order to induce ovulation and/or achieve pregnancy in women with polycystic ovarian syndrome.

## Case Description

A 36-year-old married gravida 0 sees her OB/GYN after stopping oral contraceptive pills (OCPs) in order to get pregnant. She started using OCPs while in college to help with acne. Her weight, since her wedding 5 years ago, has steadily increased by 4–5 pounds per year. While her menstrual cycles on OCPs were regular, every 25 days since OCP discontinuation, her cycles became irregular coming every 6–9 weeks lasting 8 days. Her periods are free of cramps but can be heavy warranting a change in sanitary napkin every hour for the first day. She is otherwise healthy without medical problems and sees her gynecologist on an annual basis. She has never had an abnormal PAP smear and takes no medications other than a daily multivitamin. She is 5′7″ tall and weighs 180 pounds (BMI 28.2 kg/m$^2$). Her physical examination is notable for a blood pressure of 134/88, increased hair growth on her chin and posterior thighs, and she has a skin tag in her left axilla. The following test results are reported in a workup for anovulation: hCG <1.0 mIU/ml; FSH 5.6 mIU/ml; TSH 1.480 mIU/L; FT4 1.21 ng/dL; Prolactin 9.3 ng/mL; 17-OHP 120 ng/dl; DHEAS 240 ug/dl; Total Testosterone 55 ng/dl; HgbA1c 6.0 %; fasting glucose 88 mg/dl;

D. Frankfurter, M.D. (✉)
George Washington University School of Medicine and Health Sciences,
2150 Pennsylvania Avenue, Washington, DC 20037, USA
e-mail: dfrankfurter@mfa.gwu.edu

© Springer Science+Business Media New York 2015
T.F. Davies (ed.), *A Case-Based Guide to Clinical Endocrinology*,
DOI 10.1007/978-1-4939-2059-4_38

fasting insulin 21 uU/ml; transvaginal ultrasound demonstrates an endometrial lining of 1.2 cm and bilateral ovarian diffuse enlargement with multiple peripheral cysts in a "string of pearls" configuration.

## Introduction

Affecting between 6 % and 15 % of women, polycystic ovarian syndrome (PCOS) is the most common female endocrine disorder [1]. Commonly, PCOS presents during adolescence and continues throughout a woman's reproductive life [2]. The clinical features typically include a combination of ovulatory disturbance and hyperandrogenism with or without characteristic polycystic ovaries [3]. There remains no unifying theory as to the pathophysiologic basis of PCOS and the phenotype can be highly variable. Two distinct conventions regarding the requisite diagnostic findings when considering PCOS remain [3, 4]. The NIH criteria include a combination of ovulatory disturbance and hyperandrogenism in the absence of other conditions that share clinical findings. Because of the marked heterogeneity amongst PCOS presentations, the Rotterdam criteria included any two of the three classic features: oligo-ovulation, hyperandrogenism (clinical or biochemical) or sonographic findings [3]. Management of PCOS involves an understanding of the various aspects of women's health including hirsutism, pregnancy, anovulation, cancer, metabolic, and cardiac well being. *This patient's history of hyperandrogenism began shortly after adolescence and, while controlled by OCPs, returned after she discontinued OCPs. This presentation will focus on diagnosing PCOS and interventions aimed at achieving pregnancy.*

## Clinical Features

Typically, PCOS is associated with of hyperandrogenism, the most distinctive feature of which is hirsutism [2, 5]. Hirsutism can be mild to severe and in patients with PCOS it is usually of a gradual onset [6]. Rapid onset of severe hirsutism with thick pigmented hair is suggestive of a neoplastic source of androgens [7, 8]. In PCOS, the areas most commonly involved include the sides of the face, chin, upper lip, neck, posterior thigh, and the upper abdomen with extension from the pubic escutcheon. In severe cases, sexual hair can be seen on the chest and may be associated with temporal balding [6].

Menstrual bleeding is usually irregular and may be absent. In many cases, the menstrual pattern never becomes regular and may transition from irregular cycles to intervals of amenorrhea. While nearly 20 % of women with PCOS have no menses, those with very heavy periods should be followed for endometrial hyperplasia or carcinoma [7].

Roughly half of women with PCOS are obese [9]. Obese women with PCOS commonly have an increased waist-to-hip ration and android fat pattern. Such increased visceral fat is commonly seen in individuals with insulin resistance and may serve as a marker of metabolic dysfunction [7]. Both thin and obese women with PCOS commonly exhibit insulin resistance [10–12]. Insulin resistance may lead to a reduction in sex hormone-binding globulin (SHBG) leading to more bio-available androgens for receptor binding [12, 13]. High concentrations of peripheral insulin can lead to an insulin action on the insulin-like growth factor I (IGF-I) receptor in the ovary. IGF-I receptor activation leads to enhanced ovarian testosterone production. Women with insulin resistance may demonstrate hyperpigmentation in areas of skin folds like the axillae and groin (acanthosis nigricans) and they can be prone to developing skin tags [7, 14].

Women with PCOS are at an increased risk for both gestational and nongestational diabetes [15, 16]. By improving glucose metabolism and amelioration of insulin resistance, androgen levels can be reduced and ovulation restored in some patients with PCOS. This can be accomplished with weight loss, insulin lowering medications, or a combination of the two [15, 17, 18].

Women with PCOS demonstrate arrested development of antral follicles. Such cysts persist for a period of time only to undergo atresia and replacement by similar peripherally situated mid-antral cysts. The cysts are nested in a hyperplastic stroma that exhibits enhanced androgen production [7]. The morphologic characteristics of the PCOS ovary seem to derive from enhanced ovarian androgen exposure. Therefore the PCOS ovary both reflects and creates a hyperandrogenic environment [5]. Peripherally, androgens are converted to estrogens by aromatase expressing adipose tissue. Chronic exposure to unopposed estrogens results in multiple physiologic changes [5].

Polycystic ovarian syndrome is notable for an alteration in LH secretion. Women with PCOS demonstrate both increased pituitary LH pulse frequency and amplitude [19]. The underlying cause of this pituitary malfunction is not known, but it may be partially driven by chronic exposure of the pituitary gonadotroph to elevated estrogen levels [7]. Such exposure may alter the gonadotroph's sensitivity to GnRH leading to increased LH pulse amplitude, frequency or both. Increased pituitary LH release leads to enhanced ovarian androgen production further exacerbating both the local follicular dysfunction with follicular arrest and the peripheral hormonal environment with chronically elevated peripheral estrogen levels [19].

Unopposed estrogen exposure leads to chronic proliferation of the endometrial lining with the potential for hyperplasia and carcinoma. Endometrial carcinoma has been reported in young women with ovulatory disturbances and young women with endometrial cancer have been noted to have a high frequency of anovulatory menstrual irregularities. Polycystic ovarian syndrome does not appear to increase the risk for either breast or ovarian cancer [7].

The combination of obesity, hyperandrogenism and insulin resistance increases the potential that women with PCOS develop heart disease [20]. It is unknown if PCOS is an independent risk factor for heart disease. Women with PCOS exhibit dyslipidemia with high levels of LDL and triglycerides and low levels of HDL. The combined effects of obesity, dyslipidemia, insulin resistance, and hyperandrogen-emia increase the potential for plaque formation on coronary vessels. Hypertension maybe more common among PCOS individuals further exacerbating cardiac risk. However, whether hypertension is independently associated with PCOS or if it is related to obesity remains unclear [20].

## Diagnosing PCOS

Central to the diagnosis of PCOS is the exclusion of other conditions that share clinical findings. Congenital adrenal hyperplasia (CAH) leads to increased serum androgens as a result of a relative block in cortisol production. 21 hydroxylase defi-ciency can mimic PCOS. It results in an increased production of cortisol precursors which include androgens. One can rule out CAH prior to diagnosing PCOS by assessing serum 17-OHP levels. Women with CAH exhibit an elevation in 17-OHP, a cortisol precursor, and normal 17-OHP levels (<200) exclude CAH from the dif-ferential diagnosis [3].

It is also important to exclude androgen producing neoplasms as the cause of the hyperandrogenemia. Androgen producing neoplasms usually exhibit rapid acuity and markedly elevated androgens. Sudden onset or severely virilizing symptoms suggest a neoplastic process. Measurement of serum total testosterone and DHEAS can both establish the presence of an androgen producing tumor and localize its etiology. Testosterone is made both by the ovaries and adrenal glands while DHEAS is made exclusively by the adrenal glands. The presence of markedly elevated tes-tosterone and normal DHEAS levels suggest an ovarian etiology while elevations in both reveal an adrenal source.

Excluding nonovarian causes of ovulatory dysfunction is also critical in estab-lishing PCOS as a diagnosis. Normal FSH levels rule out ovarian failure as a cause of anovulation. Both thyroid dysfunction and hyperprolactinemia can be easily excluded with a routine blood draw.

Finally pelvic sonography can be helpful by assessing for the presence of mul-tiple peripherally located small follicular cysts. These must be differentiated from ovaries with multiple nonperipherally distributed follicular cysts. The latter is a normal variant seen in the youthful fertile ovary [3, 8]. In PCOS, the ovarian volume is increased. Furthermore, a thickened endometrial lining can be suggestive of endometrial hyperplasia.

Hyperandrogenemia leads to continuous peripheral conversion of testosterone to estrogen by aromatase containing tissue including muscle and adipose. The general lack of ovulation translates to a lack of progesterone production and unopposed estrogen action on the endometrium. This increases the risks of meno-metrorrhagia, endometrial hyperplasia and endometrial adenocarcinoma. In patients with irregular menses and a thickened endometrial stripe (>5 mm), endometrial sampling fol-lowed by histological assessment is warranted.

## PCOS and Fertility

Owing to reduced ovulation, women with PCOS demonstrate reduced fertility. Furthermore, an increase in early fetal wastage is noted in women with PCOS [15, 17]. The increased miscarriage rate may be related to obesity. It has been suggested that both hyperandrogenemia and hyperinsulinemia may contribute to fetal wastage, however the exact mechanism by which these effect early pregnancy remains unclear [9].

## Managing Infertility in PCOS

The strategies for fertility intervention in the setting of PCOS are directed at well health and a restoration of ovulation. The goal should be to minimize the risk of a multiple gestation.

## Lifestyle Modification

Because of the association between PCOS and cardiac health as well as the desire to optimize health prior to and during pregnancy, it is extremely important for PCOS patients to stop smoking. Weight management is also critical and may serve as the sole intervention needed to establish ovulation. A loss of 5–10 % of body weight can improve insulin resistance, increase SHBG, decrease both total and free testosterone, reduce peripheral androgen aromatization and lower circulating estrogen levels [18]. The combination of these effects can restore a normal ovulatory pattern. While effective, this approach requires active commitment, time and patience from the PCOS patient [7, 18].

## Ovulation Induction

### *Metformin*

Metformin is an oral insulin-sensitizing agent that improves hyperglycemia [21]. In addition to lowering serum insulin, it may act to lower ovarian androgen production directly. That being said, metformin's ability to restore ovulation is modest. Randomized clinical trials fail to demonstrate an improvement in live birth rates beyond that seen with classic ovulation inducing agents. Women treated with metformin demonstrated higher miscarriage rates than women treated with clomiphene citrate. Such data imply that metformin may actually reduce live birth rates [17, 22]. Therefore the use of metformin strictly for fertility reasons has been called into question [2].

## Clomiphene Citrate

Clomiphene is a synthetic, very weak estrogen agonist that when used in eu-estrogenic individuals acts as an antiestrogen. This antiestrogenic action blocks estrogen's negative feedback at the level of the hypothalamus allowing for enhanced pituitary FSH release. Enhanced FSH release allows the ovaries to initiate follicular maturation and subsequent ovulation. Clomiphene is used for a short course, of typically 2–5 days following menses. Roughly 80 % of PCOS patients placed on clomiphene will ovulate on a dose of 150 mg or less [17]. Of these, nearly half will conceive within six ovulatory cycles. Approximately 90 % of clomiphene gestations are singleton and almost all clomiphene multiple pregnancies are twins [23, 24]. Its shortcomings are related to its antiestrogenic effects, which are not limited to the hypothalamus and pituitary. Clomiphene thins the endometrial lining and thickens the viscosity of cervical mucus [23].

## Gonadotropins

Urinary derived or recombinant FSH is available to induce follicular maturation and subsequent ovulation. These agents are subcutaneously administered and very potent requiring close monitoring of the ovarian response. Their potency confers high efficacy. Numerous regimens had been promoted for gonadotropin use in the setting of PCOS. These agents are nearly 100 % effective for ovulation induction. However, they commonly lead to polyovulation [25]. The observed pregnancy rate with injectable gonadotropin is approximately 20 % per attempt. However, upwards of 40 % of pregnancies are multiple with 30 % of these resulting in triplets or higher [26]. Moreover, approximately 2–5 % of gonadotropin ovulation induction cycles are associated with severe ovarian hyperstimulation syndrome (OHSS), a potentially fatal iatrogenic complication. For these reasons, as well as improvements in in vitro fertilization (IVF), gonadotropin ovulation induction is no longer commonly used in PCOS patients [27].

## In Vitro Fertilization

Women with PCOS who fail first-line treatment with clomiphene, commonly proceed to treatment with IVF. Combined with gonadotropin stimulation, the ability to retrieve oocytes, fertilize them extracorporally and transfer a limited number of embryos, IVF provides a highly efficacious means of treating PCOS. IVF protocols must be adjusted to account for the potential for hyper-response to gonadotropin stimulation. The combination of low-dose gonadotropin stimulation, close monitoring, the use of a GnRH agonist to induce oocyte maturation and single embryo transfer (SET) minimize the most significant risks associated with ovulation induction. Undertaken as described, IVF affords a 20–40 % pregnancy rate with no risk of fraternal multiples and <1.0 % risk of severe OHSS [28, 29]. Further, IVF allows for the cryopreservation of residual embryos to provide a means of fertility preservation.

The patient presented in the case description demonstrated classic findings in PCOS. She was oligo-ovulatory, mildly hirsute, overweight, and demonstrated findings consistent with insulin resistance, i.e., skin tags. She was hyperandrogenemic and based upon an elevated hemoglobin A1c and a glucose to insulin ration of <4.5, she was hyperinsulinemic. Her ultrasound was confirmatory. She went on to attempt ovulation with clomiphene after which she conceived and had an early miscarriage. She delivered a baby girl after her first attempt with IVF and single embryo transfer. Her pregnancy was complicated with diet controlled gestational diabetes. She has four cryopreserved embryos and will attempt a pregnancy with them after she stops breastfeeding.

## Summary

Polycystic ovarian syndrome is a condition with unclear etiology. It is associated with oligo-ovulation, hyperandrogenism, hyperinsulinemia, and chronic unopposed estrogen exposure. Women with PCOS are at risk for diabetes, coronary artery disease, endometrial carcinoma, and are infertile. Interventions are aimed at optimizing well cardiac and metabolic health and inducing ovulation for those seeking pregnancy. Simple lifestyle modification plays an important role in the management of PCOS.

## Lessons Learned

1. PCOS is noted for at least two of the following: reduced ovulation, hyperandrogenism or sonographic findings of polycystic ovaries.
2. PCOS findings must exist in the absence of another clear etiology, i.e., androgen producing tumor, congenital adrenal hyperplasia, pituitary microadenoma (hyperprolactinemia), or significant hypothyroidism.
3. PCOS is commonly associated with obesity, insulin resistance, increased risk of coronary artery disease, and infertility.
4. Management of PCOS includes optimizing well health and allowing for follicular maturation to cause pregnancy.

## Multiple Choice Questions

1. Women with polycystic ovarian syndrome are at increased risk for which of the following endocrinology disorders:

   a. Hypothyroidism
   b. Type-2 diabetes mellitus
   c. Primary Hyperparathyroidism
   d. 21 hyroxylase deficiency
   e. Cushing's disease

2. All of the following are consistent with the diagnosis of polycystic ovarian syndrome except which of the following:

   a. Hyperandrogenism
   b. Insulin resistance
   c. Sudden onset of virilizing symptoms
   d. Acanthosis nigricans
   e. Elevated levels of LDL and triglycerides

3. Which of the following fertility treatments is rarely used nowadays in women with polycystic ovarian syndrome because of an increased risk of hyperstimulation syndrome

   a. Clomiphene citrate
   b. In vitro fertilization
   c. Metformin
   d. Gondotropin ovulation induction

## Answers to Questions

1. b
2. c
3. d

## References

1. Hull MG. Epidemiology of infertility and polycystic ovarian disease: endocrinological and demographic studies. Gynecol Endocrinol. 1987;1(3):235–45.
2. Amsterdam, E.A.-S.r.P.C.W.G. Consensus on women's health aspects of polycystic ovary syndrome (PCOS). Hum Reprod. 2012;27(1):14–24.
3. Rotterdam, E.A.-S.P.C.W.G. Revised 2003 consensus on diagnostic criteria and long-term health risks related to polycystic ovary syndrome. Fertil Steril. 2004;81(1):19–25.

4. Zawadski J, Dunaif A. Diagnostic criteria for polycystic ovary syndrome: towards a rationale approach. In: Dunaif A, editor. Polycystic ovary syndrome. Boston, MA: Blackwell Scientific; 1992. p. 377–84.

5. Dunaif A, et al. The effects of continuous androgen secretion on the hypothalamic-pituitary axis in woman: evidence from a luteinized thecoma of the ovary. J Clin Endocrinol Metab. 1984;59(3):389–93.

6. Hatch R, et al. Hirsutism: implications, etiology, and management. Am J Obstet Gynecol. 1981;140(7):815–30.

7. Strauss III JF, Williams CJ. In: Strauss III JF, Barbieri RL, editors. Yen and Jaffe's reproductive endocrinology: physiology, pathophysiology and clinical management. 5th ed. Philadelphia, PA: Elsevier Saunders; 2004.

8. Polson DW, et al. Polycystic ovaries–a common finding in normal women. Lancet. 1988; 1(8590):870–2.

9. Al-Azemi M, Omu FE, Omu AE. The effect of obesity on the outcome of infertility management in women with polycystic ovary syndrome. Arch Gynecol Obstet. 2004;270(4):205–10.

10. Gambineri A, et al. Glucose intolerance in a large cohort of mediterranean women with polycystic ovary syndrome: phenotype and associated factors. Diabetes. 2004;53(9):2353–8.

11. Li M, et al. Decreased insulin receptor (IR) autophosphorylation in fibroblasts from patients with PCOS: effects of serine kinase inhibitors and IR activators. J Clin Endocrinol Metab. 2002;87(9):4088–93.

12. Wijeyaratne CN, et al. Clinical manifestations and insulin resistance (IR) in polycystic ovary syndrome (PCOS) among South Asians and Caucasians: is there a difference? Clin Endocrinol (Oxf). 2002;57(3):343–50.

13. Hogeveen KN, et al. Human sex hormone-binding globulin variants associated with hyperandrogenism and ovarian dysfunction. J Clin Invest. 2002;109(7):973–81.

14. Mathur SK, Bhargava P. Insulin resistance and skin tags. Dermatology. 1997;195(2):184.

15. Boomsma CM, et al. A meta-analysis of pregnancy outcomes in women with polycystic ovary syndrome. Hum Reprod Update. 2006;12(6):673–83.

16. Legro RS, et al. Prevalence and predictors of risk for type 2 diabetes mellitus and impaired glucose tolerance in polycystic ovary syndrome: a prospective, controlled study in 254 affected women. J Clin Endocrinol Metab. 1999;84(1):165–9.

17. Legro RS, et al. Clomiphene, metformin, or both for infertility in the polycystic ovary syndrome. N Engl J Med. 2007;356(6):551–66.

18. Holte J, et al. Restored insulin sensitivity but persistently increased early insulin secretion after weight loss in obese women with polycystic ovary syndrome. J Clin Endocrinol Metab. 1995;80(9):2586–93.

19. Taylor AE, et al. Determinants of abnormal gonadotropin secretion in clinically defined women with polycystic ovary syndrome. J Clin Endocrinol Metab. 1997;82(7):2248–56.

20. Talbott E, et al. Coronary heart disease risk factors in women with polycystic ovary syndrome. Arterioscler Thromb Vasc Biol. 1995;15(7):821–6.

21. Kirpichnikov D, McFarlane SI, Sowers JR. Metformin: an update. Ann Intern Med. 2002; 137(1):25–33.

22. Palomba S, et al. Effect of preconceptional metformin on abortion risk in polycystic ovary syndrome: a systematic review and meta-analysis of randomized controlled trials. Fertil Steril. 2009;92(5):1646–58.

23. Kousta E, White DM, Franks S. Modern use of clomiphene citrate in induction of ovulation. Hum Reprod Update. 1997;3(4):359–65.

24. Deaton JL, et al. Clomiphene citrate ovulation induction in combination with a timed intrauterine insemination: the value of urinary luteinizing hormone versus human chorionic gonadotropin timing. Fertil Steril. 1997;68(1):43–7.

25. De Leo V, et al. Effects of metformin on gonadotropin-induced ovulation in women with polycystic ovary syndrome. Fertil Steril. 1999;72(2):282–5.

26. Ganesh A, et al. Comparison of letrozole with continuous gonadotropins and clomiphene-gonadotropin combination for ovulation induction in 1387 PCOS women after clomiphene citrate failure: a randomized prospective clinical trial. J Assist Reprod Genet. 2009;26(1): 19–24.

27. Homburg R. Pregnancy complications in PCOS. Best Pract Res Clin Endocrinol Metab. 2006;20(2):281–92.

28. Engmann L, et al. The use of gonadotropin-releasing hormone (GnRH) agonist to induce oocyte maturation after cotreatment with GnRH antagonist in high-risk patients undergoing in vitro fertilization prevents the risk of ovarian hyperstimulation syndrome: a prospective randomized controlled study. Fertil Steril. 2008;89(1):84–91.

29. Gerris J, et al. A real-life prospective health economic study of elective single embryo transfer versus two-embryo transfer in first IVF/ICSI cycles. Hum Reprod. 2004;19(4):917–23.

# Chapter 39
# Thyrotoxicosis in Pregnancy

Elizabeth N. Pearce

## Objectives

1. To understand the differential diagnosis of thyrotoxicosis in early pregnancy and how to determine the etiology.
2. To understand how to treat and monitor women with Graves' hyperthyroidism throughout pregnancy.

## Case Description

A 27-year-old woman presents for evaluation of abnormal thyroid function tests; she is currently 10 weeks pregnant. She has previously been healthy and is taking no medications except a prenatal multivitamin. A serum thyroid-stimulating hormone (TSH) was obtained and was <0.01 mIU/l. Follow-up peripheral thyroid hormone tests were: total thyroxine (T4) 18 µg/dl (nonpregnancy reference range 4.5–10.5 µg/dl), free thyroxine index (FT4I) 6.2 (nonpregnancy reference range 1.0–4.0), and total triiodothyronine (T3) 390 ng/dl (nonpregnancy reference range 60–181 ng/dl). She complains of nausea with frequent emesis that started about 3 weeks ago. She also complains of fatigue, anxiety, occasional palpitations, and heat intolerance. She has lost 2 lbs. over the past 3 weeks. Her family history is significant for hypothyroidism in a maternal grandmother. She has no lid lag, exophthalmos, or stare. Her thyroid is easily palpable, without nodules or tenderness.

A thyroid hormone receptor antibody (TRAb) is 310 % of controls (normal <140 %). She is diagnosed with Graves' disease and propylthiouracil (PTU) 50 mg

E.N. Pearce, M.D., M.Sc. (✉)
Boston University School of Medicine, 88 East Newton Street, H3600,
Boston, MA 02118, USA
e-mail: elizabeth.pearce@bmc.org

© Springer Science+Business Media New York 2015
T.F. Davies (ed.), *A Case-Based Guide to Clinical Endocrinology*,
DOI 10.1007/978-1-4939-2059-4_39

327

three times daily is started. She is also started on propranolol. Four weeks later (at 14 weeks gestation), she reports that symptoms are much improved. Her thyroid function tests are as follows: serum TSH <0.01 mIU/l, total T3 265 ng/dl, total T4 16 µg/dl, and FT4I 4.3. She is changed from PTU to methimazole (MMI) 15 mg daily, and the propranolol is stopped. Thyroid function is measured again at 4-week intervals and remains normal for pregnancy. The MMI dose is decreased to 10 mg daily at 22 weeks gestation and to 5 mg daily at 28 weeks; she remains on this dose until delivery. A repeat serum TRAb value is obtained at 22 weeks gestation and is 150 % of controls. An ultrasound performed at 28 weeks gestation demonstrates a fetal heart rate of 140 bpm and a no sign of fetal goiter or growth retardation. Six weeks after uneventful delivery of a full-term infant, thyroid function is again measured and remains normal on MMI; the patient is breastfeeding.

## Introduction

Thyrotoxicosis occurs in up to 3 % of pregnancies and poses significant diagnostic and therapeutic challenges. The most common causes in pregnant women are Graves' disease and gestational hyperthyroidism. Close cooperation between obstetricians, endocrinologists, and neonatologists is required.

## Determining the Etiology of Thyrotoxicosis in Pregnancy

Thyrotoxicosis is diagnosed by the presence of a suppressed serum TSH concentration. Peripheral thyroid hormones (free T4 and/or total T3) are elevated in overt hyperthyroidism, but remain within the normal range in subclinical hyperthyroidism. Importantly, serum thyroid hormone levels change over the course of normal gestation and nonpregnant reference ranges do not apply in pregnancy [1, 2]. TSH is the most sensitive indicator of thyroid status. Human chorionic gonadotropin (hCG) is a weak thyroid stimulator, binding to the TSH receptor. During the first trimester, when hCG levels are highest, serum TSH concentrations are often slightly below or at the low end of the non-pregnant normal range. High estrogen levels in pregnant women induce increased concentrations of circulating thyroxine-binding globulin (TBG). Therefore, total T3 and T4 levels are increased throughout pregnancy. Where trimester-specific assay-specific normal ranges are not available, the upper limit for total T3 and T4 levels in pregnancy can be estimated as 1.5 times the upper limit of the assay reference range for nonpregnant individuals [3]. Free T4 levels typically are highest in the first trimester and decline later in gestation [4].

Thyrotoxicosis in pregnancy is most frequently caused by gestational thyrotoxicosis (transient hyperthyroidism caused by elevated serum hCG levels) or Graves' disease. Toxic nodular goiter is a less common cause. Symptoms such as fatigue, heat intolerance, and tachycardia are common to both pregnancy and all forms of thyrotoxicosis. Definitive diagnosis can also be more difficult in pregnancy because radioactive iodine thyroid scans are contraindicated. Several clinical clues may help to elucidate the diagnosis. A history of hyperthyroid symptoms that began prior to the pregnancy makes gestational thyrotoxicosis less likely. The presence of a diffuse goiter favors Graves' disease. Ophthalmopathy or pretibial myxedema may be present only in Graves' disease. Gestational thyrotoxicosis is more common with multiple gestation, where peak serum hCG concentrations are far higher than in single pregnancies. Gestational thyrotoxicosis is also more common in women with morning sickness, particularly in those with the most severe form, hyperemesis gravidarum (defined as persistent vomiting, ketonuria, and at least 5 % weight loss) [5]. Serum thyroid hormone receptor antibody (TRAb) is frequently positive in Graves' disease, and may be helpful in determining the etiology of thyrotoxicosis.

## Management of Thyrotoxicosis in Pregnancy

Gestational thyrotoxicosis does not require antithyroid drug treatment and resolves spontaneously as hCG levels fall after the 11th week of gestation [1, 2, 6]. Care is supportive, with antiemetics and management of dehydration. Subclinical hyperthyroidism, regardless of cause, is not associated with adverse maternal or fetal outcomes [7], and therefore requires monitoring, but not treatment.

Women with untreated overt Graves' hyperthyroidism during pregnancy are at increased risk for having low birth weight infants, stillbirths, preterm delivery, severe preecclampsia, congestive heart failure, placental abruption, and possibly for having infants with congenital malformations [1]. The antithyroid drugs PTU and MMI are the mainstay of Graves' therapy. Small amounts of both PTU and MMI cross the placenta and may decrease fetal thyroid function. Therefore, treatment with relatively low doses of anti-thyroid drugs to keep the free T4 of pregnant women in the high–normal to slightly thyrotoxic range is recommended [1, 2]. MMI has been associated with congenital anomalies including cutis aplasia and esophageal and choanal atresia in several case reports [8]. A recent registry study demonstrated that both MMI and PTU were associated with an increased prevalence of birth defects, although birth defects were less frequent with PTU [9]. For this reason, PTU may be preferable to MMI for the treatment of hyperthyroidism in the first trimester, during the period of organogenesis [10]. However, because PTU has been associated with a risk for fulminant hepatic failure [11], changing from PTU to MMI after the first trimester is currently recommended [1, 2]. Frequent monitoring of thyroid function tests (approximately every 4 weeks) is required throughout pregnancy in women taking anti-thyroid drugs. In 20–30 % of women, Graves' disease remits spontaneously in the last trimester of pregnancy, and antithyroid drugs can be discontinued [12]. However, they often need to be restarted postpartum.

Most beta blockers are rated pregnancy class C by the FDA (risk cannot be ruled out; human studies are lacking). Beta blockers do cross the placenta and have been associated with intrauterine growth restriction. However, short-term use of beta blockers, such as propranolol, to control the symptoms of thyrotoxicosis is generally considered safe [6].

Thyroidectomy is only rarely required for the treatment of refractory hyperthy-roidism, medication noncompliance, or when severe side effects of antithyroid drugs are present. When necessary, thyroidectomy is safest when performed in the second trimester [1, 2].

Graves' disease frequently improves throughout gestation due to the immuno-suppressive effects of pregnancy. However, TRAb cross the placenta (even in euthy-roid pregnant women with Graves' disease who have undergone thyroidectomy or radioactive iodine thyroid ablation prior to pregnancy) and should be routinely measured in all patients between 20 and 24 weeks of pregnancy [1, 2]. Values greater than 300 % of controls raise concern for the development of fetal hyperthy-roidism. In addition, fetal ultrasound may be considered in order to assess for signs of fetal hyperthyroidism such as fetal tachycardia, intrauterine growth restriction, fetal goiter, and accelerated bone maturation [13].

Moderate doses of antithyroid drugs are considered safe during lactation. MMI is preferred over PTU due to the concerns about PTU-induced hepatotoxicity [1, 2].

## Lessons Learned

1. A suppressed serum TSH concentration is the hallmark of thyrotoxicosis, but thyroid function tests must be interpreted with caution in pregnancy, as nonpreg-nant reference ranges do not apply.
2. It is important to determine the etiology of thyrotoxicosis in pregnancy.
3. Gestational thyrotoxicosis requires supportive care, but not antithyroid drug treatment.
4. Overt hyperthyroidism caused by Graves' disease or toxic nodular goiter should be treated with anti-thyroid drugs: PTU is preferred in the first trimester, while MMI is the first-line drug pre-pregnancy and in trimesters two and three.
5. The goal of antithyroid drug therapy is a serum free T4 concentration at or just above the upper limit of normal; the lowest possible doses should be used and monitoring thyroid hormone levels at least every 4 weeks is required.
6. Short-term use of beta blockers may be helpful to reduce hyperthyroid symptoms.
7. In women with Graves' disease, TRAb should be measures between 20 and 24 weeks gestation to gauge risk for fetal and neonatal hyperthyroidism.
8. Moderate doses of MMI are safe during lactation.

## Questions

1. Which statement about antithyroid drugs is correct:

    a. Methimazole has been associated with an embryopathy
    b. Propylthiouracil is preferred in trimesters two and three of pregnancy

   c. The goal of therapy is normalization of the serum TSH concentration

   d. Antithyroid drugs should not be used during lactation

2. Gestational thyrotoxicosis is:

   a. An autoimmune disease

   b. Typically diagnosed by radioactive iodine uptake and scan

   c. Best treated with propylthiouracil

   d. Treated with supportive care

3. Which of the following is true about Graves' hyperthyroidism in pregnancy:

   a. Hyperthyroidism usually resolves as serum hCG levels decline.

   b. TRAb should be measured at 20–24 weeks gestation.

   c. Overt hyperthyroidism from Graves' disease can be managed with supportive care and does not require antithyroid drugs.

   d. Thyroidectomy, if required, is best performed in the first trimester.

## Answers to Questions

1. a. Methimazole has been associated with an embryopathy
2. d. Treated with supportive care
3. b. TRAb should be measured at 20–24 weeks gestation.

## References

1. Stagnaro-Green A, Abalovich M, Alexander E, Azizi F, Mestman J, Negro R, Nixon A, Pearce EN, Soldin OP, Sullivan S, Wiersinga W, American Thyroid Association Taskforce on Thyroid Disease During Pregnancy and Postpartum. Guidelines of the American Thyroid Association for the diagnosis and management of thyroid disease during pregnancy and postpartum. Thyroid. 2011;21(10):1081–125.
2. De Groot L, Abalovich M, Alexander EK, Amino N, Barbour L, Cobin RH, Eastman CJ, Lazarus JH, Luton D, Mandel SJ, Mestman J, Rovet J, Sullivan S. Management of thyroid dysfunction during pregnancy and postpartum: an Endocrine Society clinical practice guideline. J Clin Endocrinol Metab. 2012;97(8):2543–65.
3. Mandel SJ, Spencer CA, Hollowell JG. Are detection and treatment of thyroid insufficiency in pregnancy feasible? Thyroid. 2005;15:44–53.
4. Soldin OP, Tractenberg RE, Hollowell JG, Jonklaas J, Janicic N, Soldin SJ. Trimester-specific changes in maternal thyroid hormone, thyrotropin, and thyroglobulin concentrations during gestation: trends and associations across trimesters in iodine sufficiency. Thyroid. 2004; 14(12):1084–90.
5. Goodwin TM, Montoro M, Mestman JH. Transient hyperthyroidism and hyperemesis gravidarum: clinical aspects. Am J Obstet Gynecol. 1992;167:648–52.
6. American College of Obstetricians and Gynecologists. ACOG Practice Bulletin. Clinical management guidelines for obstetrician-gynecologists. Thyroid disease in pregnancy. Obstet Gynecol. 2002;100:387–96.

 7. Casey BM, Dashe JS, Wells CE, McIntire DD, Leveno KJ, Cunningham FG. Subclinical hyperthyroidism and pregnancy outcomes. Obstet Gynecol. 2006;107(2 Pt 1):337–41.
 8. Clementi M, Di Gianantonio E, Cassina M, Leoncini E, Botto LD, Mastroiacovo P, SAFE-Med Study Group. Treatment of hyperthyroidism in pregnancy and birth defects. J Clin Endocrinol Metab. 2010;95(11):E337–41.
 9. Andersen SL, Olsen J, Wu CS, Laurberg P. Birth defects after early pregnancy use of antithyroid drugs: a Danish nationwide study. J Clin Endocrinol Metab. 2013:98(11):4373–81.
10. Mandel SJ, Cooper DS. The use of antithyroid drugs in pregnancy and lactation. J Clin Endocrinol Metab. 2001;86:2354–9.
11. Bahn RS, Burch HS, Cooper DS, Garber JR, Greenlee CM, Klein IL, Laurberg P, McDougall IR, Rivkees SA, Ross D, Sosa JA, Stan MN. The Role of Propylthiouracil in the Management of Graves' Disease in Adults: report of a meeting jointly sponsored by the American Thyroid Association and the Food and Drug Administration. Thyroid. 2009;19(7):673–4.
12. Hamburger JL. Diagnosis and management of Graves' disease in pregnancy. Thyroid. 1992;2:219–24.
13. Polak M, Le Gac I, Vuillard E, Guibourdenche J, Leger J, Toubert ME, Madec AM, Oury JF, Czernichow P, Luton D. Fetal and neonatal thyroid function in relation to maternal Graves' disease. Best Pract Res Clin Endocrinol Metab. 2004;18(2):289–302.

# Chapter 40
# Gestational Diabetes

Carol J. Levy

## Objectives

1. To understand the criteria for diagnosis of Gestational Diabetes (GDM)
2. To understand the pathophysiology of normal and abnormal glucose metabolism during pregnancy
3. To learn management guidelines during pregnancy and post-delivery for patients with GDM

## Case Description

A 34-year-old Asian female presented for a visit at 26 weeks to her obstetrician for follow-up care. This was her second pregnancy. The patient's pregnancy had been uncomplicated except for some mild morning sickness in the first trimester which resolved. Her last pregnancy went smoothly and she delivered an 8 lb 6 oz baby at 40 weeks gestation. She expressed concern about her weight gain and mentioned that her mother has type-2 diabetes. Her weight at this visit is 162 lbs (pre-pregnancy 135 lbs ) her height was 5 ft 2 in. Her blood pressure was 105/68 and she had no edema and a gravid abdomen. The patient underwent a 2 h 75 g oral glucose tolerance test which came back with the following values:

Fasting—91 mg/dl (normal <92 mg/dl)
1 h—194 mg/dl (normal < 180 mg/dl)
2 h—162 mg/dl (153 mg/dl)

C.J. Levy, M.D., C.D.E. (✉)
Division of Endocrinology, Diabetes, and Metabolism, Mount Sinai School of Medicine, New York, NY, USA
e-mail: carol.levy@mssm.edu

© Springer Science+Business Media New York 2015
T.F. Davies (ed.), *A Case-Based Guide to Clinical Endocrinology*,
DOI 10.1007/978-1-4939-2059-4_40

Based on these results the patient was diagnosed with gestational diabetes mellitus. The patient was referred to a diabetes educator (RD, CDE) and given a meal plan containing 40 % carbohydrate, 20 % protein, and 40 % fat (1,900 calories) with three meals and two snacks. She was also taught home glucose monitoring and was instructed to test fasting and 1 h postprandially. Her Hba1c came back at 5.5 %.

The patient returned 1 week later for follow-up at 27 weeks and has showed good dietary compliance (with detailed food records) and appropriate testing intervals. Fasting values were 97–100 mg/dl and 1 h readings 145–158 mg/dl postmeals. Urine ketones were negative and the patient had lost 2 lbs.

The patient was started on NPH insulin 7 units at night (weight based approx 0.8 units kg). She followed up 1 week later and her fasting glucose was down to 88 mg/dl on most mornings. Postmeal readings were now in the 125–130 range. Continued weekly follow-up revealed increasing postprandial fingersticks and lispro was added at breakfast, lunch, and dinner at 30 weeks. Total pregnancy weight gain was 30 lbs and the patient delivered a healthy baby at 39 weeks weighing 8 lbs. No hypoglycemia was noted for mom or baby during labor and delivery or postpartum. Mom was planning to breast feed.

At postpartum follow-up at 6½ weeks, mom and baby were doing well with breastfeeding. Follow-up 2 h 75 g oral glucose tolerance test was performed and revealed:

FBS-88
2 h 132.

## Normal Pregnancy Glucose Physiology

Normal pregnancy is characterized by mild fasting hypoglycemia, postprandial hyperglycemia, and elevated serum insulin levels. This increased basal level of plasma insulin (insulin resistance) is associated with several unique responses to glucose ingestion. For example, after an oral glucose meal, gravid women demonstrate prolonged hyperglycemia and hyperinsulinemia as well as lower glucagon levels [1].

The factors responsible for insulin resistance are not completely understood. Progesterone and estrogen may act, directly or indirectly, to mediate this resistance. Plasma levels of placental lactogen increase with gestation, and this protein hormone is characterized by growth hormone-like action that may result in increased lipolysis with liberation of free fatty acids [2]. Other diabetogenic hormones including growth hormone, corticotropin-releasing hormone, placental lactogen, and progesterone, as well as increased maternal adipose deposition, decreased exercise, and increased caloric intake likely contribute to the resistance. The increased concentration of circulating free fatty acids also may aid increased tissue resistance to insulin [3].

Insulin resistance reaches maximal levels in the third trimester and thus guidelines for screening are typically at this point in pregnancy (24–28 weeks gestation). Women with higher degrees of risk for GDM include the following: strong family history of type-2 DM, prior personal history of GDM, history of a large baby at delivery, member of a higher risk ethnic group, obesity, and polycystic ovarian syndrome [4].

## Prevalence of Gestational Diabetes

The prevalence of gestational diabetes is typically quoted as 3–5 % but in some studies higher percentages are reported. The prevalence varies worldwide and among racial and ethnic groups, generally in step with the prevalence of type-2 diabetes. In the USA, prevalence rates are higher in African American, Hispanic American, Native American, and Asian women than in white women [5]. Prevalence also varies because of differences in screening practices (universal versus selective screening), population characteristics (e.g., average age and body mass index (BMI) of pregnant women), testing method, and diagnostic criteria. Prevalence has been increasing over time, possibly related to increases in mean maternal age and weight.

## Risks Associated with Gestational Diabetes

Identifying pregnant women with diabetes is important because diagnosis with appropriate therapy can decrease fetal and maternal morbidity, particularly macrosomia. A study was performed which included 1,000 women with mild gestational diabetes in which subjects were randomly assigned to a group in which patients and providers were informed of the diagnosis and treatment was initiated or to a group in which patients and providers were blinded to the diagnosis and thus routine care was provided . Infants of women in the treatment group had significantly lower rates of perinatal complications (e.g., death, shoulder dystocia, bone fracture, nerve palsy; 1 % vs. 4 %) and a lower rate of macrosomia (10 % vs. 21 %) [5].

## Screening

The purpose of screening is to identify asymptomatic individuals with a high probability of having or developing a specific disease. Screening for GDM is usually performed in the United States as a two-step process Step one identifies individuals at increased risk for the disease so that step two, diagnostic testing, which is definitive but usually more complicated or costly than the screening test, can be limited to individuals with a positive initial screen. Alternatively, a diagnostic test can be administered to all individuals, which is a one-step process. Currently different organizations have different approaches to screening as listed below and procedure choice is continuing to be debated:

- *Two-step approach*—The two-step approach is the most widely used approach for identifying pregnant women with diabetes in the USA and is recommended by the ACOG (American College of Obstetrics and Gynecology). This approach uses a 50 g nonfasting screening test and if the value is >130–140 mg/dl, a 3 h 100 g test is performed. Abnormal values in the 3 h test are as follows: fasting 0.95 mg/dl, 1 h > 180 mg/dl, 2 h > 155 mg/dl, and 3 h > 140 mg/dl). A diagnosis of GDM is made when two abnormal values are present [6].
- *One-step approach*—The one-step approach has been proposed by the International Association of Diabetes in Pregnancy Study Group and endorsed by the American Diabetes Association) [4], but not by ACOG as it is a more costly approach. The one step approach consists of a 75 g 2 h oral GTT with glucose sampling at fasting and 1 and 2 h following ingestion of the 75 g. A diagnosis of GDM is made if one of the values exceeds the following cutoffs: fasting > 92 mg/dl, 1 h > 180 mg/dl, 2 h > 153 mg/dl [7].

Universal screening is recommended because 90 % of pregnant women have risk factors for glucose impairment during pregnancy.

## Treatment

The mainstay of treatment of GDM remains nutritional counseling and dietary intervention.

Most commonly carbohydrate intake is recommended to be about 40 % of total calories [8].

In clinical practice, women often require 1,800–2,500 kcal/day. For women who are at ideal body weight during pregnancy, the caloric requirement is 30 kcal/kg/day; for women who are overweight, the caloric requirement is 22–25 kcal/kg/day; and for morbidly obese women, the caloric requirement is 12–14 kcal/kg/day (present pregnant weight). For those women who are underweight, the caloric requirement may be up to 40 kcal/kg/day to achieve recommended weight gains, blood glucose goals, and nutrient intake. Weight gain for obese women (BMI > 30) is now recommended at 11–20 lbs reduced from 15 lbs [9].

Glucose targets for pregnancy range vary depending on literature reviewed but fasting numbers should be less than 90–95 mg/dl and 1 h readings postmeal between 120 and 140 mg/dl. The reason for the variable recommendations is based on recent reviews of what is normal for women without GDM during pregnancy [10].

Insulin has been the preferred medication for women with GDM who fail to achieve satisfactory glucose control with dietary intervention. Typical starting doses is generally 0.7–1.0 units/kg and shorter acting analogs (Lispro and Aspart) are safe and superior to regular insulin at reducing postprandial glucose excursions.

Oral agents (glyburide and metformin) have emerged as treatment alternatives to insulin however glyburide poses risk of hypoglycemia and in some patients is not effective in reaching goals. In addition questions have been raised recently on whether it may cross the placenta [11]. Metformin crosses the placenta and often patients require insulin as well as metformin to reach glucose targets [12]. All medication for gestational diabetes should be carefully discussed with patients with a focus on the risks and benefits.

## Postpartum Follow-Up

Women with GDM have a sevenfold increased risk of developing type-2 DM relative to women who do not have diabetes in pregnancy [12]. Factors influencing risk include body weight, family history, *glucose* levels, and the need for insulin treatment during pregnancy and lifestyle after pregnancy. Current recommendations for follow-up of women with prior GDM are a 2 h 75 g OGTT 6–12 weeks postpartum. The American Diabetes Association Recommends follow up testing for patients at least every 3 years [13].

## Lessons Learned

1. Insulin resistance becomes more pronounced in all pregnant women in the third trimester of pregnancy. Any woman (SHOULD THIS BE ALL WOMEN) with identifiable risk for Gestational diabetes should be screened with a glucose tolerance test at 24–28 weeks gestation. Different organizations recommend different testing guidelines using either a 50 g screening followed by 100 g OGTT (ACOG) or a 75 g OGTT in all subjects (ADA, IADPSG).
2. Diet and glucose monitoring is recommended treatment for all patients with GDM.
3. Medication is recommended for glucose values greater than 90 mg/dl fasting or over 120–140 mg/dl at 1 h postmeal. Treatments options should be carefully chosen and titrated to ensure safety to both the mother and fetus.
4. Postpartum screening of all patients with GDM is recommended at 6–12 weeks after delivery with a 2 h 75 g OGTT . Continued follow-up in this population is recommended due to the significant risk of developing diabetes in the future.

## Questions

1. The time of greatest insulin resistance in pregnancy is

   a. The first trimester
   b. The second trimester
   c. The third trimester*
   d. Immediately postpartum

2. Offspring born to mothers with untreated gestational diabetes have a higher risk of

   a. Shoulder dystocia
   b. Macrosomia
   c. Hypothyroidism
   d. a and b*

3. Management of Gestational diabetes includes all of the following except:

   a. Glucose testing with specific outlined targets
   b. Exercise as deemed safe during pregnancy
   c. Medication if glucose goals not achieved
   d. Strict carbohydrate restriction to less than 20 % dietary calories*

4. Postpartum women with Gestational Diabetes mellitus soon after delivery:

   a. Only require follow-up glucose testing if in a high risk group
   b. Should be screened for diabetes after delivery at 1 week postpartum with a 2 h 75 g oral glucose tolerance test
   c. Should be screened postpartum at 6–12 weeks after delivery with an HBA1C test
   d. Should be screened postpartum at 6–12 weeks after delivery with a 2 h 75 g oral glucose tolerance test*

## Answers to Questions

1. c
2. d
3. d
4. d

## References

1. Phelps RL, Metzger BE, Freinkel N. Carbohydrate metabolism in pregnancy, 17. Diurnal profiles of plasma glucose, insulin, free fatty acids, triglycerides, cholesterol, and individual amino acids in late normal pregnancy. Am J Obstet Gynecol. 1981;140:730.
2. Freinkel N. Banting lecture 1980: Of pregnancy and progeny. Diabetes. 1980;29:1023.
3. Freemark M. Regulation of maternal metabolism by pituitary and placental hormones: roles in fetal development and metabolic programming. Horm Res. 2006;65:41.
4. Metzger BE, Coustan DR. Summary and recommendations of the Fourth International Workshop-Conference on Gestational Diabetes Mellitus. The Organizing Committee. Diabetes Care. 1998;21 Suppl 2:B161–7.

5. Anna V, van der Ploeg HP, Cheung NW, et al. Sociodemographic correlates of the increasing trend in prevalence of gestational diabetes mellitus in a large population of women between 1995 and 2005. Diabetes Care. 2008;31:2288.

6. Crowther CA, Hiller JE, Moss JR, et al. Effect of treatment of gestational diabetes mellitus on pregnancy outcomes. N Engl J Med. 2005;352:2477.

7. Carpenter MW, Coustan DR. Criteria for screening tests of gestational diabetes. Am J Obstet Gynecol. 1982;144:768–73.

8. International Association of Diabetes in Pregnancy Study Group Consensus Panel, Metzger BE, Gabbe SG, Persson B, Buchanan TA, Catalano PA, et al. International Association of Diabetes in Pregnancy Study Group recommendations on the diagnosis and classification of diabetes in pregnancy. Diabetes Care. 2010;33:676–82.

9. Moses RG, Barker M, Winter M, Petocz P, Brand-Miller JC. Can a low glycemic diset reduce the need for insulin in gestational diabetes mellitus? A randomized trial. Diabetes Care. 2009;32:996–1000.

10. Rasmussen KM, Yaktine AL, editors. Weight gain during pregnancy: reexamining the recommendations. Washington, DC: The National Academic Press; 2009.

11. Yogev Y, Ben Hanoush A, Chen R, Rosenn B, Hod M, Langer O. Diurnal glycemic profile in obese and normal weight nondiabetic pregnant women. Am J Obstet Gynecol. 2004;191:949–53.

12. Hebert MF, Ma X, Naraharisetti SB, Krudys KM, Urmans JG, Hankins GD, et al. Are we optimizing gestational diabetes treatment with glyburide? The pharmacologic basis for better clinical practice. Clin Pharmacol Ther. 2009;85(6):607–14.

13. Rowan JA, Hague WM, Gao W, Battin MR, Moore MP, MiG Trial Investigators. Metformin versus insulin for treatment of gestational diabetes. N Engl J Med. 2008;358:2003–15.

# Part X
# Diabetes

# Chapter 41
# Introduction: Type-2 Diabetes

Susana A. Ebner

There are over 25 million people in the USA with diabetes, representing 8.3 % of the US population. The worldwide prevalence of diabetes was 347 million in 2010 and it is estimated to rise to 439 million by 2030. This diabetes epidemic can be largely attributed to rise in worldwide obesity [1].

Type-2 diabetes is characterized by insulin resistance and progressive beta cell failure. Obesity is associated with the state of insulin resistance seen in diabetes. The underlying metabolic abnormalities that lead to the development of insulin resistance in obese individuals are poorly understood. Accumulation of lipids in liver and skeletal muscle may play a contributing role. Beta cell failure (decrease beta cell mass and beta cell dysfunction) may also occur in genetically susceptible individuals [2].

Type-2 diabetes is associated with a number of microvascular and macrovascular complications and is the most common cause of chronic renal failure and blindness in US adults. The risk of coronary artery disease and stroke is 2–4 times higher in patients with diabetes as compared to nondiabetic individuals; macrovascular complications are the leading cause of death.

Aggressive glycemic control has been shown to decrease microvascular complications in patients with both type-1 and type-2 diabetes [3–5]. Tight glycemic control has also been shown to improve macrovascular complications in patients with type-1 diabetes [6]. However, clinical trials have thus far been inconclusive on the potential benefits of intensive glycemic control on the development macrovascular complications in patients with type-2 diabetes. Treatment of cardiovascular risk factors such as HTN and dyslipidemia may be more important for the prevention of vascular complications in patients with type-2 diabetes [7].

S.A. Ebner, M.D. (✉)
Department of Medicine, Division of Endocrinology, Columbia University Medical Center,
180 Fort Washington Avenue, Room 904, New York, NY 10032, USA
e-mail: sae2103@columbia.edu

© Springer Science+Business Media New York 2015                                      343
T.F. Davies (ed.), *A Case-Based Guide to Clinical Endocrinology*,
DOI 10.1007/978-1-4939-2059-4_41

Over the past decade, there has been a rapid growth in the number of type of therapeutic modalities designed to treat hyperglycemia. However, lifestyle modification, including dietary recommendations to promote weight loss in overweight and obese individuals and increased physical activity, forms the foundation in the management of patients with type-2 diabetes [8, 9]. Over 80 % of patients with type-2 diabetes are obese. A modest weight loss of approximately 4 kg has been associated with significant improvement in insulin sensitivity and glycemic control [10, 11]. Moreover, weight loss associated with gastric bypass surgery has recently been shown to significantly improve glycemic control in patients with diabetes [12, 13].

The cases described in this chapter present three clinical scenarios that allow for discussion of areas critical to type-2 diabetes management. Within the context of pertinent clinical practice guidelines, glycemic goals, medication classes, transition to insulin therapy, and risk factor modification are all emphasized. In particular, we stress the importance of empowering patients, individualizing treatment goals, and tailoring pharmacologic therapies based on contemporary approaches to patient-centered diabetes care [14].

# References

1. Centers for Disease Control (CDC). 2011 National Diabetes Fact Sheet [Internet]. Available at: http://www.cdc.gov/diabetes/pubs/pdf/ndfs_2011.pdf.
2. Muoio DM, Newgard CB. Molecular and metabolic mechanisms of insulin resistance and [beta]-cell failure in type 2 diabetes. Nat Rev Mol Cell Biol. 2008;9(3):193–205.
3. Effect of intensive blood-glucose control with metformin on complications in overweight patients with type 2 diabetes (UKPDS 34). UK Prospective Diabetes Study (UKPDS) Group. Lancet. 1998;352(9131):854–65.
4. Intensive blood-glucose control with sulphonylureas or insulin compared with conventional treatment and risk of complications in patients with type 2 diabetes (UKPDS 33). UK Prospective Diabetes Study (UKPDS) Group. Lancet. 1998;352(9131):837–53.
5. The effect of intensive treatment of diabetes on the development and progression of long-term complications in insulin-dependent diabetes mellitus. The Diabetes Control and Complications Trial Research Group. N Engl J Med. 1993;329(14):977–86.
6. Nathan DM, Cleary PA, Backlund JY, Genuth SM, Lachin JM, Orchard TJ, et al. Intensive diabetes treatment and cardiovascular disease in patients with type 1 diabetes. N Engl J Med. 2005;353(25):2643–53.
7. Mannucci E, Dicembrini I, Lauria A, Pozzilli P. Is glucose control important for prevention of cardiovascular disease in diabetes? Diabetes Care. 2013;36(8):S259–63.
8. Nathan DM, Buse JB, Davidson MB, Ferrannini E, Holman RR, Sherwin R, et al. Medical management of hyperglycemia in type 2 diabetes: a consensus algorithm for the initiation and adjustment of therapy: a consensus statement of the American Diabetes Association and the European Association for the Study of Diabetes. Diabetes Care. 2009;32(1):193–203.
9. Standards of medical care in diabetes–2013. Diabetes Care. 2013;36 Suppl 1:S11–66.
10. Lindstrom J, Ilanne-Parikka P, Peltonen M, Aunola S, Eriksson JG, Hemio K, et al. Sustained reduction in the incidence of type 2 diabetes by lifestyle intervention: follow-up of the Finnish Diabetes Prevention Study. Lancet. 2006;368(9548):1673–9.
11. Tuomilehto J, Lindstrom J, Eriksson JG, Valle TT, Hamalainen H, Ilanne-Parikka P, et al. Prevention of type 2 diabetes mellitus by changes in lifestyle among subjects with impaired glucose tolerance. N Engl J Med. 2001;344(18):1343–50.

12. Mingrone G, Panunzi S, De Gaetano A, Guidone C, Iaconelli A, Leccesi L, et al. Bariatric surgery versus conventional medical therapy for type 2 diabetes. N Engl J Med. 2012; 366(17):1577–85.
13. Schauer PR, Kashyap SR, Wolski K, Brethauer SA, Kirwan JP, Pothier CE, et al. Bariatric surgery versus intensive medical therapy in obese patients with diabetes. N Engl J Med. 2012;366(17):1567–76.
14. Inzucchi SE, Bergenstal RM, Buse JB, Diamant M, Ferrannini E, Nauck M, et al. Management of hyperglycemia in type 2 diabetes: a patient-centered approach: position statement of the American Diabetes Association (ADA) and the European Association for the Study of Diabetes (EASD). Diabetes Care. 2012;35(6):1364–79.

# Chapter 42
# Evaluation and Management of the Newly Diagnosed Patient with Type-2 Diabetes

Joshua D. Miller

## Objectives

1. To learn the diagnostic criteria for type-2 diabetes.
2. To understand the components of the initial evaluation of an individual with type-2 diabetes.
3. To learn how to manage newly diagnosed individuals with type-2 diabetes.

## Case Description

A 57-year-old Caucasian man was self-referred for assistance with glycemic management. He was diagnosed with type-2 diabetes 3 months prior by his primary care physician. Laboratory data at that time revealed a hemoglobin A1c (HbA1c) level of 9.7 % with a fasting plasma glucose of 258 mg/dL. The patient had noticed increased urination with increased thirst for a few weeks preceding this laboratory assessment. He also endorsed a 15-pound unintentional weight loss over the preceding 3 months. The patient was started on metformin ER 500 mg once daily by his primary care doctor. Since then, he has had occasional loose stools and bloating. He has been monitoring his blood glucose twice daily with fasting numbers ranging from 105 to 140 mg/dL and bedtime numbers as high as 184 mg/dL. The patient denies hypoglycemia.

His past medical history is significant for nephrolithiasis and he underwent a cholecystectomy 8 years ago. His family history is notable for a mother diagnosed

J.D. Miller, M.D., M.P.H. (✉)
Department of Medicine, Division of Endocrinology and Metabolism,
Stony Brook University Medical Center, 26 Research Way, Setauket,
NY 11733, USA
e-mail: joshua.miller@stonybrookmedicine.edu

© Springer Science+Business Media New York 2015                                      347
T.F. Davies (ed.), *A Case-Based Guide to Clinical Endocrinology*,
DOI 10.1007/978-1-4939-2059-4_42

with type-2 diabetes in her 50s now using insulin as well as a maternal grandfather with type-2 diabetes. His father was diagnosed with coronary artery disease at age 53. He denies any history of tobacco or illicit drug use and drinks one 8 ounce glass of red wine 2–3 times weekly. He is married and works as a teacher.

The patient's current medications include aspirin 81 mg daily, hydrochlorothiazide 25 mg daily, metformin ER 500 mg once daily, omeprazole 20 mg daily, and vitamin D3 2,000 units daily. He has no known drug allergies.

In addition to occasional loose stools and bloating, he endorses a slightly decreased energy level and occasional difficulty staying asleep. He denies polyuria, polydipsia, or polyphagia.

He is 5′10″ and weighs 233 pounds (Body Mass Index 33.4 kg/m$^2$). His blood pressure is 145/91 mmHg with a heart rate of 75 beats/min. On physical exam he is a well-appearing, obese man. He does not appear Cushingoid. Fundoscopic exam is without evidence of retinopathy. Cardiopulmonary exam is unremarkable. Abdominal exam reveals obesity, a well-healed right upper quadrant scar and no striae. Pedis dorsalis pulses were 2+ bilaterally. No peripheral edema was noted. Laboratory data from 3 months prior is remarkable for a HbA1c of 9.7 %, fasting plasma glucose of 258 mg/dL, serum creatinine of 1.0 mg/dL, LDL cholesterol of 126 mg/dL, triglycerides 209 mg/dL, HDL cholesterol 37 mg/dL, and TSH of 2.0 μIU/mL. His liver function tests and spot urine microalbumin were within normal limits. He also had a normal resting electrocardiogram. Point of care A1c at this visit is 8.6 %.

The patient was counseled extensively on the importance of healthy lifestyle and regular physical activity. After discussion of glycemic and lipid goals and medication side effects, the patient's metformin ER dose was increased to 750 mg twice daily; he was also started on simvastatin 5 mg at bedtime. He was advised to check fingerstick blood glucose more frequently. The patient was referred to an ophthalmologist for a dilated screening eye exam and to a nutritionist for further counseling.

## How Was the Diagnosis of Diabetes Made?

In 2010, the American Diabetes Association (ADA) adopted the use of HbA1c in the diagnosis of diabetes [1]. HbA1c measurement has some advantages, including no need for pretest fasting and less day-to-day variability due to stress or illness. Follow-up data has shown HbA1c testing to be both reliable and valid [2–5]. Certain conditions can falsely elevate (iron or vitamin B12 deficiency, alcoholism, uremia) or lower (hemolysis, recent blood transfusion, certain hemoglobinopathies, chronic liver disease, acute blood loss) HbA1c test results [6]. According to the ADA, diagnosis of diabetes is established in individuals with HbA1c ≥ 6.5 % or fasting plasma glucose (FPG) ≥126 mg/dL or 2-h plasma glucose ≥200 mg/dL after a 75 g oral glucose tolerance test (OGTT) or a random plasma glucose ≥200 mg/dL in individuals with classic signs/symptoms of hyperglycemia (polyuria, polydipsia,

**Table 42.1** Initial evaluation of the newly diagnosed patient with type-2 diabetes

| Laboratory studies | Basic metabolic profile, fasting lipid panel, hepatic function panel, hemoglobin A1c (HbA1c), urine microalbumin-to-creatine ratio, anti-GAD/anti-insulin antibodies[a] |
|---|---|
| Clinician referrals | Ophthalmologist, Nutritionist and/or Certified Diabetes Educator, Dentist, Mental Health Professional (when indicated) |
| *Treatment goals for most adult patients with type-2 diabetes*[b] | |
| HbA1c | <7.0 %[c] |
| Preprandial blood glucose | 70–130 mg/dL |
| 2-h postprandial blood glucose | <180 mg/dL |
| Systolic blood pressure | <140 mmHg |
| Diastolic blood pressure | <80 mmHg |
| LDL-cholesterol (high risk patients[d]) | <100 mg/dL |
| LDL-cholesterol (highest risk patients[e]) | <70 mg/dL |
| Exercise goals | ≥150 min/week of moderate activity |

*GAD* glutamic acid decarboxylase antibodies

[a]If clinical suspicion for autoimmune disease, especially in thin individuals, presence of other autoimmune diseases, or family history of type-1 diabetes

[b]According to the American Diabetes Association, diagnosis of diabetes is established in individuals with HbA1c ≥ 6.5 % or fasting plasma glucose ≥126 mg/dL or 2-h plasma glucose ≥200 mg/dL after a 75 g oral glucose tolerance test (OGTT) or a random plasma glucose ≥200 mg/dL in individuals with classic signs/symptoms of hyperglycemia (polyuria, polydipsia, unintentional weight loss) [1]

[c]In older patients, particularly those with established cardiovascular disease or risk for hypoglycemia, a less strict glycemic goal of HbA1c 7.5–8 % may be more appropriate

[d]Those without diabetes or known cardiovascular disease (CVD) but ≥2 additional major risk factors or those with diabetes and no other major CVD risk factors

[e]Those with known CVD or diabetes and one more major CVD risk factor

unintentional weight loss) (Table 42.1) [1, 7]. Our patient experienced polyuria in the setting of unintentional weight loss. His HbA1c of 9.7 % combined with FPG of 258 mg/dL further confirmed the diagnosis of diabetes.

## What Initial Clinical and Laboratory Evaluation Is Recommended for This Patient with Newly Diagnosed Type-2 Diabetes?

Initial laboratory evaluation of the patient with diabetes includes HbA1c level (if not available within the previous 3 months), fasting lipid profile, liver function tests, evaluation of urine albumin excretion (urine microalbumin-to-creatinine ratio), and assessment of renal function. Patients should undergo baseline and annual dilated eye exam by an ophthalmologist; blindness due to diabetic retinopathy is preventable with early laser photocoagulation surgery [8]. It is also recommended that individuals receive regular and comprehensive dental care and be referred to a mental health professional when indicated (Table 42.1) [7].

If there is any clinical suspicion for autoimmune disease in a person with newly diagnosed diabetes, especially in thin individuals, presence of other autoimmune diseases, or family history of type-1 diabetes, testing for insulin autoantibodies and glutamic acid decarboxylase (GAD) antibodies to rule out latent autoimmune diabetes (LADA) would be advised [9].

This patient's primary care physician appropriately sent baseline laboratory tests including HbA1c, basic metabolic profile, hepatic function panel, fasting lipids, and spot urine microalbumin.

## What Are Appropriate Glycemic Goals for This Patient?

Multiple large prospective randomized studies have demonstrated the beneficial effects of glycemic control on the development or progression of microvascular complications in patients with diabetes. Both the Diabetes Control and Complications Trial (DCCT) in patients with type-1 diabetes and the United Kingdom Prospective Diabetes Study (UKPDS) in patients with type-2 diabetes showed decreasing rates of microvascular disease (retinopathy, neuropathy, and nephropathy) in individuals who received intensive blood glucose control management [10, 11].

Although epidemiological data in patients with type-2 diabetes has shown an association between macrovascular complications and poor glycemic control, there is a lack of definitive evidence from available randomized studies of the benefits of tight glycemic control on macrovascular complications. Data from the Action in Diabetes and Vascular Disease—Preterax and Diamicron Modified Release Controlled Evaluation (ADVANCE) and Veterans Affairs Diabetes Trial (VADT) studies showed no significant decrease in cardiovascular morbidity and mortality with intensive blood glucose management [12, 13]. However, the Action to Control Cardiovascular Risk in Diabetes (ACCORD) study revealed increased mortality in subjects receiving intensive glycemic control [14]. There has since been much debate about the role of intensive glycemic control in managing patients with diabetes.

In light of the challenges presented by this conflicting data, the ADA has emphasized the importance of tailoring glycemic goals to individual patients with regards to age, established cardiovascular disease, functional status, risk for hypoglycemia, and life expectancy [15]. The ADA recommends achieving a HbA1c <7.0 % with preprandial glucose 70–130 mg/dL and peak postprandial glucose <180 mg/dL in most nonpregnant adults with diabetes (Table 42.1). In older individuals, particularly those with established cardiovascular disease or risk for hypoglycemia, a less strict glycemic goal (HbA1c 7.5–8 %) may be more appropriate [7].

In this newly diagnosed middle-aged patient with obesity and a family history of cardiovascular disease, it was reasonable to target an HbA1c <7 %. After 3 months of metformin therapy, his HbA1c had decreased from 9.7 % to 8.6 %. Thus, in addition to counseling regarding the importance of physical activity and lifestyle change, the patient's metformin ER dose was increased on this visit.

## What Are the Various Treatment Options for Newly Diagnosed Patients with Type-2 Diabetes?

Care for individuals with diabetes should be provided in collaboration with the patient's primary care physician, nutritionist, ophthalmologist, diabetes educator, and when indicated, a mental health professional. It is vital that patients take an active role in diabetes self-management.

Recent collaboration between the ADA and the European Association for the Study of Diabetes (EASD) established the importance of individualized treatment goals in the management of type-2 diabetes [16]. Among the issues to consider when developing a diabetes treatment plan are medication side-effect profiles and cost, risk of hypoglycemia, patient's attitude, and expected treatment efforts and patients' functional status.

All patients should be offered basic education about diabetes self-management. The mainstay of treatment in type-2 diabetes is attention to lifestyle change, including dietary counseling and increasing physical activity (ideally, at least 150 min/week of moderate activity) [7]. The American College of Sports Medicine and the ADA both endorse increased physical activity for its role in improving glycemic control, positively affecting lipids and blood pressure and preventing cardiovascular mortality in patients with diabetes [17].

Metformin has been the first-line pharmacologic therapy of choice for patients with type-2 diabetes for some time. The UKPDS demonstrated the benefits of metformin on cardiovascular outcomes in diabetes-related endpoints [18]. On the cellular level, metformin, a biguanide, is thought to activate AMP-kinase thereby decreasing hepatic gluconeogenesis [19]. Newer data suggests that it may also act by suppressing hepatic glucagon signaling [20]. Metformin does not cause hypoglycemia and is weight neutral. While it has been shown to cause lactic acidosis, this side effect is exceedingly rare. As such, metformin is not recommended in patient with renal insufficiency or a history of alcohol abuse. Common side effects of the medication include bloating and gastrointestinal upset [21, 22]. Gastrointestinal side effects tend to resolve in most patients over a short period of time and individuals should be counseled about their occurrence. Metformin is available in immediate and extended-release formulations. While the extended-release formulation can be dosed once daily, many clinicians prefer dosing the medication twice daily.

When patients fail to achieve glycemic goals with metformin alone, another agent should be considered. Treatment options are varied and include multiple classes of medications such as sulfonylureas/insulin secretogogues, thiazolidinediones (TZDs), and the newer incretin-mimetics/GLP-1 receptor agonists, and oral dipeptidyl peptidase 4 (DPP-4) inhibitors. Choice of drug is dependent on multiple patient-specific factors including age, renal function, and functional status, as well as medication-specific factors such as cost, pharmacokinetics, and side-effect profile [7].

Sulfonylureas have the potential to cause hypoglycemia and weight gain and secondary failure with this class of medications is common; thus, their use is limited [23]. TZDs activate peroxisome proliferator-activated receptor-γ (PPAR-γ) causing improvement in peripheral insulin sensitivity [24]. They also decrease hepatic gluconeogenesis [25]. Unfortunately, TZDs have been associated with increased risk of bladder cancer and myocardial infarction [26, 27]. Combined with the known side-effects of fluid retention, weight gain, and increased risk of bone fracture, TZDs have generally fallen out of favor among many diabetologists as second-line agents and have been replaced by some of the newer diabetes medication classes.

The newer incretin mimetics enhance pancreatic insulin secretion, suppress glucagon output, and delay gastric emptying by mimicking the effects of endogenous glucagon-like-peptide 1 (GLP-1) [28]. Exenatide, liraglutide, and long-acting exenatide can also cause nausea and vomiting in some patients and are both injectable medications. Overall however, many patients experience weight-loss, making GLP-1 agonists an appealing addition to existing diabetes treatment regimens.

Oral DPP-4 inhibitors/gliptins act similarly to incretin mimetics by upregulating insulin and decreasing glucagon secretion [29]. They do so by increasing circulating levels of GLP-1 and gastric inhibitory peptide (GIP). In addition to their oral formulation, these medications tend to be weight-neutral, adding to their appeal.

It was appropriate for this patient's primary care physician to initiate metformin therapy at time of diagnosis. Now, 3 months after treatment, combined with attention to lifestyle management, it is reasonable to consider up-titration of his metformin dose. If he were not to experience improvement in HbA1c at future visits, one might consider further titration of his metformin or consider adding another oral agent to his regimen at that time.

## Should This Patient Be Screened for Cardiovascular Disease?

Diabetes is widely recognized as a cardiovascular disease equivalent and it is important to risk stratify individuals with the disease. The ultimate goal of cardiovascular risk stratification is to identify high cardiac risk patients who might benefit from increased surveillance or coronary revascularization. The ADA, however, does not recommend routine screening of asymptomatic patients for cardiovascular disease [7, 30]. Data from the Bypass Angioplasty Revascularization Investigation 2 Diabetes (BARI 2-D) trial found no significant difference in rates of death from major cardiovascular events between patients undergoing coronary revascularization and those undergoing medical therapy [31]. Thus, aggressive cardiac risk factor modification should be pursued in patients with diabetes.

Our patient's baseline laboratory evaluation revealed normal renal function and resting ECG and a fundoscopic examination was without evidence of retinopathy.

He does not endorse any cardiac symptoms. His family history is significant for a father with premature coronary disease. Therefore, modifiable risk factors such as elevated LDL cholesterol and obesity should be aggressively managed. He is already on low dose antiplatelet therapy. In the absence of cardiac symptoms, he should not be referred for cardiac testing at this time.

## Should This Patient with an LDL Cholesterol of 126 mg/dL Be Treated with Cholesterol-Lowering Therapy?

LDL cholesterol is a major predictor of cardiovascular disease, especially in patients with diabetes. LDL-lowering therapies, particularly statins, are beneficial in both primary and secondary prevention of cardiovascular disease. The ADA recommends that patients with diabetes have annual fasting lipid profiles [7]. In highest risk patients (those with known cardiovascular disease), it is reasonable to target an LDL cholesterol goal of <70 mg/dL and a non-HDL cholesterol goal of <100 mg/dL (Table 42.1). Patients with diabetes over the age of 40 without overt cardiovascular disease should target an LDL cholesterol goal of <100 mg/dL and a non-HDL cholesterol goal of <130 mg/dL [7, 32]. The Framingham risk score has been widely validated in assessing an individual's risk of major coronary event (fatal or nonfatal myocardial infarction) over a 10-year period [33, 34]. Experts consider a 10-year risk of major coronary event ≥20 % to be an appropriate cut-off for aggressive intervention directed at the abnormal prognostic factors. This patient has multiple cardiovascular disease risk factors including a history of hypertension as well as a family history of cardiovascular disease. His Framingham risk score is 15 %. Hence, he was started on statin therapy with a target LDL cholesterol of <100 mg/dL. Treatments aimed at addressing elevated triglyceride and low HDL cholesterol levels are generally considered of less import [32]. Moreover, statins are the initial therapy of choice for patients with elevated triglycerides and low HDL cholesterol. Our patient's HDL cholesterol of 37 mg/dL is slightly below the ADA recommended cutoff of 40 mg/dL. His triglyceride level of 209 mg/dL is also slightly above the ADA recommended cutoff of 150 mg/dL. Thus, statin therapy was initiated.

## Should We Continue This Patient's Low Dose Aspirin Therapy?

There are numerous studies examining the role of antiplatelet therapy in primary and secondary prevention of cardiovascular disease in patients with diabetes. The Antithrombotic Trialists' (ATT) collaboration conducted a meta-analysis of available data on the evidence of aspirin for the prevention of vascular disease in high risk patients [35]. In their analysis, data from primary prevention trials revealed a

12 % reduction in serious vascular events (mainly myocardial infarction). Secondary prevention data revealed that aspirin use conferred a significant absolute risk reduction in serious vascular events (6.7 % vs. 8.2 %, $p < 0.0001$). In 2010, a collaborative effort between the ADA, American Heart Association and American College of Cardiology further examined the existing data (inclusive of ATT trials) for the use of aspirin in prevention of cardiovascular disease [36]. Data from their meta-analysis revealed a reduction in risk of cardiovascular events of 9 % (myocardial infarction) and reduction in risk of stroke of 10 %, though neither was statistically significant.

The ADA now recommends low-dose aspirin (75–162 mg/day) for primary prevention of cardiovascular disease in men over age 50 years and women over age 60 years with one other major risk factor (HTN, tobacco use, dyslipidemia, family history of early cardiovascular disease, or albuminuria) [7, 36]. Caution should be exercised in patients at increased risk for gastrointestinal and intracranial bleeding as these are the main adverse events associated with aspirin use. In the absence of the above contraindications, it is appropriate for this patient to continue taking low-dose aspirin.

## What Are the Target Blood Pressure Goals for This Patient with Newly Diagnosed Type-2 Diabetes?

Blood pressure control is an integral part of comprehensive diabetes management. Poorly controlled hypertension can lead to increased risk of macrovascular complications such as myocardial infarction and stroke as well as microvascular diabetes-associated complications such as nephropathy, retinopathy, and autonomic neuropathy [37]. Recent data from the ACCORD and ADVANCE trials support the establishment of target systolic blood pressure of <140 mmHg and diastolic blood pressure <80 mmHg in most individuals with type 2 diabetes [7, 38, 39]. More aggressive systolic endpoints can be appropriately targeted in younger individuals in whom longer term blood pressure control might provide an added renal protective benefit. Additionally, the importance of lifestyle modification through diet and exercise cannot be overemphasized. Amidst the numerous antihypertensive agents available, several studies have shown an added benefit to angiotensin converting enzyme inhibitors (ACE-i) and angiotensin receptor blockers (ARBs) in patients with diabetes, especially those with evidence of renal disease or albuminuria [40, 41].

On this visit, our patient's systolic blood pressure is slightly above goal (145 mmHg) while on 25 mg of hydrochlorthiazide daily. If on follow-up visit his blood pressure is still above goal, one might consider adding a second antihypertensive agent to his regimen. Given his history of diabetes, an ACE-I would be a reasonable choice at that time.

## Questions

1. Which of the following statements concerning incretin mimetics is correct?

    a. They can worsen pre-existing heart failure in some patients.
    b. They improve insulin sensitivity in skeletal muscle.
    c. They can cause hypoglycemia and weight gain.
    d. They delay gastric emptying and enhance pancreatic insulin secretion.

2. In which of the following patients with diabetes is cardiac testing indicated?

    a. An asymptomatic 43-year-old woman with microalbuminuria.
    b. A 67-year-old man with dyspnea on exertion and a remote smoking history.
    c. A 59-year-old woman with a Body Mass Index of 39 kg/m$^2$ and HbA1c of 8.7 %.
    d. A 49-year-old male business executive with hypoglycemia unawareness.

3. Which of the following sets of laboratory analyses is most appropriate for a patient newly diagnosed with diabetes?

    a. Basic metabolic profile, HbA1c, fasting lipid panel, urinalysis, and hepatic function panel.
    b. Basic metabolic profile, HbA1c, thyroid-stimulating hormone, and fasting insulin levels.
    c. Hepatic function panel, HbA1c, thyroid-stimulating hormone, and AM cortisol.
    d. Basic metabolic profile, HbA1c, anti-GAD antibody, and c-peptide of insulin.

## Answers to Questions

1. d.
2. b.
3. a.

## References

1. Diagnosis and classification of diabetes mellitus. Diabetes Care. 2013;36 Suppl 1:S67–74.
2. International Expert Committee report on the role of the A1C assay in the diagnosis of diabetes. Diabetes Care. 2009;32(7):1327–34.
3. Nathan DM, Singer DE, Hurxthal K, Goodson JD. The clinical information value of the glycosylated hemoglobin assay. N Engl J Med. 1984;310(6):341–6.
4. Rohlfing CL, Wiedmeyer HM, Little RR, England JD, Tennill A, Goldstein DE. Defining the relationship between plasma glucose and HbA(1c): analysis of glucose profiles and HbA(1c) in the Diabetes Control and Complications Trial. Diabetes Care. 2002;25(2):275–8.

5. Nathan DM, Turgeon H, Regan S. Relationship between glycated haemoglobin levels and mean glucose levels over time. Diabetologia. 2007;50(11):2239–44.
6. Sacks DB, Arnold M, Bakris GL, Bruns DE, Horvath AR, Kirkman MS, et al. Position statement executive summary: guidelines and recommendations for laboratory analysis in the diagnosis and management of diabetes mellitus. Diabetes Care. 2011;34(6):1419–23.
7. Standards of medical care in diabetes–2013. Diabetes Care. 2013;36 Suppl 1:S11–66.
8. Photocoagulation for diabetic macular edema. Early Treatment Diabetic Retinopathy Study report number 1. Early Treatment Diabetic Retinopathy Study research group. Arch Ophthalmol. 1985;103(12):1796–806.
9. Stenstrom G, Gottsater A, Bakhtadze E, Berger B, Sundkvist G. Latent autoimmune diabetes in adults: definition, prevalence, beta-cell function, and treatment. Diabetes. 2005;54 Suppl 2:S68–72.
10. Effect of intensive blood-glucose control with metformin on complications in overweight patients with type 2 diabetes (UKPDS 34). UK Prospective Diabetes Study (UKPDS) Group. Lancet. 1998;352(9131):854–65.
11. The effect of intensive treatment of diabetes on the development and progression of long-term complications in insulin-dependent diabetes mellitus. The Diabetes Control and Complications Trial Research Group. N Engl J Med. 1993;329(14):977–86.
12. Duckworth W, Abraira C, Moritz T, Reda D, Emanuele N, Reaven PD, et al. Glucose control and vascular complications in veterans with type 2 diabetes. N Engl J Med. 2009;360(2): 129–39.
13. Patel A, MacMahon S, Chalmers J, Neal B, Billot L, Woodward M, et al. Intensive blood glucose control and vascular outcomes in patients with type 2 diabetes. N Engl J Med. 2008; 358(24):2560–72.
14. Gerstein HC, Miller ME, Genuth S, Ismail-Beigi F, Buse JB, Goff Jr DC, et al. Long-term effects of intensive glucose lowering on cardiovascular outcomes. N Engl J Med. 2011;364(9):818–28.
15. Lund SS, Vaag AA. Intensive glycemic control and the prevention of cardiovascular events: implications of the ACCORD, ADVANCE, and VA diabetes trials: a position statement of the American Diabetes Association and a scientific statement of the American College of Cardiology Foundation and the American Heart Association: response to Skyler et al. Diabetes Care. 2009;32(7):e90–1; author reply e2–3.
16. Inzucchi SE, Bergenstal RM, Buse JB, Diamant M, Ferrannini E, Nauck M, et al. Management of hyperglycemia in type 2 diabetes: a patient-centered approach: position statement of the American Diabetes Association (ADA) and the European Association for the Study of Diabetes (EASD). Diabetes Care. 2012;35(6):1364–79.
17. Colberg SR, Albright AL, Blissmer BJ, Braun B, Chasan-Taber L, Fernhall B, et al. Exercise and type 2 diabetes: American College of Sports Medicine and the American Diabetes Association: joint position statement. Exercise and type 2 diabetes. Med Sci Sports Exerc. 2010;42(12):2282–303.
18. Holman R. Metformin as first choice in oral diabetes treatment: the UKPDS experience. Journ Annu Diabetol Hotel Dieu. 2007;13–20.
19. Zhou G, Myers R, Li Y, Chen Y, Shen X, Fenyk-Melody J, et al. Role of AMP-activated protein kinase in mechanism of metformin action. J Clin Invest. 2001;108(8):1167–74.
20. Miller RA, Chu Q, Xie J, Foretz M, Viollet B, Birnbaum MJ. Biguanides suppress hepatic glucagon signalling by decreasing production of cyclic AMP. Nature. 2013;494(7436): 256–60.
21. Bailey CJ, Turner RC. Metformin. N Engl J Med. 1996;334(9):574–9.
22. Product information: Glucophage. New Brunswick, NJ: Bristol-Myers Squibb Company. http://packageinserts.bms.com/pi/pi_glucophage.pdf
23. Gangji AS, Cukierman T, Gerstein HC, Goldsmith CH, Clase CM. A systematic review and meta-analysis of hypoglycemia and cardiovascular events: a comparison of glyburide with other secretagogues and with insulin. Diabetes Care. 2007;30(2):389–94.
24. Yki-Jarvinen H. Thiazolidinediones. N Engl J Med. 2004;351(11):1106–18.

25. Kahn CR, Chen L, Cohen SE. Unraveling the mechanism of action of thiazolidinediones. J Clin Invest. 2000;106(11):1305–7.
26. Colmers IN, Bowker SL, Majumdar SR, Johnson JA. Use of thiazolidinediones and the risk of bladder cancer among people with type 2 diabetes: a meta-analysis. CMAJ. 2012;184(12): E675–83.
27. Kaul S, Bolger AF, Herrington D, Giugliano RP, Eckel RH. Thiazolidinedione drugs and cardiovascular risks: a science advisory from the American Heart Association and American College of Cardiology Foundation. Circulation. 2010;121(16):1868–77.
28. Bloomgarden ZT, Blonde L, Garber AJ, Wysham CH. Current issues in GLP-1 receptor agonist therapy for type 2 diabetes. Endocr Pract. 2012;18 Suppl 3:6–26.
29. Demuth HU, McIntosh CH, Pederson RA. Type 2 diabetes–therapy with dipeptidyl peptidase IV inhibitors. Biochim Biophys Acta. 2005;1751(1):33–44.
30. Bax JJ, Young LH, Frye RL, Bonow RO, Steinberg HO, Barrett EJ. Screening for coronary artery disease in patients with diabetes. Diabetes Care. 2007;30(10):2729–36.
31. Dagenais GR, Lu J, Faxon DP, Bogaty P, Adler D, Fuentes F, et al. Prognostic impact of the presence and absence of angina on mortality and cardiovascular outcomes in patients with type 2 diabetes and stable coronary artery disease: results from the BARI 2D (Bypass Angioplasty Revascularization Investigation 2 Diabetes) Trial. J Am Coll Cardiol. 2013;61(7):702–11.
32. Brunzell JD, Davidson M, Furberg CD, Goldberg RB, Howard BV, Stein JH, et al. Lipoprotein management in patients with cardiometabolic risk: consensus conference report from the American Diabetes Association and the American College of Cardiology Foundation. J Am Coll Cardiol. 2008;51(15):1512–24.
33. Third Report of the National Cholesterol Education Program (NCEP) Expert Panel on Detection, Evaluation, and Treatment of High Blood Cholesterol in Adults (Adult Treatment Panel III) final report. Circulation. 2002;106(25):3143–421.
34. Wilson PW, D'Agostino RB, Levy D, Belanger AM, Silbershatz H, Kannel WB. Prediction of coronary heart disease using risk factor categories. Circulation. 1998;97(18):1837–47.
35. Baigent C, Blackwell L, Collins R, Emberson J, Godwin J, Peto R, et al. Aspirin in the primary and secondary prevention of vascular disease: collaborative meta-analysis of individual participant data from randomised trials. Lancet. 2009;373(9678):1849–60.
36. Pignone M, Alberts MJ, Colwell JA, Cushman M, Inzucchi SE, Mukherjee D, et al. Aspirin for primary prevention of cardiovascular events in people with diabetes: a position statement of the American Diabetes Association, a scientific statement of the American Heart Association, and an expert consensus document of the American College of Cardiology Foundation. Circulation. 2010;121(24):2694–701.
37. Adler AI, Stratton IM, Neil HA, Yudkin JS, Matthews DR, Cull CA, et al. Association of systolic blood pressure with macrovascular and microvascular complications of type 2 diabetes (UKPDS 36): prospective observational study. BMJ. 2000;321(7258):412–9.
38. Cushman WC, Evans GW, Byington RP, Goff Jr DC, Grimm Jr RH, Cutler JA, et al. Effects of intensive blood-pressure control in type 2 diabetes mellitus. N Engl J Med. 2010;362(17): 1575–85.
39. Patel A, MacMahon S, Chalmers J, Neal B, Woodward M, Billot L, et al. Effects of a fixed combination of perindopril and indapamide on macrovascular and microvascular outcomes in patients with type 2 diabetes mellitus (the ADVANCE trial): a randomised controlled trial. Lancet. 2007;370(9590):829–40.
40. Tatti P, Pahor M, Byington RP, Di Mauro P, Guarisco R, Strollo G, et al. Outcome results of the Fosinopril Versus Amlodipine Cardiovascular Events Randomized Trial (FACET) in patients with hypertension and NIDDM. Diabetes Care. 1998;21(4):597–603.
41. Effects of ramipril on cardiovascular and microvascular outcomes in people with diabetes mellitus: results of the HOPE study and MICRO-HOPE substudy. Heart Outcomes Prevention Evaluation Study Investigators. Lancet. 2000;355(9200):253–9.

# Chapter 43
# Transition to Insulin in Patients with Type-2 Diabetes

**Susana A. Ebner and Joshua D. Miller**

## Objectives

1. To gain an appreciation for the progressive nature of glucose deterioration in patients with type-2 diabetes.
2. To learn about the different oral treatment options for patients with type-2 diabetes.
3. To learn when and how to transition patients with type-2 diabetes to insulin therapy.

## Case Description

A 65-year-old Caucasian woman presented to our clinic for management of her type-2 diabetes. The patient was diagnosed with diabetes 8 years prior to her presentation by routine blood work. She was initially started on metformin 500 mg twice daily at the time of diagnosis. Metformin dose was increased to 1,000 mg twice daily 3 years after diagnosis. She had experienced good glycemic control until

S.A. Ebner, M.D. (✉)
Department of Medicine, Division of Endocrinology, Columbia University Medical Center, 180 Fort Washington Avenue, Room 904, New York, NY 10032, USA
e-mail: sae2103@columbia.edu

J.D. Miller, M.D., M.P.H.
Department of Medicine, Division of Endocrinology and Metabolism,
Stony Brook University Medical Center, 26 Research Way, Setauket, NY 11733, USA

© Springer Science+Business Media New York 2015                                      359
T.F. Davies (ed.), *A Case-Based Guide to Clinical Endocrinology*,
DOI 10.1007/978-1-4939-2059-4_43

1 year ago. Her hemoglobin A1c (HbA1c) level was 6.8 % 1 year prior to this visit. The patient was feeling well. She denied polyuria, polydipsia, visual changes, or hypoglycemia. She further denied burning pain in her lower extremities or distal paresthesias. Her fasting blood glucose levels ranged from 170 to 190 mg/dL.

Her past medical history was significant for hypertension, dyslipidemia, and nephrolithiasis. She experienced surgical menopause at age 40 for history of endometriosis. She was never placed on estrogen replacement therapy. Her family history was positive for maternal type-2 diabetes, osteoporosis, and coronary artery disease (CAD). Her medications included atorvastatin 10 mg daily, fenofibrate 145 mg daily, valsartan 160 mg daily, and metformin ER 1,000 mg twice daily. On physical examination, she was 5′3″ and weighed 163 lbs (Body Mass Index 28.9 kg/m$^2$). Her blood pressure was 140/80 mmHg and heart rate was 72 beats/min and regular. Her neck showed no evidence of acanthosis or thyromegaly. Her fundoscopic exam did not reveal retinopathy. Her foot exam showed 2+ distal pulses and normal monofilament testing. On laboratory tests, her creatinine level was 0.9 mg/dL, LDL cholesterol was 65 mg/dL, HDL cholesterol was 37 mg/dL, and triglycerides were 139 mg/dL. Her HbA1c was 8.2 %. Spot urine did not reveal evidence of microalbuminuria.

Because of her elevated fasting blood glucose and HbA1c, our plan on her first visit was to add glipizide ER 5 mg daily and to continue metformin. At her 3-month follow-up visit, the patient complained of episodic mid-morning hypoglycemia. Glipizide ER was discontinued and glimepiride 0.5 mg daily was started. Episodes of symptomatic mid-day hypoglycemia (with blood glucose levels ranging from 47 to 63 mg/dL) persisted. Glimepiride was stopped and metformin ER 1,000 mg twice daily continued. She continued to have fasting hyperglycemia. Her HbA1c was 8.1 %. Sitagliptin 100 mg daily was then added to her regimen.

At a second 3-month follow-up visit, the patient reported nausea and headaches following initiation of sitagliptin. These symptoms resolved after discontinuing the medication. She had an intentional weight loss of 10 lbs over a 6-month period as a result of healthier eating and lifestyle change. The patient was testing her glucose at home and her average blood glucose level was 190 mg/dL. Her HbA1c was now 8.3 %. A spot urine microalbumin/creatinine ratio was elevated at 72 mg/g. A repeat urinalysis confirmed her microalbuminuria. Consideration was given to adding pioglitazone to her regimen; however, the patient was reluctant due to fear of potential weight gain. After discussing the advantages and disadvantages of insulin treatment, the patient agreed to initiate insulin. The patient was educated about how to self-administer insulin via insulin pen delivery and insulin glargine, 10 units subcutaneously at bedtime was added to metformin ER 1,000 mg twice daily.

At her most recent follow-up visit, she reported feeling well. Her weight increased by 2 lbs. Her fasting blood glucose levels were mostly <130 mg/dL. Her bedtime blood glucose levels ranged from 200 to 220 mg/dL. Her HbA1c was 7.6 %. Aspart insulin was added before dinner. The patient was taught to count carbohydrates and a ratio of 1:10 (units of insulin:grams of carbohydrates) was used to calculate her dinnertime aspart bolus dose.

# What Are Some of the Pharmacologic Treatment Approaches to Type-2 Diabetes?

Type-2 diabetes is characterized by progressive blood glucose deterioration due to progressive pancreatic beta cell failure in the presence of persistent insulin resistance [1]. The patient reported in this case is typical of many patients with type-2 diabetes who need to be transitioned from oral antihyperglycemic agents to insulin. The number of different antidiabetic medications has grown exponentially in the past decade. There are currently six main classes of antihyperglycemic oral medications (Table 43.1). Patients with diabetes are best treated with an individualized approach, not only in terms of the medication choice but also specific glycemic goals [2]. Understanding the mechanism of action, advantages, medication interactions, side effects, and contraindications is key to designing an acceptable and effective diabetes treatment. Prescription cost may also play a role in deciding treatment options.

Although insulin can be added as an initial step in the hyperglycemic patient with type-2 diabetes, patients and physicians are usually reluctant to or fearful of starting injectable medications. Most commonly, insulin treatment is initiated after a combination of two or three oral medications have failed to achieve adequate glycemic control [2]. However, insulin should be recommended as initial therapy in patients with type-2 diabetes if they are symptomatic with polyuria and polydipsia and particularly if they are glucotoxic (blood glucose levels >300 mg/dL) or if they present in a catabolic state (i.e., ketosis).

In addition to lifestyle modification, metformin (the only medication of the biguanide class) is usually the first therapeutic intervention recommended to patients with type-2 diabetes [3]. Metformin is an insulin sensitizer that reduces fasting hyperglycemia by decreasing hepatic glucose production. Its HbA1c lowering effect is between 1 and 1.5 % when given as monotherapy. It can also promote mild weight loss in some patients. Furthermore, metformin has been shown to have cardioprotective effects, independent of glycemic improvement. This drug may cause gastrointestinal symptoms (in up to 50 % of patients), including bloating and diarrhea, but these are usually transient and less than 10 % of patients discontinue the medication due to side effects. Metformin is contraindicated in patients with advanced renal dysfunction and decompensated heart failure due to the potential yet rare life-threatening side effect of lactic acidosis [4]. The patient in this case was able to tolerate metformin, and her glycemic control improved. Unfortunately, however, her glycemic control deteriorated with time.

If glycemic endpoints have not been reached with metformin alone, sulfonylureas can be added [3]. The risk of hypoglycemia increases with this combination therapy, as observed in this case. Longer acting sulfonylureas (i.e., glyburide) are more likely to cause hypoglycemia, especially in the elderly and in patients with renal dysfunction [5]. Glipizide is mainly metabolized by the liver and is therefore a safer drug to use in patients with impaired renal function. Weight gain may also occur in patients taking sulfonylureas. Secondary failure with this class of medication is

**Table 43.1** Oral antihyperglycemic and non-insulin injectable medications

| Generic name | Brand name | Starting dose | Max. dose | Duration of action |
|---|---|---|---|---|
| *Sulfonylureas* | | | | |
| Glimepiride 1, 2, 4 mg | Amaryl® | 1–2 mg qd | 8 mg qd | 24 h |
| Glipizide 5,10 mg | Glucotrol® | 5 mg qd elderly: 2.5 mg | 20 mg bid | 12–24 h |
| Glipizide extended release 2.5, 5, 10 mg | Glucotrol XL® | 5 mg qd elderly: 2.5 mg | 20 mg qd | 24 h |
| Glyburide 1.25, 2.5, 5 mg | Diabeta®, Micronase® | 2.5–5 mg qd | 10 mg bid | 16–24 h |
| *Metiglinides* | | | | |
| Repaglinide 0.5, 1, 2 mg | Prandin® | 0.5 mg tid with meals | 4 mg tid | 2–4 h |
| Nateglinide 60, 120 mg | Starlix® | 60 mg tid with meals | 120 mg tid | 2–4 h |
| *Thiazolidinediones* | | | | |
| Pioglitazone 15, 30, 45 mg | Actos® | 15 mg qd | 45 mg qd | 24 h |
| Rosiglitazone 2, 4, 8 mg | Avandia® | 4 mg qd | 8 mg qd | 12–24 h |
| *Biguanides* | | | | |
| Metformin 500, 850, 1,000 mg, or 500 mg/5 mL | Glucophage®, Riomet® oral solution | 500 mg qd | 2,500 mg qd | 12–18 h |
| Metformin extended release 500, 750 mg | Glucophage® XR | 500 mg qd | 2,000 mg/day | 24 h |
| *Alpha-glucosidase inhibitors* | | | | |
| Acarbose 25, 50, 100 mg | Precose® | 25 mg tid with meals | 100 mg tid | |
| Miglitol 25, 50, 100 mg | Glyset® | 25 mg tid with meals | 100 mg tid | |
| *Dipeptidyl peptidase-IV inhibitors (DDP-4)* | | | | |
| Sitagliptin 25, 50, 100 mg | Januvia® | 100 mg qd 25–50 mg in CRI | 100 mg qd | 24 h |
| Saxagliptin 2.5, 5 mg | Onglyza® | 2.5–5 mg qd | 5 mg qd | 24 h |
| Linagliptin 5 mg | Tradjenta® | 5 mg | 5 mg qd | 24 h |
| Alogliptin 6.25, 12.5, 25 mg | Nesina® | 25 mg 6.25–12.5 mg in CRI | 25 mg qd | 24 h |
| *Incretin mimetics (GLP-1 receptor agonists)* | | | | |
| Exenatide 5 mcg/0.02 mL or 10 mcg/0.04 mL | Byetta® | 5 μg SQ bid | 10 μg SQ bid | 12 h |
| Liraglutide 6 mg/mL | Victoza® | 0.6 mg qd | 1.8 mg | 24 h |
| Exenatide extended release 2 mg/0.65 mL | Bydureon® | 2 mg | 2 mg | 7 days |

common. This patient was unable to tolerate the lowest dose available of glimepiride and the medication needed to be discontinued.

Meglitinides (i.e., repaglinide) enhance insulin secretion by a similar mechanism to sulfonylureas, but have a shorter half-life and lesser incidence of hypoglycemia [6]. Given with meals, they are useful for addressing postprandial hyperglycemia. However, the lowering effect on fasting glucose levels is minimal. Because our patient had fasting hyperglycemia, this class of medication would not have been helpful.

Thiazolidinediones (TZDs) are agonists for the peroxisome proliferator-activated receptor (PPAR) gamma and increase insulin action in liver and skeletal muscle [7]. Pioglitazone and rosiglitazone belong to this class of drugs, but rosiglitazone is currently only available through a special program, owing to its increase cardiovascular risk. TZDs lower HbA1c levels by 1.5–2 %. They are associated with weight gain and edema and may exacerbate congestive heart failure. Additionally, increased rates of fractures have been reported with TZDs. The patient in this case was trying to lose weight and has risk factors for osteoporosis; therefore, this class of medication would not have been an ideal choice for this patient.

DPP-4 inhibitors are a newer class of oral antihyperglycemic agents [8, 9]. There are four available drugs on this class: sitagliptin, saxagliptin, linagliptin, and the recently FDA-approved alogliptin. Medications in this group increase incretin (glucagon-like peptide-1) action by inhibiting the dipeptidylpeptidase-4 (DPP-4) enzyme, resulting in enhanced insulin secretion suppression of glucagon production. Medications in this class are considered weight neutral and are unlikely to cause hypoglycemia when used as monotherapy. They primarily address postprandial hyperglycemia (via increase of glucose-stimulated insulin release); a mild improvement of fasting hyperglycemia is also mediated by glucagon suppression. The HbA1c decrease obtained with DPP-4 inhibitors ranges from 0.6 % to 1 %. Of note, upper respiratory infections, nasopharyngitis and headaches are reported side effects. Acute pancreatitis has been associated with this class of medications. Our patient experienced headaches, which resolved with discontinuation of the medication.

GLP-1 receptor agonists also target the incretin system. Available medications in this class include exenatide (dosed twice daily), liraglutide, (dosed once daily), and the newer once weekly extended-release exenatide [10]. These are injectable medications that bind to the GLP-1 receptor and stimulate insulin release in a glucose-dependent manner. They also decrease glucagon secretion and gastric emptying. Their HbA1c lowering effect is between 0.5 and 1.5 %. GLP-1 receptor agonist is associated with significant weight loss. They can sometimes cause minor hypoglycemia as monotherapy. Commonly, they can initially cause nausea and vomiting. They may be associated with pancreatitis and should be used with caution in patients with renal dysfunction [11]. The patient in the case was already successfully losing weight through lifestyle change. She struggled with postprandial hypoglycemia when taking sulfonlyureas. Thus, this medication class was not recommended.

# When to Consider Transitioning to Insulin Therapy?

Insulin therapy was the most appropriate next step toward helping this patient improve her glycemic control. In addition to deteriorating glycemic control above goal, the patient started to show evidence of diabetes-related microvascular complications (microalbuminuria); inaction would be unacceptable in her case. Although absolute insulin deficiency is uncommonly seen in patients with type-2 diabetes, there is progressive loss of beta cell function and insulin production with subsequent deterioration of glucose control. The United Kingdom Prospective Diabetes Survey (UKPDS) provided evidence that the gradual worsening of glycemic control in patients with type-2 diabetes was likely a result of progressive loss of insulin producing pancreatic beta cells [12]. Thus, the need for insulin therapy after a diabetes duration of 10–15 years is common.

Insulin therapy has no maximal dose. There are no contraindications to insulin, except for insulin allergies, which are exceedingly rare with use of human insulins produce by recombinant DNA technology and the newer insulin analogues. Initiation of insulin may cause weight gain and fluid retention. When starting insulin therapy in patients with type-2 diabetes, basal insulin is either initiated alone or added to one or more oral medications (most commonly metformin). Insulin NPH (intermediate-acting), glargine or detemir (long-acting insulins) may be added at a dose of 0.15–0.25 units/kg at night. Periodic up-titration of the bedtime insulin dose by ~10–20 % at a time is done based on fasting blood glucose levels to a predetermined goal, optimally <130 mg/dL [13, 14]. Previous data comparing the benefits of NPH versus glargine insulin at bedtime, added to one or two oral medications showed similar effects in terms of blood glucose target and HbA1c [15, 16]. However, NPH insulin at bedtime was associated with increased incidence of hypoglycemia. A Cochrane Review published in 2007 compared long-acting insulin analogues with NPH insulin in patients with type-2 diabetes [17]. The authors found that there was no significant benefit of long-acting insulins over NPH, except for a slight decrease in incidence of nocturnal hypoglycemia. Obese patients with type-2 diabetes who failed oral antihyperglycemic agents and are uncontrolled with escalating doses of long-acting insulin analogs may benefit from switching to NPH insulin twice daily. All basal insulins can cause hypoglycemia in patients with renal dysfunction; glargine insulin, in particular, should be dosed with caution in patients with end-stage renal disease.

If a discrepancy emerges between near-goal fasting blood glucose levels and above goal HbA1c, one must examine postprandial glycemic control. Two-hour postprandial glucose levels in upwards of >200 mg/dL can contribute substantially to poor overall glycemic control. In this case, rapid acting insulin analogs (aspart, lispro, or glulisine) can initially be added before the largest meal of the day, usually breakfast or dinner. The rapid acting insulin dose can be based on the carbohydrate content of each meal by using an insulin-to-carbohydrate ratio, or it can be a fixed weight-based dose (usually 0.1 units/kg/meal). When using the former strategy (as we did in our case), the patient should be educated about carbohydrate counting.

A referral to a nutritionist or diabetes educator is generally necessary. One often-used mathematical formula for calculating the insulin-to-carbohydrate ratio is commonly known as "the 500 rule" [18]. The result of dividing 500 by the total daily insulin dose represents the grams of carbohydrate covered by approximately by 1 unit of rapid-acting insulin. The use of regular insulin for prandial coverage is generally discouraged. Regular insulin has a less physiologic pharmacokinetic profile with slower absorption and longer duration of action as compared to that of rapid-acting insulins. It may provide inadequate prandial coverage and cause late postprandial hypoglycemia. Once a patient is placed on a combination of basal and bolus insulin, oral secretagogues should be discontinued since they will not contribute to improving glycemic control and may, in fact, lead to hypoglycemia.

If a more simplified regimen is needed (for reasons of patient preference or capability to self-manage their diabetes), the use of premixed insulin may be helpful (Table 43.2). Premixed insulins combine intermediate acting insulin with rapid-acting insulin in a fixed ratio (75/25, 70/30, or 50/50). Premixed insulins provide both basal and prandial coverage in one injection. They are usually given before breakfast and dinner. Three randomized clinical trials comparing the effects of basal insulins alone versus premixed insulin injections twice daily each showed a significant improvement in HbA1c [15]. Premixed insulins, however, did produce increased incidence of minor hypoglycemia. Mixed insulin regimens are generally less flexible regimen and require patients to eat similar amounts of carbohydrates at each meal and at fixed time intervals. Motivated patients and/or those with more advanced disease may benefit from multiple daily insulin injections (MDII), with basal insulin given once daily and bolus insulin injections before each meal (and snacks).

# Questions

1. In which of the following patients with type-2 diabetes is insulin therapy the best therapeutic modality?

   A. An 89-year-old woman with HbA1c of 7.2 %
   B. A 62-year-old obese man with recently diagnosed type-2 diabetes and HbA1c of 8 %
   C. A 58-year-old woman with a 20 year-history of type-2 diabetes treated with three oral antihyperglycemic medications and HbA1c of 10 %
   D. An 80-year-old man with established cardiovascular disease treated with sitagliptin and a HbA1c 7.5 %

2. Which of the following clinical situations is one in which insulin use is contraindicated?

   A. Blindness
   B. End-stage renal disease

**Table 43.2** Insulin formulations

| Type | Generic name | Brand name | Onset | Peak | Duration of action | Administration time |
|---|---|---|---|---|---|---|
| Rapid-acting | Lispro | Humalog | 5–15 m | 0.5–2 h | 3–5 h | With meals (within 15 min before or after) |
|  | Aspart | NovoLog | 5–15 m | 0.5–2 h | 3–5 h |  |
|  | Glulisine | Apidra | 5–15 m | 0.5–2 h | 3–5 h |  |
| Short-acting | Regular | Novolin R; humulin R | ½–1 h | 2–3 h | 4–8 h | With meals (30 min before) |
| Intermediate-acting | NPH | Novolin N; humulin N | 2–3 h | 4–12 h | 12–18 h | q 12–24 h |
| Long-acting | Glargine | Lantus | 2–3 h | None | 20–24 h | q 12–24 h |
|  | Detemir | Levemir | 1 h | None | 12–24 h | q 12–24 h |
| Premixed | 75 % lispro protamine/25 % lispro | Humalog mix 75/25 | 5–15 min | – | – | Before breakfast and dinner |
|  | 50 % lispro protamine/50 % lispro | Humalog mix 50/50 | 5–15 min |  |  |  |
|  | 70 % aspart protamine/30 % aspart | NovoLog mix 70/30 | 5–15 min |  |  |  |
|  | 70 % NPH/30 % regular | Novolin or humulin 70/30 | ½–1 h |  |  |  |

C. Liver failure
D. None of the above

3. Which of the following statements best describes the effects of basal insulin on patients with type-2 diabetes?

   A. NPH insulin is associated with increased risk of nocturnal hypoglycemia as compared with insulin glargine given at bedtime.
   B. NPH insulin is more effective than insulin detemir when given at bedtime.
   C. Glargine insulin is more effective than NPH insulin when given at bedtime.
   D. None of the above

## Answers to Questions

1. C
2. D
3. A

## References

1. Muoio DM, Newgard CB. Molecular and metabolic mechanisms of insulin resistance and [beta]-cell failure in type 2 diabetes. Nat Rev Mol Cell Biol. 2008;9(3):193–205. doi:10.1038/nrm2327.
2. Inzucchi SE, Bergenstal RM, Buse JB, Diamant M, Ferrannini E, Nauck M, et al. Management of hyperglycemia in type 2 diabetes: a patient-centered approach: position statement of the American Diabetes Association (ADA) and the European Association for the Study of Diabetes (EASD). Diabetes Care. 2012;35(6):1364–79. Practice Guideline Review.
3. Nathan DM, Buse JB, Davidson MB, Ferrannini E, Holman RR, Sherwin R, et al. Medical management of hyperglycemia in type 2 diabetes: a consensus algorithm for the initiation and adjustment of therapy: a consensus statement of the American Diabetes Association and the European Association for the Study of Diabetes. Diabetes Care. 2009;32(1):193–203. Consensus Development Conference Practice Guideline.
4. Bailey CJ, Turner RC. Metformin. N Engl J Med. 1996;334(9):574–9.
5. Gangji AS, Cukierman T, Gerstein HC, Goldsmith CH, Clase CM. A systematic review and meta-analysis of hypoglycemia and cardiovascular events: a comparison of glyburide with other secretagogues and with insulin. Diabetes Care. 2007;30(2):389–94.
6. Moses RG. Repaglinide/metformin fixed-dose combination to improve glycemic control in patients with type 2 diabetes: an update. Diabetes Metab Syndr Obes. 2010;3:145–54.
7. Kahn CR, Chen L, Cohen SE. Unraveling the mechanism of action of thiazolidinediones. J Clin Invest. 2000;106(11):1305–7.
8. Demuth HU, McIntosh CH, Pederson RA. Type 2 diabetes–therapy with dipeptidyl peptidase IV inhibitors. Biochim Biophys Acta. 2005;1751(1):33–44.
9. Dicker D. DPP-4 inhibitors: impact on glycemic control and cardiovascular risk factors. Diabetes Care. 2011;34 Suppl 2:S276–8. Review.

10. Garber AJ. Long-acting glucagon-like peptide 1 receptor agonists: a review of their efficacy and tolerability. Diabetes Care. 2011;34 Suppl 2:S279–84. Review.
11. Bloomgarden ZT, Blonde L, Garber AJ, Wysham CH. Current issues in GLP-1 receptor agonist therapy for type 2 diabetes. Endocr Pract. 2012;18 Suppl 3:6–26.
12. Intensive blood-glucose control with sulphonylureas or insulin compared with conventional treatment and risk of complications in patients with type 2 diabetes (UKPDS 33). UK Prospective Diabetes Study (UKPDS) Group. Lancet. 1998;352(9131):837–53, Clinical Trial Comparative Study Randomized Controlled Trial Research Support, Non-U.S. Gov't Research Support, U.S. Gov't, P.H.S.
13. Swinnen SG, Hoekstra JB, DeVries JH. Insulin therapy for type 2 diabetes. Diabetes Care. 2009;32 Suppl 2:S253–9. Review.
14. Vaag A, Lund SS. Insulin initiation in patients with type 2 diabetes mellitus: treatment guidelines, clinical evidence and patterns of use of basal vs premixed insulin analogues. Eur J Endocrinol. 2012;166(2):159–70. Comparative Study Evaluation Studies Research Support, Non-U.S. Gov't Review.
15. Ilag LL, Kerr L, Malone JK, Tan MH. Prandial premixed insulin analogue regimens versus basal insulin analogue regimens in the management of type 2 diabetes: an evidence-based comparison. Clin Ther. 2007;29 Spec No:1254–70, Comparative Study Review.
16. Riddle MC, Rosenstock J, Gerich J. The treat-to-target trial: randomized addition of glargine or human NPH insulin to oral therapy of type 2 diabetic patients. Diabetes Care. 2003;26(11):3080–6. Clinical Trial Multicenter Study Randomized Controlled Trial Research Support, Non-U.S. Gov't.
17. Horvath K, Jeitler K, Berghold A, Ebrahim SH, Gratzer TW, Plank J, et al. Long-acting insulin analogues versus NPH insulin (human isophane insulin) for type 2 diabetes mellitus. Cochrane Database Syst Rev. 2007(2):CD005613, Meta-Analysis Review.
18. Davidson PC, Hebblewhite HR, Steed RD, Bode BW. Analysis of guidelines for basal-bolus insulin dosing: basal insulin, correction factor, and carbohydrate-to-insulin ratio. Endocr Pract. 2008;14(9):1095–101.

# Chapter 44
# Inpatient Management of Type 2 Diabetes

**Dorothy A. Fink and Kim T. Nguyen**

## Objectives

1. To understand the goals for inpatient glycemic control in patients with type 2 diabetes.
2. To learn the treatment options of hyperglycemia in the inpatient setting.
3. To gain an appreciation for inpatient diabetes management in special situations in the hospitalized patient.

## Case Presentation

A 69-year-old woman with type 2 diabetes, hypertension, dyslipidemia, and chronic kidney disease was admitted following a fall at home and sustained a right hip fracture. She underwent a right hip arthroplasty on the day of admission. Her blood glucose levels were noted to be in the range of 200-300 mg/dL after her surgery. The orthopedic team ordered a preset aspart sliding scale with meals. Due to persistent hyperglycemia over the following 24 h, an endocrine consult was requested.

D.A. Fink, M.D. (✉)
Department of Medicine, Division of Endocrinology, Columbia University College
of Physicians and Surgeons, 630 West 168th Street, Ph-864, New York, NY 10032, USA
e-mail: Dorothy.Fink@nyumc.org

K.T. Nguyen, M.D.
Department of Medicine, Division of Endocrinology, Columbia University College
of Physicians and Surgeons, 630 West 168th Street, Ph-864, New York, NY 10032, USA

Division of Endocrinology at Columbia University/New York Presbyterian Hospital,
630 W. 168th St., PH 8W Rm 864, New York, NY 10032, USA
e-mail: ktnguyen@post.harvard.edu

© Springer Science+Business Media New York 2015                              369
T.F. Davies (ed.), *A Case-Based Guide to Clinical Endocrinology*,
DOI 10.1007/978-1-4939-2059-4_44

The patient has had a history of diabetes for 20 years prior to this admission. She takes glyburide 5 mg daily, sitagliptin 100 mg daily, and a combination of metformin 850 mg/pioglitizone 15 mg twice daily. She denies taking insulin in the past. She does not check her blood glucose at home and denies hypoglycemic events. She reports a history of retinopathy for which she has received laser treatment in the past. She complains of right hip pain, but otherwise feels well. She denies nausea, vomiting, polydipsia, and polyuria. On physical examination, her weight is 80 kilograms (kg) and her height is 152 cm with a body mass index of 34.6 kg/m$^2$. She has acanthosis. Dorsalis pedis pulses were 2+ bilaterally and she had no lesions on her feet.

Laboratory tests showed a creatinine level of 1.77 mg/dL, GFR 29 mL/min/m$^2$, and a fasting serum glucose of 325 mg/dL. Her liver function tests were normal. Her hemoglobin A1c (HbA1c) was 10.6 %. Review of prior laboratory tests shows a GFR of 47 mL/min/m$^2$ approximately 2 years prior to this admission.

## Inpatient Goals for Hyperglycemia in Noncritical Care Settings

Controversy surrounds glycemic targets for inpatients. A critical care versus a noncritical care setting is important in defining glycemic goals in the hospital. Although poor blood glucose control has been associated with negative outcomes (infections, longer length of stay, mortality), further evidence-based data is needed to determine optimal glycemic goals for hospitalized patients in a noncritical care setting [1]. One of the main factors limiting tight glycemic control is the risk of hypoglycemia, which itself may result in increased mortality. The American Diabetes Association (ADA) and the American Association of Clinical Endocrinologists (AACE) published a Consensus Statement on inpatient glycemic control in 2009 and the ADA includes recommendations for inpatient glycemic goals in the *Standards of Medical Care in Diabetes* yearly [2, 3]. The Endocrine Society published a Clinical Practice Guideline for managing hyperglycemia in a noncritical care setting in 2012 [4]. According to guidelines, the glycemic goals for noncritically ill patients are: fasting or premeal glucose levels ≤140 mg/dL and a random blood glucose level ≤180 mg/dL. In our clinical vignette, the patient's blood glucose levels are above goal and therefore her insulin regimen should be adjusted.

## Should Oral Medications Be Continued in the Inpatient Setting?

Most oral antihyperglycemic medications are either ineffective in the inpatient setting, contraindicated, or prone to causing hypoglycemia in the unstable patient. Our patient's oral medications were discontinued. Metformin is contraindicated in women with creatinine levels >1.4. The drug is also not an ideal choice given the potential for patient exposure to contrast agents, procedures, or hemodynamic instability while she is acutely sick in the hospital. Pioglitizone is known to increase fracture risk in some patients; given that the patient recently sustained a fragility fracture, it would not be prudent to continue this oral antihyperglycemic agent. Glyburide, a secretogogue, carries a high risk of causing hypoglycemia in elderly patients, particularly in the context of renal dysfunction; Hypoglycemia would compromise safety in a patient already at high risk for falls. The dose of sitagliptin could be adjusted according to her renal dysfunction; however, the use of sitagliptin alone will be unlikely to control this patient's hyperglycemia. While a DPP-4 inhibitor could be considered at discharge, combining a DPP-4 inhibitor and insulin would also increase her risk of hypoglycemia. She will need insulin at discharge.

## How Do We Determine an Appropriate Inpatient Insulin Regimen?

There are three main factors that contribute to determining the most appropriate insulin regimen for the hospitalized patient:

1. Dietary status
2. Weight
3. Renal function

For patients who are prescribed a diet, it is important to provide both basal and prandial insulin coverage. The RABBIT-2 medicine [5] and surgery [6] trials demonstrated that basal/bolus insulin is superior to sliding scale insulin in the treatment of noncritically ill patients with type 2 diabetes. Unfortunately, it is very common to find patients only receiving "sliding scale" insulin prior to meals for several days in the hospital setting. It is important to educate healthcare professionals about the importance of basal/bolus insulin treatment.

The main component to establishing an inpatient insulin regimen is to first calculate the patient's estimated total daily dose (TDD) of insulin. On average, patients with type 2 diabetes require a TDD of 0.4–1 units/kg. For elderly patients and those with renal or hepatic dysfunction, a TDD of 0.3 units/kg is a reasonable starting dose. For obese patients or those receiving steroids, 0.5–0.6 units/kg provides additional insulin to counter the increased insulin resistance associated with these states. Generally, basal insulin requirements make up 50 % of the patient's TDD. Initial insulin requirements in the hospital may often be higher than the patient's insulin needs at home due to stress, infection, and altered eating patterns.

In our patient with renal dysfunction, we selected a formula of 0.3 units/kg to determine her total daily insulin requirements: for an 80 kg woman, TDD=0.3 units×80 kg, or 24 units. Her basal dose should be 50 % of her estimated TDD requirements or 12 units; therefore, she received 12 units of glargine insulin. The remaining 50 % of her TDD approximates the patient's prandial rapid-acting insulin dose, which is further divided by 3 to give 4 units rapid acting insulin with each meal. Her prandial dose may be supplemented by a correctional insulin scale for hyperglycemia as well.

For patients who are already receiving an established insulin regimen at home, it is common practice to initiate basal insulin at 80–100 % of their home dose in the inpatient setting. Lower insulin doses should be given to patients with decreased dietary intake, especially if the home basal insulin dose is inappropriately high and appears to be covering prandial needs as well. Patients who understand carbohydrate counting prior to their admission and are reliable at practicing diabetes self-management may be allowed (and often encouraged) to use their home insulin ratios to determine their premeal insulin dose in the hospital.

## Carbohydrate Counting: Insulin-to-Carbohydrate Ratio

The insulin-to-carbohydrate ratio is an estimate of the number of grams of carbohydrate (CHO) covered by 1 unit of rapid-acting insulin. Based on data from patients with type 1 diabetes using insulin pumps/continuous subcutaneous insulin infusion (CSII), the "500 rule" approximates insulin requirements [7]. To determine an insulin-to-CHO ratio, divide 500 by the TDD of insulin; the result is an approximation of the amount of CHO (in grams) covered by 1 unit of rapid-acting insulin (i.e., "carbohydrate ratio") [6]. An average carbohydrate ratio is 1:15, meaning that 1 unit of short-acting insulin is required for every 15 g of CHO consumed. It is important to keep in mind that insulin-to-carbohydrate ratios may vary by time of day (patients tend to be more insulin resistant in the morning). Physical activity, illness, infection, steroids, and stress also contribute to variations in insulin requirements.

## Carbohydrate Counting: Insulin Correction/Sensitivity Factor

The insulin correction factor ("sensitivity factor") helps approximate the amount of rapid-acting insulin required to account for potential premeal hyperglycemia. The insulin correction factor estimates the glucose-lowering effect (in mg/dL) of 1 unit of rapid-acting insulin. To estimate the insulin correction factor, divide 1,800 by the patient's TDD (for regular insulin, use 1,500). These equations are also based on data from patients with type 1 diabetes on CSII [7, 8]. However, this concept is helpful for treating insulin-naïve patients and confirming home insulin regimens. On average, 1 unit of rapid-acting insulin will decrease the blood glucose by 50 mg/dL. If more insulin is required to accomplish this 50 mg/dL decrease, the patient is likely more insulin resistant. For example, in a patient with a blood glucose of 240 mg/dL with a target of 140 mg/dL who requires a TDD of 36 units of insulin: 1,800/36=50, the correction factor would be 1:50 mg/dL and the patient would require approximately 2 units of rapid acting insulin to reach goal blood glucose.

The case patient's insulin regimen initially included an insulin-to-carbohydrate ratio of 1:15 and correction factor of 1:50. These ratios were adjusted throughout her hospitalization.

The insulin correction factor is also useful for correcting hyperglycemia in between meals or at bedtime. However, administering additional doses of rapid acting insulin more frequently than every 3  h should be undertaken carefully as rapid acting insulin usually lasts about 3–4 h in the serum following a subcutaneous injection and overlapping doses may result in hypoglycemia.

On hospital day #3, the patient's blood glucose levels remained in the 200 mg/dL range despite the addition of glargine; her basal insulin dose was increased by approximately 20 % to glargine 14 units at bedtime. In order to assess adequacy of basal insulin dosing, the patient's fasting evening blood glucose should be compared to the morning fasting blood glucose. If the patient's fasting glucose level is significantly higher than the glucose measured the evening prior, one should inquire about the possibility of bedtime or overnight snacking, both of which can contribute to morning hyperglycemia. The differential of fasting morning hyperglycemia also includes the Dawn phenomenon (thought to be due to release of counterregularory hormones such as cortisol and growth hormone), insufficient insulin dosing, and the Somogyi effect (rebound hyperglycemia), although this effect has not been well demonstrated.

On hospital day #4, the patient developed a fever and hypotension and was diagnosed with sepsis. The patient was transferred to the intensive care unit (ICU) for further management.

## Inpatient Goals for Hyperglycemia in Critical Care Settings

In contrast to noncritical care settings, there have been multiple studies focusing on glycemic control in the ICU [9–11]. In the largest study to date, NICE-SUGAR (Normoglycemia in Intensive Care Evaluation and Survival Using Glucose Algorithm Regulation), a multinational, multicenter, randomized controlled trial (RCT) compared the effect of intensive glycemic control (target 81–108 mg/dL) to standard glycemic control (target 144–180 mg/dL) in 6,104 critically ill patients [11]. Ninety-day mortality was significantly higher in both medical and surgical patients placed on more intensive glycemic control, as was mortality from cardiovascular causes. Essentially, the NICE-SUGAR study suggested that a highly stringent blood glucose target of <110 mg/dL may potentially be harmful to patients.

These results contrasted directly with an earlier RCT performed in surgical ICU patients [9] which suggested that intensive glycemic control to target 80–110 mg/dL was more beneficial than standard glucose control, leading to a 42 % relative reduction in mortality and morbidity. However, incidence of severe hypoglycemia was also increased in the intensively treated group. A study by the same authors comparing intensive versus standard glycemic control in medical ICU patients was unable to replicate their earlier findings [10].

A more recent meta-analysis of 26 trials, including the NICE-SUGAR data, revealed a pooled relative risk of death of 0.93 with intensive insulin therapy compared to conventional therapy [12]. There was also increased risk of severe hypoglycemia. Surgical ICU patients appeared to benefit more from intensive insulin therapy than patients in other medical and mixed critical care settings. Overall, results of this meta-analysis support the conclusion that while there may be some mortality benefit from intensive insulin therapy in surgical ICU patients, there is otherwise no overall benefit on mortality in the critically ill, and in fact, increased risk of hypoglycemia.

In light of these data, insulin infusion should be initiated for hyperglycemia in critically ill patients with a starting threshold of no higher than 180 mg/dL. For the majority of critically ill patients, a glucose range of 140–180 mg/dL is recommended once insulin is started. Greater benefit may be achieved at the lower end of this range, although this should take into account the individual circumstances for each patient. Patients should be placed on an intravenous insulin protocol that is both safe and efficacious but one that does not increase their risk of severe hypoglycemia. Frequent blood glucose monitoring ranging from every 30 min to every 2 h should be implemented to monitor for hypoglycemia during intravenous insulin infusion.

In the ICU, the case patient was unresponsive and was placed on IV insulin infusion to maintain blood glucose values between 140 and 180 mg/dL. Her subcutaneous insulin regimen was held. Forty-eight hours after her ICU admission, the patient was initiated on enteral tube feedings.

## Transitioning of the Insulin Infusion to Subcutaneous Insulin

Hyperglycemia is a common side effect in patients who are receiving enteral nutrition. Insulin regimens need to take into account the carbohydrate content of tube feed formulas as well as changes in the patient's status, such as impending NPO status or further procedures and interventions. A 2009 study showed similar glycemic control could be achieved using glargine or sliding scale regular insulin; however, up to 48 % of patients on sliding scale regular insulin required the addition of intermediate-acting insulin (NPH) to achieve glycemic targets [13]. Given the longer duration of glargine, there is an increased risk of hypoglycemia in the event of tube feed disruption due to patient instability or other mechanical factors; for this reason, use of NPH insulin is often preferred. In the event of tube feed discontinuation after NPH is given, start an intravenous solution containing 10 % dextrose at a rate equivalent to the rate of enteral nutrition to avoid hypoglycemia. In addition, adjust the aspart scale to accommodate the patient's decreased insulin needs once she is no longer receiving enteral nutrition.

For patients on enteral nutrition, weight-based insulin dosing estimates about 0.6–0.8 units/kg/day, with two-thirds given as NPH insulin and one-third given as short-acting insulin (regular or aspart). For our 80 kg patient, this means a TDD of 48 units, and therefore a total of NPH 32 units and total short-acting insulin 16 units. Because NPH starts to work in 1–3 h and peaks between 4 and 10 h, the dosing interval for patients on enteral nutrition is typically every 8 h for NPH and short-acting insulin, with the short-acting insulin "smoothing" out the peaks and troughs of the NPH insulin. Our patient should therefore be started on NPH 11 units, aspart insulin 5 units, and a correctional aspart scale for hyperglycemia every 8 h. Use of a correctional scale every 8 h can help inform further adjustments in NPH dosing, which should be titrated every few days if she remains hyperglycemic.

When transitioning a patient from continuous intravenous insulin infusion to subcutaneous insulin, the infusion should be discontinued 1–2 h after the first dose of long-acting insulin is administered. If short-acting insulin is also administered subcutaneously, this interval can be shortened.

Our patient's NPH insulin overlapped with her insulin infusion by 1 h prior to its discontinuation. She tolerated enteral nutrition well, maintaining serum glucose less than 180 mg/dL on NPH and aspart correction scale by the time of transfer to the floor. Once transferred to the general medicine floor, the patient's diet was slowly advanced to clear liquids and then to a cardiac and diabetic diet and enteral nutrition was discontinued. NPH and sliding scale insulin were discontinued and the patient resumed her prior glargine and aspart regimen. She was discharged to a subacute care center on glargine insulin 14 units at bedtime and aspart insulin 5 units three times daily with meals.

## Questions

1. Which trial demonstrates the importance of basal-bolus insulin regimens?

    a. ACCORD trial
    b. NICE-SUGAR
    c. DIGAMI
    d. RABBIT 2 surgery trial

2. In order to determine an insulin regimen, you need to take into account all of the following except?

    a. Weight
    b. Diet
    c. Renal dysfunction
    d. Number of oral agents at home

3. Which of the following is false about prandial, rapid-acting insulin dosages?

    a. Insulin–carbohydrate ratio and correction factor both must be accounted for when determining a prandial insulin dose for a patient who is tolerating oral intake
    b. A correction factor can be estimated by dividing 1,800/TDD

   c.  An insulin–carbohydrate ratio can be estimated by dividing 1,500/TDD

   d.  It is not prudent to use a sliding scale for inpatient glycemic control

## Answers to Questions

1. d
2. d
3. c

## References

1. Murad MH, Coburn JA, Coto-Yglesias F, Dzyubak S, Hazem A, Lane MA, et al. Glycemic control in non-critically ill hospitalized patients: a systematic review and meta-analysis. J Clin Endocrinol Metab. 2012;97(1):49–58.
2. Moghissi ES, Korytkowski MT, DiNardo M, Einhorn D, Hellman R, Hirsch IB, et al. American Association of Clinical Endocrinologists and American Diabetes Association consensus statement on inpatient glycemic control. Endocr Pract. 2009;15(4):353–69.
3. Standards of medical care in diabetes–2014. Diabetes Care. 2014;37 Suppl 1:S14–80.
4. Umpierrez GE, Hellman R, Korytkowski MT, Kosiborod M, Maynard GA, Montori VM, et al. Management of hyperglycemia in hospitalized patients in non-critical care setting: an endocrine society clinical practice guideline. J Clin Endocrinol Metab. 2012;97(1):16–38.
5. Umpierrez GE, Smiley D, Zisman A, Prieto LM, Palacio A, Ceron M, et al. Randomized study of basal-bolus insulin therapy in the inpatient management of patients with type 2 diabetes (RABBIT 2 trial). Diabetes Care. 2007;30(9):2181–6.
6. Umpierrez GE, Smiley D, Jacobs S, Peng L, Temponi A, Mulligan P, et al. Randomized study of basal-bolus insulin therapy in the inpatient management of patients with type 2 diabetes undergoing general surgery (RABBIT 2 surgery). Diabetes Care. 2011;34(2):256–61.
7. Davidson PC, Hebblewhite HR, Steed RD, Bode BW. Analysis of guidelines for basal-bolus insulin dosing: basal insulin, correction factor, and carbohydrate-to-insulin ratio. Endocr Pract. 2008;14(9):1095–101.
8. Walsh J, Roberts R, Bailey T. Guidelines for optimal bolus calculator settings in adults. J Diabetes Sci Technol. 2011;5(1):129–35.
9. van den Berghe G, Wouters P, Weekers F, Verwaest C, Bruyninckx F, Schetz M, et al. Intensive insulin therapy in critically ill patients. N Engl J Med. 2001;345(19):1359–67.
10. Van den Berghe G, Wilmer A, Hermans G, Meersseman W, Wouters PJ, Milants I, et al. Intensive insulin therapy in the medical ICU. N Engl J Med. 2006;354(5):449–61.
11. Investigators N-SS, Finfer S, Chittock DR, Su SY, Blair D, Foster D, et al. Intensive versus conventional glucose control in critically ill patients. N Engl J Med. 2009;360(13):1283–97.
12. Griesdale DE, de Souza RJ, van Dam RM, Heyland DK, Cook DJ, Malhotra A, et al. Intensive insulin therapy and mortality among critically ill patients: a meta-analysis including NICE-SUGAR study data. CMAJ. 2009;180(8):821–7.
13. Korytkowski MT, Salata RJ, Koerbel GL, Selzer F, Karslioglu E, Idriss AM, et al. Insulin therapy and glycemic control in hospitalized patients with diabetes during enteral nutrition therapy: a randomized controlled clinical trial. Diabetes Care. 2009;32(4):594–6.

# Part XI
# Lipid Abnormalities

# Chapter 45
# Introduction

Neil J. Stone

This section includes three cases with challenging lipid management. Lipids and lipoproteins are often viewed separately in atherosclerosis or pancreatitis risk assessment but an understanding of lipid and lipoprotein physiology is required to understand fully the basis for thoughtful management. It's been more than half a century since John Gofman focused our attention on lipoproteins that were defined by their physical and chemical characteristics in the analytical ultracentrifuge. Further work at the National Institutes of Health by researchers such as Don Fredrickson, Richard Havel, Robert Levy, and Dan Steinberg enlarged our understanding of the structure and function of lipoproteins and their relationship to atherosclerosis and hypertriglyceridemic pancreatitis.

By way of brief review, the major classes of lipoproteins include chylomicrons that transport dietary triglycerides (TG), very low density lipoproteins (VLDL) that transport TG of mainly hepatic origin, TG rich remnant lipoproteins, low-density lipoproteins (LDL) that transport two-thirds of the plasma cholesterol, and high-density lipoproteins (HDL). Lipoproteins vary not only in their lipid loads but also in the types of apolipoproteins (apo) that they carry. For example, apoA1 is the predominant apoprotein on HDL. One apo B is seen on every molecule of VLDL and LDL. Apo B levels can be used for both diagnosis of genetic lipid disorders as well as to convey an accurate appraisal of atherosclerosis risk. Non-HDL cholesterol (Total minus HDL cholesterol) was used as an entry criterion in the primary prevention Helsinki randomized clinical trial of gemfibrozil versus placebo. Non-HDL Cholesterol (HDL-C) was later recommended as a secondary target for risk reduction when LDL was at goal and triglycerides were ≥200 mg/dl.

N.J. Stone, M.D., M.A.C.P., F.A.H.A., F.A.C.C. (✉)
Bonow Professor of Medicine, Feinberg School of Medicine,
Northwestern University, Suzanne and Milton Davidson Distinguished Physician and
Medical Director, Vascular Center of the Bluhm Cardiovascular Institute of Northwestern
Memorial Hospital, Chicago, Illinois
e-mail: n-stone@northwestern.edu

© Springer Science+Business Media New York 2015                                    379
T.F. Davies (ed.), *A Case-Based Guide to Clinical Endocrinology*,
DOI 10.1007/978-1-4939-2059-4_45

Low values for HDL cholesterol (HDL-C) are useful in risk assessment for atherosclerotic cardiovascular disease, but recent genetic and clinical trial data have not supported use of HDL-C as a risk reduction target. This has led to a focus on HDL function that should provide important insights into how to use measurements of HDL in lipid management.

Each case in this section highlights pathophysiology that is important to address to avoid complications of atherosclerotic vascular disease or hyperlipidemic pancreatitis.

The first case is one of refractory hypercholesterolemia owing to an inherited defet in LDL receptors. Although statin drugs interfere with the rate-limiting step of cholesterol synthesis in the liver and thus upregulate LDL receptors, they are not highly effective in cases where two mutant copies of the LDL gene are present. Liver transplantation is a definitive treatment for severe homozygous familial hypercholesterolemia (FH), but is not as practical or as available as LDL apheresis. The case report in this section describes this well. As a historical note, I saw a double heterozygous (phenotypically homozygous) case of severely affected FH who presented with angina, xanthomas, and total cholesterol greater than 800 mg/dl, who underwent regular plasma exchange (later changed to LDL apheresis) and survived for four decades before dying of a noncadiac cause.

The second case illustrates the importance of accurate diagnosis. Type III can be suggested clinically by almost equivalent raised levels of cholesterol and triglyceride and especially if accompanied by palmar xanthomas. The mixed hyperlipidemia seen is characteristically carbohydrate sensitive. As indicated in the case, the diagnosis is made by demonstrating a cholesterol rich VLDL that is accompanied by an apoE2/E2 genotype. Secondary causes often exacerbate or make clinically obvious, genetic hyperlipidemia and this can be seen in type-III cases that have associated hypothyroidism. It's important to note that in type-III cases measuring LDL-C by the Friedewald equation or even using apolipoprotein B measurements are not as accurate as following the non-HDL cholesterol levels.

Finally, this section concludes with a well-characterized case of a young patient with very high levels of triglycerides. Managing severe hypertriglyceridemia requires special knowledge and several principles must be kept in mind. First, it has been long recognized that cases of severe hypertriglyceridemia represent almost invariably the effects of both an acquired cause of hypertriglyceridemia as well as an underlying genetic cause. Overweight and insulin resistance, alcohol excess, steroid, estrogen, retinoic acid or l-asparaginase therapy, insulinopenic diabetes, and hypothyroidism can all exacerbate genetic hypertriglyceridemia and result in patients who present with hypertriglyceridemic pancreatitis. Second there is no specific level above which hypertriglyceridemia produces pancreatitis. Third, when TGs rise above approximately 1,000 mg/dl, chylomicrons, and VLDL both compete for removal by lipoprotein lipase action. This enzyme requires both insulin and thyroid as cofactors. Knowledge of this saturation kinetics can inform thoughtful therapeutic recommendations. Fourth, the very high levels of triglycerides can cause measurement artifacts such as "pseudohyponatremia" that should not go unnoticed to avoid unneeded and risky attempts to raise artifactually low sodium levels. And it is important to keep in mind that normal range amylase values are seen often with severe hypertriglyceridemia and should not discourage imaging to uncover strong evidence of associated pancreatitis.

All of the cases have in common the need to understand underlying lipid and lipoprotein physiology. Also we would underscore the need for family screening in those with genetic lipid disorders so that prevention efforts can be extended to affected relatives. Whether it be knowledge of how excess levels of LDL or triglyceride develop and then how they can be efficiently removed from the bloodstream or appreciating the need to recognize abnormal VLDL metabolism, the thoughtful approaches emphasized in these chapters will serve the clinician well in dealing with difficult lipid clinical problems.

# Chapter 46
# LDL-Apheresis Therapy for Refractory Familial Hypercholesterolemia

Binh An P. Phan

## Objectives

1. To understand the pathophysiology, clinical presentation, and treatment of familial hypercholesterolemia.
2. To recognize the role of LDL-apheresis in the treatment of refractory severe hypercholesterolemia.

## Case Presentation

A 53-year-old woman presents with a history of premature coronary artery disease (CAD) and severe hypercholesterolemia. She experienced a myocardial infarction (MI) at the age of 37 years old. At that time her total cholesterol (TC) was above 400 mg/dL and her LDL cholesterol (LDL-C) was above 300 mg/dL. She was first started on atorvastatin but developed severe transaminitis requiring discontinuation. She was next treated with simvastatin and then lovastatin but both statins caused similar elevations in her liver enzymes. Subsequent trials of pravastatin and then low dose rosuvastatin resulted in severe myalgias and leg weakness that prompted discontinuation. At 42 years old, she presented with recurrent chest pain and found to have restenosis of her coronary stent in her left anterior descending artery (LAD) requiring repeat coronary stenting. With her statin intolerance and continued elevations in her LDL-C above 300 mg/dL, she was started on ezetimibe and colesevelam. Six years later, she presented with recurrent chest pain, found to have diffuse 3-vessel CAD on cardiac catheterization, and underwent coronary artery bypass grafting (CABG).

B.A.P. Phan, M.D. (✉)
Division of Cardiology, University of California, San Francisco,
1001 Potrero Ave, Room 5G1, San Francisco, CA 94110

© Springer Science+Business Media New York 2015
T.F. Davies (ed.), *A Case-Based Guide to Clinical Endocrinology*,
DOI 10.1007/978-1-4939-2059-4_46

She has a family history of premature CAD and severe hypercholesterolemia. Her father died suddenly at the age of 45 years old; presumed due to sudden cardiac death (SCD) from an acute MI. She has two brothers, both of whom have elevated LDL-C above 300 mg/dL and have had MIs in their late 30s.

Her physical exam reviewed normal blood pressure and heart rate. Her body mass index (BMI) was 32 kg/m$^2$. She had corneal arcus and tendon xanthomas located on her hands. Her lipid profile showed a TC 408 mg/dL, LDL-C 285 mg/dL, high-density lipoprotein cholesterol (HDL-C) 42 mg/dL, and triglycerides (TG) 157 mg/dL. Her thyroid function and liver laboratories were within normal limits.

After placement of a central venous catheter, she was started on LDL-apheresis. Immediately post-LDL-apheresis, her lipid panel showed TC 125 mg/dL, LDL-C 51 mg/dL, TG 140 mg/dL, and HDL-C 39 mg/dL. For the past 5 years she has had twice monthly LDL-apheresis. She has not had recurrence of chest pain nor required additional coronary interventions since the initiation of LDL-apheresis.

## How the Diagnosis Was Made

Familial hypercholesterolemia (FH) is an autosomal codominant genetic condition characterized by absent or defective hepatic LDL receptors [1, 2]. Given that LDL receptors function to clear serum LDL cholesterol, FH patients have severely elevated cholesterol levels. More than 1,500 mutations have been identified in the LDL receptor gene that alter the production, delivery, or function of the LDL receptor. In heterozygous FH patients who have inherited a genetic defect from one parent, they have total cholesterol in the 300–500 mg/dL range and have a prevalence of 1 in 300–500 people. Homozygous FH patients who inherited two abnormal genetic defects from both parents generally have total cholesterol above 500 mg/dL and have a prevalence of 1 in a million people. Due to the severely elevated cholesterol levels, untreated heterozygous FH patients have early diagnosis of symptomatic atherosclerotic heart disease between 30 and 50 years old, while homozygous patients can present with clinical cardiac events in their first decade of life.

Since genetic testing does not change clinical management and the known receptor mutations are not present in 20 % of cases, FH can be diagnosed clinically by identifying a severely elevated LDL-C level and a family history of hypercholesterolemia and premature CHD in a first degree relative. Secondary causes of elevated cholesterol must be excluded such as severe liver disease, hypothyroidism, and renal disease. The diagnosis can be supported by the presence of characteristic physical exam findings including early onset corneal arcus less than 40 years old, and tendon xanthomas located in the Achilles tendon and tendons of the hand. Though helpful if present, the absence of these exam findings does not rule out a diagnosis of FH. Once a patient is diagnosed with FH, cascade screening of all first-degree relatives is recommended by testing cholesterol levels.

Cholesterol therapy is paramount to lowering the very high lifetime risk for CHD in FH patients [3]. Statins are the recommended first line agents with dose titration to achieve a LDL-C goal of <160 mg/dL for all FH patients and <100 mg/dL for higher risk patients with established atherosclerotic cardiovascular disease or multiple CHD risk factors. In patients not reaching these goals with statins or who have significant statin intolerance, alternative cholesterol lowering therapies including niacin, bile acid binders, and ezetimibe can be considered [4].

## Lessons Learned

While statins and other cholesterol lowering medications are usually successful in treating hypercholesterolemic patients, some patients are not able to reach recommended LDL-C targets despite being on maximal drug doses. At the highest available dose of the most potent statin, rosuvastatin at 40 mg daily can only lower LDL-C by up to 60 %. For FH patients with baseline LDL-C levels >250–300 mg/dL who have established CHD or multiple cardiac risk factors, achieving a recommended target of <100 mg/dL would not be feasible with current statin drugs. Additionally, statin therapy is less efficacious in homozygous FH patients; achieving only 20–25 % reduction in LDL-C. Statins lower serum LDL-C by inhibiting HMG-CoA reductase enzyme, a rate-limiting step in cholesterol production, and leading to less hepatic cholesterol concentration. The decrease in hepatic cholesterol triggers the production of LDL receptors which results in increased uptake of serum cholesterol and lowering LDL-C levels. Given that homozygous FH patients have nearly absent functional hepatic LDL receptors, the LDL-C lowering effect of statins is significantly impaired. Apart from issues with efficacy, many patients, including those with FH, have significant statin-related side effects such as myalgias and muscle weakness that limit the initiation and escalation to maximal doses of statins. Some observational studies estimate that 10–15 % of patients on statins have such symptoms while patient surveys often report higher incidences closer to 30 %. Nonstatin-based agents such as niacin, ezetimibe, and bile acid sequestrants are often used to augment or replace statins in FH patients, but are all less effective in lower LDL-C compared to statins and also can have a number of side effects.

LDL-apheresis is indicated for FH patients who have persistently and severely elevated cholesterol levels despite optimal diet and maximal tolerated drug therapy with LDL-C >300 mg/dL or >200 mg/dL with established CHD [4–6]. In clinical use now for the approximately the past 25 years, LDL-apheresis systems use several different mechanisms to remove serum LDL-C. With the immunoadsorption technique, plasma is filtered through sepharose columns coated with LDL-associated apolipoprotein B antibodies that bind to LDL-C-based antigen. In the heparin-induced LDL precipitation (HELP) method, the acidification of plasma and subsequent addition of heparin cause precipitation of LDL-C into insoluble precipitates which then can be separated from the plasma. A third technique, dextran sulfate LDL absoroption or liposorber, uses low-molecular weight dextran sulfate, which has high affinity for apolipoprotein B containing molecules, to bind and remove LDL-C. Typically, each LDL-apheresis session lasts for 2–4 h and is done every

1–2 weeks. Regardless of the apheresis technique used, LDL-C is lowered on average by 50–70 %. After each session, LDL-C slowly increases near baseline pretreatment levels and therefore many FH patients on LDL-apheresis will continue for lifelong treatment.

The clinical efficacy and cardiovascular benefits of LDL-apheresis have been evaluated in a number of small randomized controlled trials involving both homozygous and heterozygous FH patients. Data suggest that cholesterol lowering by LDL-apheresis plus drug therapy as compared to drug therapy alone is associated with greater antiatherosclerotic effects as defined by improvements in carotid intima-media thickness by ultrasound or coronary atherosclerosis by angiogram. Additionally, significant reductions in CHD events have been observed with LDL-apheresis.

## Questions

1. Which one of the following statements is true regarding the pathophysiology and diagnosis of FH?

    A. In order to acquire FH, patients must inherit two abnormal LDL receptor gene mutations, one from each parent.
    B. The clinical diagnosis of FH can be confirmed in all patients using genetic testing.
    C. Homozygous FH patients typically have total cholesterol range from 300 to 500 mg/dL.
    D. Heterozygous FH patients have early onset symptomatic CHD in the fourth to fifth decade of life, while homozygous patients have CHD diagnosed in their first decade of life.

2. Which one of the follow statements is true regarding the treatment of FH?

    A. Drug therapies including statins are not effective in lowering LDL-C in FH patients given the abnormal LDL receptors.
    B. Statin therapy lowers LDL-C levels by approximately 20 % in both homozygous and heterozygous FH patients.
    C. In a FH patient without CHD but diabetes and hypertension, the LDL-C goal is less than 100 mg/dL.
    D. Usually drug treatment with high dose statins in combination with ezetimibe, niacin, and bile acid sequestrants is effective for most homozygous FH patients to reach their cholesterol targets.

3. Which of the following statements is true regarding LDL-apheresis?

    A. LDL-apheresis is recommended for asymptomatic FH patients who despite optimal drug therapies and maximal dietary interventions have LDL-C greater than 200 mg/dL.

B. LDL-C levels after apheresis generally rebound back to pretreatment levels within 1–2 weeks.

C. Similar to high dose statin therapy, LDL-apheresis can lower LDL-C by up to 20 % in homozygous FH patients who have nearly absent LDL-receptors.

D. While LDL-apheresis can lower LDL-C levels, randomized control trials have not shown a vascular or clinical benefit.

## Answers to Questions

1. D
2. C
3. B

## References

1. Ito MK, McGowan MP, Moriarty PM. Management of familial hypercholesterolemias in adult patients: recommendations from the National Lipid Association Expert Panel on Familial Hypercholesterolemia. J Clin Lipidol. 2011;5:S38–45.
2. Goldstein JL, Hobbs HH, Brown MS. Familial hypercholesterolemia. In: Scriver CR, Beaudet AL, Sly WS, Valle D, editors. The metabolic and molecular basis of inherited disease. New York, NY: McGraw Hill; 2001. p. 2863–913.
3. Grundy SM, Cleeman JI, Merz CNB, Brewer HB, Clark LT, Hunninghake DB, Pasternak RC, Smith SC, Stone NJ. Implications of recent clinical trials for the national cholesterol education program adult treatment panel III guidelines. Circulation. 2004;110:227–39.
4. Kroon AA, Aengevaeren WR, van der Werf T, Uijen GJ, Reiber JH, Bruschke AV, Stalenhoef AF. LDL-Apheresis Atherosclerosis Regression Study (LAARS). Effect of aggressive versus conventional lipid lowering treatment on coronary atherosclerosis. Circulation. 1996; 93(10):1826–35.
5. Mabuchi H, Koizumi J, Shimizu M, Kajinami K, Miyamoto S, Ueda K, Takegoshi T. Long-term efficacy of low-density lipoprotein apheresis on coronary heart disease in familial hypercholesterolemia. Hokuriku-FH-LDL-Apheresis Study Group. Am J Cardiol. 1998;82(12): 1489–95.
6. Thompson GR. LDL apheresis. Atherosclerosis. 2003;167:1–13.

# Chapter 47
# Familial Type III Hyperlipoproteinemia (Familial Dysbetalipoproteinemia)

Conrad B. Blum

## Objective

To understand the pathophysiology, clinical presentation, and modes of therapy for familial type-III hyperlipoproteinemia.

## Case Presentation

RK is a 54-year-old woman with recent presentation of mixed hyperlipidemia at a routine examination. At that time, she complained of increased difficulty with weight control, and she noticed that leg fatigue, particularly involving the left calf, was causing some difficulty with stair climbing.

She had treated hypothyroidism, but otherwise been in good health. She had no history of hospitalizations except for childbirth when she was in her 20s. Her medications were L-thyroxine 75 µg daily and a multivitamin with mineral preparation which she had initiated several months prior to her recent routine physical examination.

Her father developed type-2 diabetes in his mid-40s. He was overweight. He died suddenly at age 55 years; there had been no previous history of cardiovascular disease. He was reported to have had elevated cholesterol and triglyceride levels.

She had not used tobacco since she was 22 years of age. Alcohol consumption averaged one glass of wine 3 nights weekly. She gained 16 pounds during the past 2 years to a current weight of 135 pounds (height 61 in.; BMI 25.5 kg/m$^2$). Menopause occurred at age 52 years.

C.B. Blum, M.D. (✉)
Professor of Medicine at Columbia University Medical Center,
Columbia University College of Physicians & Surgeons,
51 West 51st Street, NY 10019, New York, USA
e-mail: cbblum@gmail.com

© Springer Science+Business Media New York 2015
T.F. Davies (ed.), *A Case-Based Guide to Clinical Endocrinology*,
DOI 10.1007/978-1-4939-2059-4_47

**Table 47.1** Laboratory data—patient RK

| Time | CHOL | HDL | Tri-glyceride | Non-HDLc | ApoB | Non-HDLc/apoB | TSH | Weight | Treatments |
|------|------|-----|---------------|----------|------|---------------|-----|--------|------------|
| Baseline | 352 | 35 | 478 | 317 | – | | 5.8 | 135 | Baseline |
| 2 weeks | 340 | 34 | 452 | 306 | 87 | 3.5 | 5.6 | – | None |
| 3 months | 220 | 39 | 267 | 181 | 62 | 2.9 | 0.82 | 128 | Diet, ↑ L-thyroxine |
| 5 months | 114 | 40 | 192 | 74 | 32 | 2.3 | – | 126 | Atorvastatin 20 mg/day |

Lipid, lipoprotein, and apoB concentrations reported as mg/dl; TSH as µIU/ml; weight as pounds

On examination, she was 135 pounds. BP was 125/75, and heart rate was 75/min with a regular rhythm. There was yellowish discoloration of palmar creases.

Fasting blood testing showed her to have cholesterol 352 mg/dl, HDL cholesterol (HDLc) 35 mg/dl, and triglyceride 478 mg/dl. Non-HDLc was 317 mg/dl. TSH was 5.8 mcIU/ml. She had no proteinuria, and she had normal values for blood tests of renal function at hepatic function.

Two weeks later, she had confirmatory and additional blood testing: total cholesterol was 340 mg/dl, HDLc 34 mg/dl, and triglyceride 452 mg/dl; thus, non-HDLc was 306 mg/dl. TSH was 5.6 mcIU/ml. ApoB was 87 mg/dl. The ratio of non-HDLc/apoB was 3.5. Following this, apoE genotyping showed her to be homozygous for the ε2 allele of the APOE gene.

She was treated with dietary calorie restriction and exercise in an effort to achieve weight loss. Her dose of L-thyroxine was increased to 100 µg daily.

She returned for reevaluation 10 weeks later (Table 47.1). Her weight had fallen to 128 pounds. TSH had normalized. Total cholesterol had fallen to 220 mg/dl. HDLc was 39 mg/dl, and triglyceride was 267 mg/dl. Non-HDLc was 181 mg/dl. She was advised to continue with exercise and dietary efforts to achieve weight loss. Additionally, she initiated treatment with atorvastatin 20 mg daily. At follow-up, 5 months after her presentation, she weighed 126 pounds. Total cholesterol was 114 mg/dl, HDLc 40 mg/dl, and triglyceride 192 mg/dl. Non-HDLc was 74 mg/dl.

She underwent lower extremity arterial plethysmography and was found to have moderately reduced perfusion of the left lower extremity at the infrapopliteal artery level. Pharmacologic stress myocardial perfusion study gave normal results.

Her left calf claudication was treated with an exercise program and lipid management with diet and atorvastatin. Claudication resolved 6–9 months after initiation of these therapies.

## How the Diagnosis Was Made

The diagnosis of type-III hyperlipoproteinemia was suggested by the elevation of cholesterol and triglyceride levels and also by yellowish discoloration of her palmar creases. It was further suggested by an elevation of the ratio of non-HDL cholesterol to apolipoprotein B; values above 2.5 indicating likelihood of type-III hyperlipoproteinemia. The diagnosis was confirmed by apoE genotyping which showed homozygosity for the ε2 allele of apoE.

The genetic defect allowing expression of type III hyperlipoproteinemia is mutation of the gene for apolipoprotein E [1]. ApoE is the receptor recognition site on partially catabolized remnants of VLDL and chylomicrons responsible for their clearance by LDL receptors or by the high capacity low affinity heparan sulfate proteoglycans receptors involved in clearance of these remnants from the plasma. The mutant apoE protein of type III hyperlipoproteinemia, termed apoE2, is poorly bound by the LDL receptor and by the heparan sulfate proteoglycans receptors for remnants of triglyceride-rich lipoproteins. The commonest mutation causing the apoE2 isoform of apoE is arg158→cys; this results from the ε2 allele of the APOE gene. This amino acid substitution in the apoE protein results in impaired clearance of these remnant lipoproteins and their accumulation in plasma causing elevation of plasma levels of both cholesterol and triglyceride. The ε2 allele of the gene for apoE is by far the commonest mutation of APOE that causes type-III hyperlipoproteinemia, homozygosity for this allele being present in >90 % of patients with type-III hyperlipoproteinemia. Homozygosity for ε2 occurs in about 1 % of the population. However, fewer than 5 % of patients homozygous for the ε2 allele develop type-III hyperlipoproteinemia. An additional metabolic insult causing either increased synthesis of very low density lipoprotein (VLDL) or decreased clearance is necessary for hyperlipidemia to manifest itself. These additional metabolic insults include increased age, overweight, and insulin resistance, polymorphisms of lipolysis genes, hypothyroidism, menopause, certain medications (e.g., atypical antipsychotics such as olanzapine). Pregnancy has been reported to produce such severe hypertriglyceridemia in an ε2 homozygous woman as to cause pancreatitis [2].

Laboratory diagnostic criteria for type-III hyperlipoproteinemia have evolved considerably since the early 1950s when the plasma from these patients was noted to demonstrate a characteristic lipoprotein pattern on analytical ultracentrifugation. In the 1960s, the presence of an unusually broad band of lipoproteins with beta electrophoretic mobility was noted to be associated with this condition as was the presence of VLDL with beta electrophoretic mobility (normal VLDL has prebeta mobility). Beginning in the early 1970s, abnormalities of lipoprotein composition reflecting remnant accumulation were utilized in diagnosis. In particular, a landmark 1975 analysis of the clinical, genetic, and biochemical characteristics of 49 patients with type-III hyperlipoproteinemia gave a diagnostic criterion of cholesterol/triglyceride ratio of VLDL ≥0.30 type-III hyperlipoproteinemia [3]. Since VLDL remnants are relatively cholesterol rich, this criterion may be taken as an indicator of the accumulation of these remnants. A disadvantage of this criterion is that it requires isolation of VLDL by preparative ultracentrifugation. More recently, it has been suggested that a ratio of non-HDLc/apolipoprotein B (both in mg/dl) >2.5 be used as a screening criterion for type-III hyperlipoproteinemia [4]. This ratio also is based on the cholesterol-rich nature of the remnants of VLDL and chylomicrons that accumulate in this disease.

The current gold standard diagnostic criterion for type-III hyperlipoproteinemia is based on our understanding of the role of apoE genetics in the pathophysiology of type III hyperlipoproteinemia. Type-III HLP can be diagnosed when mixed hyperlipidemia occurs in the presence of homozygosity for the ε2 allele of APOE. However, approximately 10 % of patients with type-III hyperlipoproteinemia are not homozygous for the ε2 allele of APOE; they have other far less common mutations of APOE and require more detailed genetic analysis for diagnosis. Many of these individuals with rare mutations of the APOE gene will manifest type-III hyperlipoproteinemia with only a single allele of the mutant gene; they may also develop hyperlipidemia in childhood, a very rare occurrence for typical type-III hyperlipoproteinemia [1, 3].

It is suggested that initial screening of patients with mixed hyperlipidemia for non-HDLc/apolipoprotein B ratio >2.5 be used to identify individuals who warrant apoE genotyping. This was done in the current case.

In this patient, clinical characteristics also suggested that a diagnosis of type-III hyperlipoproteinemia be entertained.

She was noted to have yellowish discoloration of her palmar creases. This is a mild form of palmar xanthomas (also called palmar planar xanthomas or *xanthoma striata palmaris*). In more pronounced form, these lesions also cause some nodularity within the palmar creases. Palmar xanthomas appear to be specific for type-III hyperlipoproteinemia and have been reported to occur in approximately 50–70 % of patients. However, other types of xanthomas can also be seen including tendon xanthomas and tuboeruptive xanthomas [3].

The patient RK gave a history suggesting intermittent claudication, and noninvasive flow studies demonstrated peripheral vascular disease (PVD) involving the left lower extremity. A summary of pooled data reporting on 181 adult patients with type-III hyperlipoproteinemia indicates a prevalence of 28 % for coronary heart disease (CHD) and 21 % for PVD [1]. The high frequency of PVD, particularly in comparison CHD prevalence, is striking. By contrast, in an analysis of 119 kindred with familial hypercholesterolemia, manifested by elevation of LDL cholesterol, Stone et al. (Circulation 1974) found a 30 % prevalence of CHD and only a 4 % prevalence of PVD [3].

Other characteristics of this patient are typical of type-III hyperlipoproteinemia: presentation in adulthood, precipitation or exacerbation of hyperlipidemia by hypothyroidism, and overweight. Presentation in childhood is very uncommon except in those individuals with the rare APOE mutations that cause an autosomal dominant form of the disease (1).

## Lessons Learned

The most important lesson to be learned from this patient is that diagnosis of type-III hyperlipoproteinemia is worthwhile because of the exquisite responsiveness of this condition to lifestyle treatments and to pharmacotherapy. RK demonstrated a

**Table 47.2** Response to diet and type III hyperlipoproteinemia: NIH experience [3]

|  | Baseline | After diet | % Change |
|---|---|---|---|
| Cholesterol | 453 | 185 | −59 |
| HDLc | 38 | 40 | 5 |
| Non-HDLc | 415 | 145 | −65 |
| Triglyceride | 699 | 131 | −81 |

Concentrations reported as mg/dl

**Table 47.3** Type III hyperlipoproteinemia: response to medications

| Drug | N | Percent reduction | | | |
|---|---|---|---|---|---|
|  |  | Cholesterol | Non-HDLc | Triglyceride | ApoB |
| Gemfibrozil 600 mg bid[a] | 10 | −17 | −21 | −55 | −11 |
| Fenofibrate 200/100 mg bid[b] | 9 | −38 | −44 | −56 | −31 |
| Gemfibrozil 600 mg bid[c] | 5 | −27 | −35 | −56 | − |
| Bezafibrate 400 mg/day[d] | 6 | −36 | −44 | −64 | −17 |
| Nicotinic acid 3 g/day (mean of 1.5 g bid and 1 g tid)[c] | 5 | −34 | −43 | −48 | − |
| Atorvastatin 10 mg/day[d] | 6 | −41 | −46 | −28 | −33 |
| Atorvastatin 20 mg/day[e] | 4 | −52 | −66 | −56 | −52 |
| Atorvastatin 40 mg/day[f] | 28 | −46 | −53 | −40 | −43 |

[a]Am Heart J 1999, 138:156–162
[b]Am J Med 1987, 83(suppl 5B):71–74
[c]Atherosclerosis 1984, 51:521–529
[d]Clin Chimica Acta 2011, 412:1068–1075
[e]Atherosclerosis 2003, 168:359–366
[f]Heart 2002, 88:234–238

large reduction in total cholesterol, non-HDLc, and triglyceride levels with diet. In the NIH series, dietary modification led to approximately 60 % reductions in total cholesterol and in non-HDLc as well as an approximately 80 % reduction in fasting plasma triglycerides (Table 47.2) [3]. Diet for patients with type-III hyperlipoproteinemia should focus on calorie restriction to achieve ideal weight and restriction of alcohol. Saturated fats, transfats, and cholesterol should be limited as advised for the general population. Because many patients will become normolipidemic with diet as the sole therapy, diet should almost always precede drug therapy for patients with type-III hyperlipoproteinemia. The exception to this rule is the patient with clinical evidence of cardiovascular disease; for such patients, diet and medication should be initiated simultaneously.

Response to treatment with statins, fibrates, or nicotinic acid has similarly been excellent. A statin should be considered the first-line drug for treating type-III hyperlipoproteinemia because of the superior efficacy of this class of drugs in controlling non-HDL and remnant cholesterol levels (Table 47.3) and because of the strong record of statins in preventing CHD events in patients with a wide range of characteristics and risk factors. Table 47.3 summarizes several reports of the effects of treatment of type-III hyperlipoproteinemia with statins, fibrates, and nicotinic acid.

LDLc levels are not shown in Table 47.1 or in Table 47.3 for technical reasons. The Friedewald formula used to calculate LDLc levels is invalid in patients with type-III hyperlipoproteinemia; it overestimates LDLc. The direct measurement of LDLc has not been validated for patients with type-III hyperlipoproteinemia. Interestingly, it has been shown to be inaccurate for hypertriglyceridemic diabetic patients.

Effective treatment of type-III hyperlipoproteinemia has been shown to improve blood flow in patients with peripheral vascular disease [5] and has been associated with resolution of xanthomas, resolution of angina pectoris, and normalization of ischemic treadmill stress test results in stable CHD [6].

## Questions

1. Which of the following statements about type-III hyperlipoproteinemia is correct:

   a. This disease usually presents in childhood.
   b. Tendon xanthomas are typical and virtually pathognomonic of type-III hyperlipoproteinemia.
   c. Dietary measures can be particularly effective in reducing plasma lipid levels in patients with type-III hyperlipoproteinemia.
   d. Bile acid sequestrants such as cholestyramine or colesevelam are the first-line medications for treatment of type-III hyperlipoproteinemia.

2. Which of the following statements is true:

   a. Most patients who are homozygous for the ε2 allele of the APOE gene will manifest type-III hyperlipoproteinemia in adulthood.
   b. Most patients with type-III hyperlipoproteinemia are heterozygous for the ε2 allele of the APOE gene.
   c. Type-III hyperlipoproteinemia is characterized by accumulation in plasma of high levels of remnants of VLDL and chylomicrons.
   d. Calculated assessment of LDL cholesterol is unreliable in type-III hyperlipoproteinemia, but direct LDL cholesterol measurement has been validated and is recommended for these patients.

3. Which of the following statements is true:

   a. The major physiological defect determining the abnormal lipoprotein pattern of type-III hyperlipoproteinemia (accumulation of remnants of VLDL and chylomicrons) involves a defect in receptors for these remnant lipoproteins.

b. Although coronary heart disease frequently occurs inpatients with type III hyperlipoproteinemia, peripheral vascular disease is almost never seen in patients with this condition.

c. In order for type-III hyperlipoproteinemia to be expressed, a second metabolic insult such as insulin resistance must be present in addition to a the presence of an abnormal apolipoprotein.

d. LDL receptors do not play a role in uptake of remnants of VLDL and chylomicrons.

## Answers to Questions

1. c
2. c
3. c

## References

1. Mahley RW, Rall SC. Type III hyperlipoproteinemia (dysbetalipoproteinemia): the role of apolipoprotein E in normal and abnormal lipoprotein metabolism. In: Scriver CR, Beaudet AL, Sly WS, Valle D, editors. The metabolic and molecular bases of inherited disease. New York, NY: McGraw-Hill; 1995. p. 1953–80.
2. Chuang TY, et al. Gestational hyperlipidemic pancreatitis caused by type III hyperlipoproteinemia with apolipoprotein E2/E2 homozygote. Pancreas. 2009;38:716–7.
3. Morganroth J, Levy RI, Fredrickson DS. The biochemical, clinical, and genetic features of type III hyperlipoproteinemia. Ann Int Med. 1975;82:158–74.
4. Murase T, Okubo M, Takeuchi I. Non-HDL cholesterol/apolipoprotein B ratio: a useful distinguishing feature in screening for type III hyperlipoproteinemia. J Clin Lipidol. 2010;4:99–104.
5. Zelis R, et al. Effects of hyperlipoproteinemias and their treatment on the peripheral circulation. J Clin Invest. 1970;49:1007–15.
6. Cho EJ, et al. Disappearance of angina pectoris by lipid lowering in type III hyperlipoproteinemia. Am J Cardiol. 2011;107:793–6.

# Chapter 48
# Severe Hypertriglyceridemia

Jessica S. Lilley and Sergio Fazio

## Objectives

1. To discuss a case of acute pancreatitis caused by severe hypertriglyceridemia.
2. To review the stressors that can cause significant hypertriglyceridemia in susceptible individuals.
3. To position the clinical presentation of pancreatitis as a corollary to diabetic
   ketoacidosis.

## Case Presentation

A 14-year-old girl presented to the emergency department with excruciating abdominal pain. She had a history of dysmenorrhea, so her family had attributed her symptoms to menstrual cramps, but when the pain escalated to intolerable levels, they
sought medical evaluation. The pain was mostly on the left upper abdominal quadrant and radiated to the back. She had vomiting and anorexia but no fever; review of
systems also revealed a 15-pound weight loss over the preceding month as well as
polyuria and polydipsia. Her medications included Zoloft and a contraceptive patch,
both to treat premenstrual dysphoric disorder. Family history was significant for

J.S. Lilley, M.D. (✉)
Assistant Professor of Pediatrics, Division of Pediatric Endocrinology,
University of Mississippi School of Medicine, 2500 North State Street,
Jackson, MS 39216, USA

S. Fazio, M.D., Ph.D.
William and Sonja Connor Chair of Preventive Cardiology, Professor of Medicine and
Physiology & Pharmacology, Director, Center of Preventive Cardiology, Knight
Cardiovascular Institute, Oregon Health and Science University,
3181 SW Sam Jackson Park Rd, Portland, 97239, Oregon, USA

© Springer Science+Business Media New York 2015
T.F. Davies (ed.), *A Case-Based Guide to Clinical Endocrinology*,
DOI 10.1007/978-1-4939-2059-4_48

**Fig. 48.1** Patient's lipemic
serum

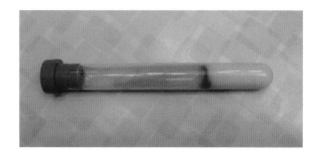

maternal Crohn's disease and type-1 diabetes mellitus. Physical exam revealed pallor, tachycardia, and abdominal tenderness with voluntary guarding. An initial lab revealed pH 7.12 and glucose 321 mg/dL with a base excess of −20.4, all consistent with new-onset diabetes mellitus with diabetic ketoacidosis (DKA). She showed an apparent severe hyponatremia.

Further laboratory evaluation was desired, so a complete metabolic panel, amylase, lipase, and complete blood count were ordered along with typical new-onset diabetes mellitus labs. The laboratory technician noted that the serum was extremely lipemic and alerted the ordering physician (Fig. 48.1). Total triglycerides were measured at 7,528 mg/dL. Lipase was extremely elevated at >800 mg/dL (normal 10–60), whereas amylase was barely elevated at 48 mg/dL (normal 5–45). C-peptide was low, antiglutamic acid decarboxylase antibodies were strongly positive, and hemoglobin A1c was measured at 11 % (normal <6.5 %). Repeat physical exam revealed no xanthomas or lipemia retinalis; there was no acanthosis nigricans. Limited abdominal ultrasound did not visualize the pancreas but identified focal fatty infiltration of the liver at the bifurcation of the portal vein.

The patient was made NPO and placed on an insulin drip at 0.1 units/kg/h along with dextrose-containing IV fluids to correct her acidosis while allowing her blood sugar to correct slowly. After 24 h, her acidosis and hyperglycemia had resolved, and her triglycerides had fallen to 4,014 mg/dL. She was started on total parenteral nutrition without lipids and multiple daily insulin injections. Within 48 h, triglycerides were 1,279 mg/dL and her abdominal pain had improved significantly. Her diet was advanced slowly until she tolerated a low-fat, low-refined carbohydrate diet, and her triglycerides were 747 mg/dL at discharge home. She was not prescribed a triglyceride-lowering medication and was encouraged to supplement her diet with 3–4 g of omega 3 fats. Upon return to the diabetes clinic 1 month later, triglycerides were 295 mg/dL with blood sugars close to goal for age. Her sodium level had normalized.

## How the Diagnosis Was Made

Given the context of the clinical presentation, with much attention placed on the DKA, the clinical suspicion for hypertriglyceridemia causing pancreatitis was not raised until the laboratory called the care team to report a lipemic sample.

At admission, this girl's severe abdominal pain had been thought to be secondary to ketosis. The differential for pancreatitis, however, must always include chylomicronemia, the condition leading to elevations in triglycerides above 1,000 mg/dL. In adult patients, pancreatitis is most commonly caused by biliary obstruction, side effect from medications, and alcohol abuse [1]. In the pediatric population, the etiology of pancreatitis is more variable and includes drug-induced pancreatitis, congenital anatomical abnormalities, infection, trauma, and cystic fibrosis [2]. Hypertriglyceridemia is a rare but important cause of pancreatitis in all ages, particularly in patients with diabetes mellitus or personal or family history of hyperlipidemia. Triglycerides elevations above 1,000 mg/dL are always caused by a failure of lipoprotein lipase (LPL) action, which can be due to genetic or environmental causes, in most cases by a combination of both. Though hypertriglyceridemia is seen in 12–22 % of patients with pancreatitis [3], the elevated triglycerides are not thought to be causative unless >1,000 mg/dL [4]; in our experience, triglyceride levels >2,000 mg/dL are usually necessary before induction of pancreatitis. It must be remembered that even forms of pancreatitis not secondary to hypertriglyceridemia are accompanied by mild to moderate elevations in triglycerides, often a puzzling finding for clinicians who have little experience in management of genetic dyslipidemia. There is no need for genetic testing or advanced lipid investigations, as the picture of pancreatitis with severe hypertriglyceridemia nails the causality link and triggers a standardized series of therapeutic maneuvers. This case is typical in showing drastic reductions in triglycerides while the patient was NPO in hospital, with an average daily drop of about 50 %. The remaining mild hypertriglyceridemia seen at follow-up suggests the presence of a genetic underpinning, maybe a heterozygous mutation in LPL.

## Lessons Learned

The pathophysiology and natural history of pancreatitis is poorly understood, irrespective of its causes. A proposed mechanism for pancreatitis due to severe hypertriglyceridemia considers escape of the end products of lipase action, lysolecithin and free fatty acids, from chylomicrons. Lysolecithin and free fatty acids are acutely toxic to the pancreas and lead to release of pancreatic lipase, resulting in acute pancreatitis [3]. Of course, the tremendous creaminess of lipemic blood also suggests that altered capillary flow in the pancreatic bed may cause perfusion and oxygenation deficits which can trigger cell death and release of pancreatic enzymes. Hypertriglyceridemia can result from obesity, physical inactivity, diabetes mellitus, hypothyroidism, and metabolic syndrome. Many pharmaceutical agents can elevate triglycerides, including corticosteroids, retinoids and rexinoids, estrogen, and thiazide and loop diuretics; several cases of asparaginase-induced hypertriglyceridemia and resultant pancreatitis have been reported. Many drugs can cause pancreatitis directly, without raising triglycerides. The most clinically significant hypertriglyceridemia is observed in patients with underlying genetic disorders leading to a phenotype compatible with a Type-I and Type-V grouping according to the Fredrickson's classification, such as homozygous LPL deficiency and associated gene defects (e.g., apoCII deficiency and mutations in apoAV or in glycosyl-phosphatidylinositol-anchored high-density lipoprotein-binding protein 1, aka GPIHBP-1). Worsening of more moderate genetic dyslipidemia (such as heterozygous LPL deficiency, familial hypertriglyceridemia, familial combined dyslipidemia, and familial dysbetalipoproteinemia) secondary to insulin resistance, comorbidities, or drugs affecting lipid metabolism can also lead to extreme triglyceride elevations and pancreatitis. Individuals who have an underlying genetic disorder are particularly susceptible to stressors such as alcohol abuse, high-estrogen states such as pregnancy, and insulin deficiency, as was the case in this patient. Alcohol abuse can also cause pancreatitis directly, without raising triglyceride levels.

Acute insulin deficiency results in increased production of very-low-density lipoproteins (VLDL) in the liver, since insulin signaling is the strongest regulator of posttranslational degradation of apoB (the main structural protein of VLDL), and in decreased clearance of triglyceride-containing lipoproteins, since insulin stimulates LPL action. Conversely, treatment with insulin corrects the acidosis and aids with lowering triglycerides by improving clearance of chylomicron remnants and decreasing VLDL output from the liver.

DKA is a common complication of new-onset and known diabetes, resulting in 100,000 inpatient admissions annually, and clinicians are most concerned about cardiovascular stability, risk for cerebral edema, possible infection triggering the acidosis, and electrolyte derangements [5]. Pancreatitis should be an additional concern; in one series, 11 % of consecutive patients presenting with DKA had CT-proven pancreatitis, though many of these cases had a self-limited hospital course [6]. Delay in diagnosis of pancreatitis can lead to shock, end-organ damage, pseudocyst formation, extended hospitalization, and even death.

The presence of pancreatitis may affect other portions of the clinical picture. This patient had severe hyponatremia upon presentation, and even following correction for hyperglycemia appeared to have dangerously low sodium. Knowing that the patient was severely hypertriglyceridemic was important for her electrolyte management since elevated triglycerides are another important cause of pseudohyponatremia. Extreme lipemia interferes with the accuracy of many laboratory tests.

This case and others reported previously resolved with intestinal rest and fluid and insulin administration. Children and adults with severe pancreatitis caused by persistent hypertriglyceridemia have been treated successfully with plasmapheresis and heparin infusions, but these interventions are not necessary if the TG levels drop as expected by about 50 % every 24 h under NPO conditions [5].

In summary, pancreatitis is a common sequela of diabetic ketoacidosis, and hypertriglyceridemia may be its cause in some patients, although triglyceride levels are moderately or severely elevated also as a consequence of pancreatitis caused by any other factor. Though the finding of a lipemic serum will lend a clue in patients with dramatic elevations in triglycerides, providers must always keep hypertriglyceridemia prominent in the differential for etiologies of pancreatitis.

## Questions

1. Which of the following conditions is NOT a potential stressor for a moderate genetic hypertriglyceridemia that can lead to triglyceride-induced pancreatitis?

   A. Pregnancy
   B. Oral contraceptive use
   C. Binge drinking
   D. Iodinated contrast

2. Which one statement is true?

   A. Pancreatitis caused by hypertriglyceridemia is more severe than that from other causes.
   B. Pancreatitis is often comorbid with diabetic ketoacidosis.
   C. All patients with TG > 2,000 mg/dL will eventually develop pancreatitis.
   D. Plasmapheresis is the standard treatment for triglyceride-induced pancreatitis.

3. A 37-year-old healthy woman without contributory medical or social history, except for a voluntary recent 30-lb weight loss, is hospitalized for acute pancreatitis after a weekend of heavy drinking. Her admission triglycerides are 550 mg/dL. Which one statement is likely correct?

   A. Her pancreatitis is caused by hypertriglyceridemia.
   B. Her hypertriglyceridemia is caused by pancreatitis.
   C. Her pancreatitis is caused by direct alcohol toxicity.
   D. Her pancreatitis is caused by biliary sludge triggered by the weight loss.

## Answers to Questions

1. D. Iodinated contrast
2. B. Pancreatitis is often comorbid with diabetic ketoacidosis.
3. B. Her hypertriglyceridemia is caused by pancreatitis.

## References

1. Wang GJ, Gao CF, Wei D, Wang C, Ding SQ. Acute pancreatitis: etiology and common pathogenesis. World J Gastroenterol. 2009;15:1427–30.
2. Minen F, De Cunto A, Martelossi S, Ventura A. Acute and recurrent pancreatitis in children: exploring etiological factors. Scand J Gastroenterol. 2012;47:1501–4.
3. Brunzell JD, Schrott HG. The interaction of familial and secondary causes of hypertriglyceridemia: role in pancreatitis. J Clin Lipidol. 2012;6:409–12.

4. Berglund L, Brunzell JD, Goldberg AC, et al. Evaluation and treatment of hypertriglyceride-mia: an Endocrine Society clinical practice guideline. J Clin Endocrinol Metab. 2012;97: 2969–89.
5. Lutfi R, Huang J, Wong HR. Plasmapheresis to treat hypertriglyceridemia in a child with diabetic ketoacidosis and pancreatitis. Pediatrics. 2012;129:e195–8.
6. Nair S, Yadav D, Pitchumoni CS. Association of diabetic ketoacidosis and acute pancreatitis: observations in 100 consecutive episodes of DKA. Am J Gastroenterol. 2000;95:2795–800.

# Part XII
# Obesity

# Chapter 49
# Introduction

Robert T. Yanagisawa and Derek LeRoith

## Epidemic of Obesity

More than 35 % of Americans are obese in the USA today and the prevalence of obesity continues to rise at an epidemic proportion. There has been a 74 % increase of obesity over the 10 years from 1991 to 2001 [1]. Over the period between 1999 and 2010, there have been observed differences between the rates of change of obesity prevalence between genders and races. Statistically significant increases are noted for non-Hispanic black women and Mexican American women as well as for men. Overall, the increases appear to be leveling off, however, there is no indication that the prevalence of obesity is declining [2]. Obesity epidemic is a reflection of the combination of excess caloric consumption with extra large portions of calorie dense food and the sedentary lifestyle that we have become accustomed to in our present society. As a consequence, obesity threatens our future with a significant increase in the prevalence of diabetes and cardiovascular morbidity and mortality. Our predisposition to obesity-related metabolic syndrome vary considerably among individuals and therefore, more personalized approaches are necessary to treat obesity. Some individuals are obese, yet they appear to be metabolically stable, while others develop many of the obesity-related metabolic complications, even with the same degree of obesity. Similar to other serious epidemic conditions, we must treat those obese individuals, with a high risk for metabolic complications, early and aggressively.

R.T. Yanagisawa, M.D. (✉) • D. LeRoith, M.D., Ph.D.
Division of Endocrinology, Diabetes, and Bone Diseases, Icahn School of Medicine at Mount Sinai, One Gustave Levy Place, Box 1055, New York, NY 10029-6574, USA
e-mail: Robert.yanagisawa@mssm.edu

© Springer Science+Business Media New York 2015
T.F. Davies (ed.), *A Case-Based Guide to Clinical Endocrinology*,
DOI 10.1007/978-1-4939-2059-4_49

# Endocrine Control of the Energy Balance System

Since the discovery of leptin in 1994, we have come to know that adipose tissue is a complex and metabolically active endocrine gland. Obesity is defined as the presence of excess adipose tissue. This excess, particularly in the visceral compartment, is associated with an increased risk for the metabolic syndrome. In addition, to metabolites such as free fatty acids (FFAs), adipose tissue secretes a variety of bioactive peptides, known as adipokines, active both at the local and systemic level [3].

These signals from adipose tissue work in concert with the rest of the energy homeostasis system. As Flier summarizes eloquently in his review, energy homeostasis involves both long-term and short-term signals [3]. Long-term afferent signals include leptin from adipose tissue and insulin from pancreatic beta cells. Short-term, meal-related afferent signals from the gut include inhibitors of appetite such as Peptide YY (PYY), Glucagon-like peptide-1 (GLP-1), and Cholecystokinin (CCK), and the stimulator of appetite such as ghrelin. These inputs are integrated within the brain, most importantly within the hypothalamic area and then processed into satiety or hunger signals as efferent output. The efferent elements of this system include those regulating the intensity of hunger and subsequent food seeking behavior. The efferent system also includes regulating the level of basal energy expenditure, energy expenditure determined by physical activity, and the levels of key circulating hormones such as insulin and glucocorticoids.

Since our survival used to be more acutely threatened by starvation than obesity, it comes as no surprise that the energy balance system is more robustly organized to respond to deficient energy intake and stores than to excess of energy. Our energy balance system is overwhelmed with the excess energy intake common in the present day, calorie-toxic environment. The system becomes more complicated when we take into account that our responses to food come not just from simple hunger or satiety, but with more variety of senses such as mood, appearance, environment, and more.

# The Present and Future of Obesity Management

A comprehensive approach should be taken to derive at an individually appropriate treatment plan for obese patients. The intensity of therapy should be scaled based on patients' degree of obesity and coexisting metabolic risk factors. In the majority of cases, relatively small reductions in weight have a significant impact on obesity-related metabolic conditions, but some require further intervention. While more than two-thirds of adults in the USA are either trying to lose or maintain weight, the majority struggle to lose any weight. One explanation is that only 17.5 % were following the basic two key recommendations, which is both to eat fewer calories and to increase physical activity [4].

There is no one dietary method that is effective for everyone, but in most cases, weight loss achieved closely approximates a mathematically estimated weight loss, by the difference between energy intake and energy requirement for the individual. There are more than 4,000 successful long-term weight loss maintainers in the National Weight Control Registry with an average weight loss of 33 kg for more than 5.7 years. They share six common behavioral strategies, and those are (1) engaging in high levels of physical activity; (2) eating a diet that is low in calories and fat; (3) eating breakfast; (4) self-monitoring weight on a regular basis; (5) maintaining a consistent eating pattern; and (6) catching "slips" before they turn into larger regains [5]. As we begin to understand some of the varied physiological mechanisms relating to obesity, we will have more options to intervene. While we are far from curing obesity, we will discuss some of the specific and successful strategies toward approaching patients with obesity.

# References

1. Ogden CL, et al. Prevalence of overweight and obesity in the United States 1999–2004. JAMA. 2006;295(13):1549–55.
2. Flegal KM, Carroll MD, Kit BK, Ogden CL. Prevalence of obesity and trends in the distribution of BMI among US adults, 1999–2010. JAMA. 2012;307(5):491–7.
3. Kershaw E, Flier JS. Adipose tissue as an endocrine organ. JCEM. 2004;89(6):2548–56.
4. Mokdad AH, et al. The continuing epidemics of obesity and diabetes in the United States. JAMA. 2001;286:1195–200.
5. Wing RR, Phelan S. Long-term weight loss maintenance. Am J Clin Nutr. 2005;82(Suppl):222S–5.

# Chapter 50
# Metabolic Syndrome Case

**Robert T. Yanagisawa, David W. Lam, and Derek LeRoith**

## Objectives

1. To review the criteria for the metabolic syndrome and the obesity assessment according to metabolic risk factors.
2. To understand the benefit of weight loss and lifestyle modification.
3. To review risk appropriate weight loss goals for individuals with the metabolic syndrome.

## Case

A 45-year-old white female presents with difficulty losing weight despite her diet and exercise program. She feels she is a setup for type-2 diabetes since her mother developed diabetes at her present age. She states she was never very "thin," but she has been gradually gaining weight over the last 10 years. She attributes her weight gain to decreased physical activity and stress-induced eating.

She has lost 15–20 lbs on several occasions on various diet programs, but she quits her diet when she does not see continued progress and then she regains her weight. The heaviest she ever weighed was 210 lbs.

Her primary physician started her on amlodipine 10 mg daily for her hypertension this past year, but she is otherwise in "good health." On physical exam, her blood pressure is controlled at 130/85 mmHg. Her weight is 200 lbs with height of 5′4″. Her waist circumference is 38″ and her hip circumference is 40″.

R.T. Yanagisawa, M.D. (✉) • D.W. Lam, M.D. • D. LeRoith, M.D., Ph.D.
Division of Endocrinology, Diabetes, and Bone Diseases,
Icahn School of Medicine at Mount Sinai, One Gustave Levy Place,
Box 1055, New York, NY 10029-6574, USA
e-mail: Robert.yanagisawa@mssm.edu

© Springer Science+Business Media New York 2015
T.F. Davies (ed.), *A Case-Based Guide to Clinical Endocrinology*,
DOI 10.1007/978-1-4939-2059-4_50

She did not have any striae, bruising, or significant hirsutism. She had a normal cervical fat pad for her weight. No acanthosis nigricans was present. Her abdomen was obese with weight distribution more typical of an android body shape. The remainder of her exam was unremarkable.

Laboratory findings were notable for impaired fasting glucose with plasma glucose of 105 mg/dl, but her Hgb A1C was normal at 5.5 %. A lipid profile reveals her total Chol of 198 mg/dl, low HDL of 39 mg/dl, high triglyceride of 200 mg/dl, and LDL of 110 mg/dl. TSH was normal at 1.6 µIU/ml as well as a 24-h urine free cortisol at 50 µg/24 h.

She wants to know what she can do to lose weight and reduce her risk of developing diabetes.

## Review of the Diagnosis

### Obesity Classification

Does she have obesity and obesity associated metabolic syndrome? Let's calculate her Body Mass Index (BMI) in order to evaluate her obesity and her metabolic risk. BMI is a standard measure of degree of obesity and it is calculated using patients' weight and height.

$$\begin{aligned} \mathrm{BMI} &= \mathrm{Weight}\left(\mathrm{kg}\right)/\mathrm{Height}\left(\mathrm{m}\right)^2 \\ &= 704 \times \mathrm{Weight}\left(\mathrm{lbs}\right)/\mathrm{Height}\left(\mathrm{in.}\right)^2 \\ &= 34.3 \,\mathrm{kg}/\mathrm{m}^2 \end{aligned}$$

In order to determine the appropriate risk of metabolic syndrome, we should use Risk-Adjusted BMI, which takes the degree of central obesity into account. Waist measure or waist to hip ratio provides the measure of central obesity. If you review the risk classification chart below, you will see by combining her BMI and central obesity, she has as much metabolic risk as someone in class II obesity (BMI 35.0–39.9) (Table 50.1).

**Table 50.1** Classification by BMI and waist circumference with associated risk for type-2 diabetes mellitus (T2DM), hypertension, and cardiovascular disease (CVD)

| Classification | BMI | Waist<br>Men <40″, Women <35″ | Circumference<br>Men >40″, Women >35″ |
|---|---|---|---|
| Overweight | 25.0–29.9 | Increased | High |
| Obesity Class I | 30.0–34.9 | High | Very high |
| Obesity Class II | 35.0–39.9 | Very high | Very high |
| Obesity Class III | >40.0 | Extremely high | Extremely high |

## Clinical Diagnosis of the Metabolic Syndrome

Central obesity is a major risk factor for metabolic syndrome. An android or an apple-shaped body weight distribution increases this risk compared to a pear body weight distribution as it is associated with increased visceral adiposity (Fig. 50.1).

Based on her waist circumference and laboratory values listed, she has all of the features of MetS. The definition was recently defined in a joint scientific statement by the International Diabetes Federation Task Force on Epidemiology and Prevention, National Heart, Lung, and Blood Institute, American Heart Association, World Heart Federation, International Atherosclerosis Society, and the International Association for the Study of Obesity. In this concerted effort to "harmonize" the definition, one major change was making central obesity just one of five components in making the diagnosis of MetS and not a prerequisite. The diagnosis of MetS is made when a patient has three of the five risk factors [1]. Because of well-described ethnic variations in the relationship of waist circumference with visceral adiposity, ethnic specific cut-offs based on population studies are recommended for use (Table 50.2).

## Obesity and Insulin Resistance

So, what role does obesity play in the metabolic syndrome? Obesity is a state of excess of body fat resulting in increased level of free fatty acid (FFA). Increased levels of FFA contribute to inhibition of insulin stimulated glucose utilization in

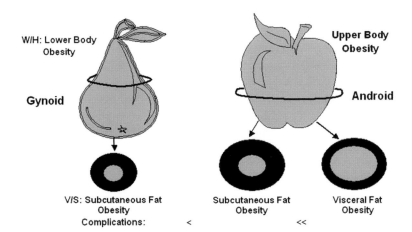

**Fig. 50.1** Classification of obesity according to fat distribution

**Table 50.2** Criteria for clinical diagnosis of the metabolic syndrome

| Measure | Categorical cut-off point |
| --- | --- |
| Elevated waist circumference | Population and country specific definition[a] |
| | Caucasian Men ≥94 cm, Women ≥80 cm |
| | Asian and Ethnic Central and South American Men ≥90 cm, Women ≥80 cm |
| Elevated triglycerides | ≥150 mg/dl (1.7 mmol/l) |
| Reduced HDL-C | <40 mg/dl (1.0 mmol/l) in males; <50 mg/dl (1.3 mmol/l) in females |
| Elevated blood pressure | Systolic ≥ 130 and/or diastolic ≥ 85 mmHg |
| Elevated fasting glucose | ≥100 mg/dl (5.5 mmol/l) |

Drug treatment for elevated triglycerides, reduced HDL-C, elevated blood pressure, and elevated glucose are considered to be an alternate indicator

Adapted from Harmonizing the metabolic syndrome: a joint interim statement of the International Diabetes Federation Task Force on Epidemiology and Prevention; National Heart, Lung, and Blood Institute; American Heart Association; World Heart Federation; International Atherosclerosis Society; and International Association for the Study of Obesity. Circulation 2009;120:1640–1645
[a]Detailed listing can be found in published joint statement

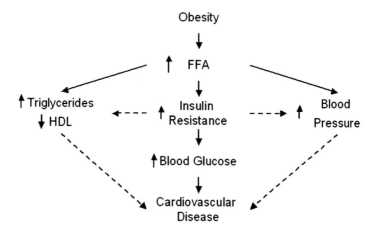

**Fig. 50.2** The role of obesity

muscle and stimulation of hepatic glucose production [2]. Visceral adipocytes are considered to be more lipolytically active than subcutaneous adipocytes and contribute to insulin resistance and its consequences (Figs. 50.2 and 50.3) [3].

## *Appropriate Weight Loss Goal*

While 5–10 % weight reduction is a significant improvement, this may not be adequate for patients with significant obesity who are considered to be at high risk for CVD. To take the weight management therapy one step further beyond the initial 5–10 %, setting a mutually agreeable goal between the patient and the treating

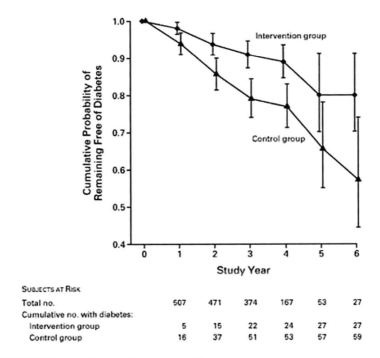

**Fig. 50.3** Weight loss by intervention prevents diabetes

physician is an important aspect of treating obesity. In order to set an appropriate goal for weight to reduce the risk of metabolic syndrome, you want the patients to have an idea of where do they stand on cardiovascular disease risk curve and see where they need to go to reduce the risk down to where it is more comparable to someone without significant obesity [4]. This is accomplished by reducing her BMI from her initial 34 kg/m$^2$ range down to 27–28 kg/m$^2$ range (Fig. 50.4).

Setting the ideal body weight range as the appropriate goal is not realistic for someone with a significant obesity. An overaggressive goal only leads to weight management failure. Many weight loss attempts fail because people do not transition well from weight loss phase to weight maintenance phase. Endocrine control of the energy balance system decreases basal energy expenditure with weight loss and counters the reduced body weight. Most people do not realize that they need to maintain both caloric restriction and exercise to increase their energy expenditure in order to maintain the weight loss.

## Lessons Learned

1. Obesity is a state of excess body fat and accumulation of more lipolytically active visceral adipocytes. Resulting increased level of FFA contributes to the metabolic syndrome.

**Fig. 50.4** Goals for risk
reduction

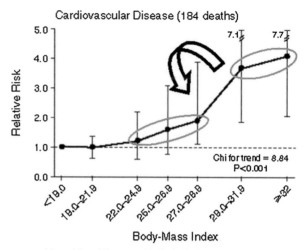

Adopted from Manson et al in Body Weight and Mortality among
Women NEJM 1999 333:677-685.

2. Metabolic risk of obesity is most commonly measured as both the degree of obesity (BMI) and regional fat distribution (Waist and Waist/Hip ratio). Increased waist circumference or central obesity is an independent risk factor for metabolic syndrome.
3. Lifestyle modification intervention, even at the modest 5–10 % total body weight reduction, has been clearly shown to have significant benefit of reducing the risk of metabolic syndrome.
4. The intensity of therapy and the appropriate goal weight should be based on patients' metabolic risk.

## Questions

1. What is her Body Mass Index (BMI) and what is her Metabolic Risk Category?

   A. BMI 30 kg/m$^2$ and increased metabolic risk
   B. BMI 34 kg/m$^2$ and high metabolic risk
   C. BMI 34 kg/m$^2$ and very high metabolic risk
   D. BMI 37 kg/m$^2$ and very high metabolic risk
   E. BMI 37 kg/m$^2$ and extremely high metabolic risk

2. What risk factors does she have for the metabolic syndrome?

   A. Central obesity
   B. Hypertriglyceridemia
   C. Reduced HDL
   D. Hypertension
   E. All of the above

3. Considering her degree of obesity and metabolic syndrome, what is her appropriate weight loss goal to reduce her metabolic risks?

   A. Her metabolic risk is normal
   B. Her metabolic risk cannot be reduced no matter what she does.
   C. Aim for the ideal body weight reaching $BMI < 24$ kg/m$^2$
   D. Start with 5–10 % total body weight loss with a goal of reaching $BMI = 27$–$28$ kg/m$^2$
   E. She needs a bariatric surgery for weight loss.

## Answers to Questions

1. C.

**Discussion**: Calculated BMI in choice A, D, E are incorrect. Metabolic risk category in Choice B is incorrect because by combining her BMI and central obesity, she has as much metabolic risk as someone in class II obesity.

2. E.

**Discussion**: Choices A–D are all determinants of metabolic syndrome. They are all part of the criteria defined in a joint scientific statement by the International Diabetes Federation Task Force on Epidemiology and Prevention, National Heart, Lung, and Blood Institute, American Heart Association, World Heart Federation, International Atherosclerosis Society, and the International Association for the Study of Obesity.

3. D.

**Discussion**: Choice A is incorrect as her metabolic risk is very high. Risk stratification was discussed with Question 1. Choice B is incorrect as several weight management intervention studies have shown that obese individuals can significantly improve their metabolic risks by reducing weight. Choice C is incorrect because setting the ideal body weight range as the appropriate goal is not realistic on someone with a significant obesity. An overaggressive goal only leads to weight management failure. This patient does not meet the NIH criteria for surgical weight loss and therefore, choice E is incorrect. (See Bariatric Surgery case discussion for details.)

# References

1. Alberti KG, Eckel RH, Grundy SM, Zimmet PZ, Cleeman JI, Donato KA, Fruchart JC, James WP, Loria CM, Smith Jr SC. Harmonizing the metabolic syndrome: a joint interim statement of the International Diabetes Federation Task Force on Epidemiology and Prevention; National Heart, Lung, and Blood Institute; American Heart Association; World Heart Federation; International Atherosclerosis Society; and International Association for the Study of Obesity. Circulation. 2009;120:1640–5.
2. Kitabchi AE, Temprosa M, Knowler WC, et al. Role of insulin secretion and sensitivity in the evolution of type 2 diabetes in the diabetes prevention program: effects of lifestyle intervention and metformin. Diabetes. 2005;54(8):2404–14.
3. Tuomilehto J, Lindstrom J, Eriksson JG, et al. Prevention of type 2 diabetes mellitus by changes in lifestyle among subjects with impaired glucose tolerance. NEJM. 2001;344:1343–50.
4. Manson JE, Willett WC, Stampfer MJ, et al. Body weight and mortality among women. NEJM. 1995;333:677–85.

# Chapter 51
# The Polycystic Ovarian Syndrome (PCOS)

**Michael Magnotti, Rachel Pessah-Pollack, and Walter Futterweit**

## Objectives

1. To review the typical presentation of a patient with PCOS
2. To examine the current diagnostic criteria for PCOS as well as the controversy surrounding these criteria
3. To learn about the link between PCOS and the metabolic syndrome
4. To understand the treatment options for PCOS
5. To discuss the long-term complications of chronic PCOS

## Background

Polycystic ovary syndrome (PCOS) is a complex and heterogeneous syndrome with an increased risk of cardiovascular morbidities and diabetes involving 6–8 % of women of reproductive age. Insulin resistance (IR) and hyperinsulinism have been known as pathogenetic mechanisms, present in 50–70 % of these women [1], whereas the metabolic syndrome (MS) prevalence is higher than in age and weight-matched controls. PCOS is defined by hyperandrogenism (clinical or biochemical), chronic anovulation, and/or polycystic ovaries, with the exclusion of adrenal, ovarian, and pituitary disorders. It is characterized by multiple metabolic aberrations,

M. Magnotti, M.D. (✉)
Diabetes, Endocrinology, Metabolism Specialties, Teaneck, NJ, USA
e-mail: mikemagnotti@yahoo.com

R. Pessah-Pollack, M.D.
Division of Endocrinology, Diabetes, and Bone Diseases,
Icahn School of Medicine at Mount Sinai, New York, NY, USA

W. Futterweit, M.D.
Division of Endocrinology, Icahn School of Medicine at Mount Sinai, New York, NY, USA

© Springer Science+Business Media New York 2015
T.F. Davies (ed.), *A Case-Based Guide to Clinical Endocrinology*,
DOI 10.1007/978-1-4939-2059-4_51

including IR and hyperinsulinemia, a high incidence of impaired glucose tolerance, visceral obesity, inflammation and endothelial dysfunction, hypertension, and dyslipidemia. These aberrations result in an increased risk for diabetes and clinical or subclinical cardiovascular disease. Even in the absence of obesity or MS, patients with PCOS may have IR and increased cardiovascular risks. Parenthetically, high insulin levels affect the hypothalamic–pituitary–ovarian axis function, as well as glucose utilization in peripheral tissues.

Obesity and excess weight are major chronic diseases in Western world countries. Obesity increases hyperandrogenism, hirsutism, infertility, and pregnancy complications both independently and by exacerbating PCOS. Likewise, in PCOS obesity worsens insulin resistance and exacerbates reproductive and metabolic features. Furthermore, women with PCOS have an increased risk of Type-2 diabetes mellitus (T2DM) and CVD. Treatment of obesity through lifestyle intervention is a key treatment strategy in PCOS and improves IR, reproductive, and metabolic features. Small, achievable goals of 5 % loss of body weight result in significant clinical improvement even if women remain clinically in the overweight or obese range.

Lean women with PCOS often, but not always have abnormalities of insulin secretion and action compared to weight-matched control subjects. In women with insulin resistance and PCOS, only a subgroup develops coexistent pancreatic insufficiency with β cell failure and subsequent DM2. In this setting, insulin output cannot overcome resistance and hyperglycemia develops. Women with PCOS are at increased risk of developing IGT and DM2 with prevalence rates of 31.3 % and 7.5 %, respectively, compared to 14 % for IGT and 0 % for DM2 in an age-matched and weight-matched non-PCOS control population. Women with PCOS also develop abnormal glucose metabolism at a younger age and may demonstrate a more rapid conversion from IGT to DM2 The rate of conversion from IGT to DM2 in a general Australian population was estimated in the large cohort Australian Diabetes, Obesity and Lifestyle (Aus Diab) study at 2.9 % per year for young females Another Australian study has reported a substantially higher conversion rate (8.7 % per year over 6.2 years) in women with PCOS; however, this has not been uniformly reported. Women with PCOS also have higher gestational diabetes risk, with a recent meta-analysis reporting an odds ratio (OR) of 2.94. The risk of GDM occurs both independent of and is exacerbated by obesity. While there are few adequately powered studies assessing the natural history of IGT, T2DM, and cardiovascular disease in PCOS, there is a need for further larger long-term studies (Fig. 51.1).

## Case

A 22-year-old Caucasian female is referred to your office for evaluation of secondary amenorrhea. She reports menarche at age 14 and irregular menses for about 1 year. Her menses became regular and occurred monthly until age 17 menstruating only once every 2–3 months. For the past 6 months she has had no menstrual periods at all, and after taking several home pregnancy tests that were normal, she presented to

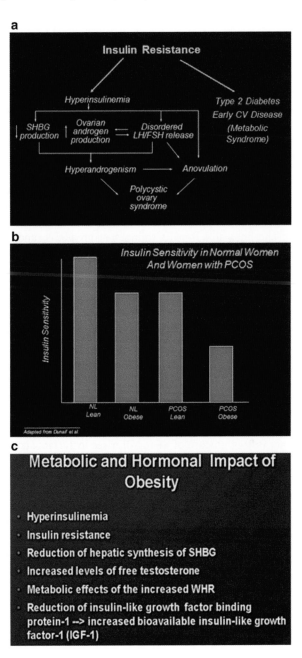

**Fig. 51.1** (**a–c**) Note the sensitivity to insulin in lean subjects with PCOS is similar to that of normal obese control. It is apparent that the extreme lowest insulin sensitivity is seen in obese women with PCOS, while the highest is present in normal lean subjects

her internist. He confirmed that she was not pregnant with a urine β-Hcg and referred her to your office for evaluation. She currently takes no medications. She notes that at age 16 she weighed 140 lbs, but gained about 40 lbs over the next 2- to 3-year period.

Her weight has been stable at 180 lbs for the past few years. She is not exercising over concern for worsening her excessive axillary perspiration. She admits to some bothersome facial and abdominal hair growth and significant facial acne. She regularly waxes her facial hair but denies any other form of hair removal. The patient tends to snore and has some degree of daytime somnolence. She has been married for 1 year and is not using any form of contraception at this time. She and her husband are very interested in having children in the future.

On physical exam, she weighs 182 lbs and is 66 in. tall, with a BMI of 29.4. Her waist circumference is 38 in., waist:hip ratio is 0.84. Her blood pressure is 125/70 mmHg and pulse is 72 beats/min. She has notable acanthosis nigricans on the back of her neck and in her axillae bilaterally; skin tags are present in the nape of the neck. There is a mild degree of excess terminal (thick, pigmented) body hair on the upper lip and chin and significant acne vulgaris on the face. In addition, moderate periareolar and linea alba thick, terminal hair growth is present. There is no thyromegaly. Heart and lung exams are unremarkable. On abdominal exam, there is central adiposity without striae and there is no peripheral edema or cliteromegaly. Her liver edge was minimally tender.

Laboratory evaluation reveals a mild microcytic anemia, normal chemistries, an elevated ALT (SGPT) of 60 U/L (normal 10–45) with otherwise normal liver function tests, fasting blood glucose of 85 mg/dL and free testosterone of 6.2. Serum testosterone is 80 pmol/L, prolactin is 17 mIU/L; DHEAS, Androstenedione, 17-hydroxyprogesterone, and 24 h urinary-free cortisol are all within normal limits. The fasting plasma insulin level is 19 μU/mL (normal is less than 12 μU/mL), and sex hormone-binding globulin (SHBG) is 12 nmol/L (normal 40–120). Lipid panel reveals a total cholesterol of 246 mg/dL, triglycerides of 190 mg/dL, HDL of 42 mg/dL, and LDL of 166 mg/dL. A standard 2 h oral glucose tolerance test is performed and her fasting glucose of 88 mg/dL rises to 180 mg/dL and her insulin to 110 μU/mL) (after 2 h). An abdominal ultrasound reveals moderate fatty infiltration suggesting nonalcoholic fatty liver disease (NAFLD), and the adrenal glands were of normal size with no nodules.

The patient is started on metformin 500 mg daily, which is titrated up over a few weeks to 1,000 mg BID with meals. She is also advised to use an effective form of birth control until she desires pregnancy. In addition, she receives extensive counseling on diet and exercise for weight loss and diabetes prevention.

## Review of Diagnosis, Treatment, and Complications

### Diagnosis

The diagnostic criteria for PCOS are the subject of continuing controversy. In 1990 after an international consensus conference, the NIH published the following criteria for the diagnosis of PCOS (all three criteria are required):

**Table 51.1**  Diagnostic criteria for PCOS[a]

| Criteria | NIH 1990 "classic" | Rotterdam 2003 | AE-PCOS |
|---|---|---|---|
| Oligomenorrhea | + | +/− | +/− |
| Clinical or biochemical hyperandrogenism | + | +/− | + |
| Polycystic ovaries on ultrasound | +/− | +/− | +/− |

[a]*AE-PCOS* Androgen Excess-Polycystic Ovarian Syndrome Society

Adopted from "Assessment of Cardiovascular Risk and Prevention of Cardiovascular Disease in Women with the Polycystic Ovary Syndrome: A Consensus Statement by the Androgen Excess and Polycystic Ovary Syndrome (AE-PCOS) Society" *J Clin Endocrinol Metab*, May 2010, 95(5): 2038-2049

1. Menstrual irregularity due to chronic anovulation
2. Evidence of clinical and/or biochemical hyperandrogenism (i.e., hirsutism, acne, or male-pattern alopecia)
3. Exclusion of other causes of hyperandrogenism and menstrual irregularities (i.e., hyperprolactinemia, Cushing's syndrome, androgen-producing tumors of the ovary or adrenal gland, adult-onset congenital adrenal hyperplasia)
4. These criteria were based mainly on "expert opinion," with limited scientific evidence. Notably, there is no mention of the presence of polycystic ovaries on ultrasonography.

In the years after the NIH criteria were released, it became apparent that there were women with normal menstrual cycles who had evidence of hyperandrogenism and polycystic ovaries on ultrasound and likely had PCOS. However, based on the NIH criteria, they would not be classified as having PCOS due to ovulatory menstrual cycles. Therefore, at a consensus conference in Rotterdam in 2003, the diagnostic criteria for PCOS were modified [6]. The new criteria require the presence of two of the following three:

1. Oligo-ovulation (fewer than nine times per year) and/or anovulation
2. Clinical and/or biochemical signs of hyperandrogenism
3. Polycystic ovaries (meeting specific criteria on transvaginal ultrasound)

The criteria specify that other etiologies of hyperandrogenism and amenorrhea must be ruled out, as PCOS is a diagnosis of exclusion. When applying the Rotterdam criteria, compared with the NIH criteria, the prevalence of PCOS in the population increases to over 20 %. A 2007 Position Paper by the Androgen Excess Society contends hyperandrogenism (clinical or biochemical), is the major criterion distinguishing PCOS from other etiologies manifesting oligo-amenorrhea, with the inclusion of polycystic ovaries on ultrasonography as a criterion [7]. Similarly, they require exclusion of other etiologies that may mimic PCOS in establishing the PCOS phenotype (Table 51.1).

Previous ultrasound criteria for polycystic ovaries included the presence of 8–10 follicles (measuring 2–8 mm in diameter), peripherally oriented with increased volume of stroma compared with the number of follicles. The Rotterdam ultrasound criteria include the presence of 12 or more follicles in each ovary (2–9 mm in diameter) and/or increased ovarian volume.

Nonetheless, sonographically apparent polycystic ovaries are not sufficient to diagnose PCOS as they can be demonstrated in many women who have other causes of hyperandrogenism or amenorrhea, as well as in up to 23 % of "normal" women. Some investigators believe the presence of a hyperandrogenic state may cause ovarian cyst formation, leading to the polycystic ovarian appearance on ultrasonography. Because of this, there continues to be controversy surrounding the inclusion of the polycystic ovarian morphology into the diagnostic criteria.

The menstrual dysfunction in PCOS typically presents around puberty with a normal or slightly delayed menarche and subsequent irregular menstrual cycles. Another pattern seen in PCOS women is initially regular cycles with subsequent menstrual irregularity associated with weight gain; often improved with weight loss. As ovulation is often infrequent, and first trimester pregnancies frequently abort, difficulty conceiving is often present.

The pathogenesis of PCOS is not completely understood. Current evidence suggests PCOS is a complex genetic trait influenced by genetic variants and environmental factors [2]. Numerous genes associated with PCOS or traits of PCOS have been identified. For example, PCOS susceptibility loci have been identified in Chinese women with PCOS and recently two of these PCOS susceptibility loci were also identified in European populations (DENND1A and THADA) [3]. Additionally, twin studies have established an inherited basis of PCOS with an increased inheritance in first-degree female relatives of women with PCOS.

In the normal ovary, the theca cells produce the androgens androstenedione and testosterone. These are converted to estrone and estradiol by aromatase activity in the granulosa cells. Androgen production by the theca cells is under the control of pituitary LH and the conversion to estrogens is under the control of FSH. LH and FSH production are in turn under the control of hypothalamic GnRH. It is the pulsatility of GnRH production that controls the relative amount of LH and FSH secreted by the pituitary. A rapid frequency of GnRH pulses favors the production of LH and slower pulse frequency favors the production of FSH. Abnormal gonadotropin secretory dynamics including altered LH action may be a component of the pathogenesis of PCOS. Women with PCOS have higher mean serum LH concentrations, possibly due to an increase in GnRH pulsatility. The serum FSH concentration may be normal or low in PCOS, causing an elevated LH/FSH production compared with young normal women in the early follicular phase with normal cycles. The likelihood of detecting an elevated serum LH depends on various factors such as last menstrual period, body mass index, and oral contraceptive pill use and as such, the diagnostic criteria for PCOS do not include an elevated serum LH and/or increased LH/FSH ratio.

The causative defect may also lie within the ovaries themselves. There may be higher LH action at the ovary in PCOS, resulting in hyperstimulation of thecal cells and premature expression of LH receptors in granulosa cells causing premature luteinization. There is evidence from several studies that the theca cells in women with PCOS may be more efficient at producing androgens than those of normal women. Therefore, these ovaries would produce a greater amount of androgen in response to a given level of LH, leading to the hyperandrogenic state of PCOS and secondary changes in GnRH pulsatility would be secondary. Of note, an elevated LH level is not mandatory in PCOS as increased ovarian androgen secretion and/or polycystic ovarian morphology can be seen without an elevated LH level. An elevated LH/FSH ratio is, however, more likely in nonobese women with PCOS. A slight elevation in prolactin may be seen, of unclear significance; however, a significant prolactin level elevation (>40 mg/dL) warrants an additional evaluation.

PCOS is also associated with the metabolic syndrome, insulin resistance, and compensatory hyperinsulinemia. The National Health and Nutrition Examination Survey (NHANES III) reported between a 40 and 50 % incidence of the metabolic syndrome (using the National Cholesterol Education/ATP III criteria) in women with PCOS. These women also have a higher incidence of insulin resistance than the general population, independent of their weight. Obesity is a frequent concomitant with PCOS and exacerbates insulin resistance, menstrual abnormalities, and higher likelihood of adverse pregnancy outcomes. Insulin resistance alone is not sufficient to develop PCOS, as hyperandrogenism is central to the disorder (via stimulation of androgen biosynthesis in the ovarian theca cell). Physical exam findings from hyperinsulinemia include the occurrence of acanthosis nigricans (darkening of skin most often on the back of the neck, in the axillae and in the groin) as was noted in our patient.

Insulin causes stimulation of theca cell secretion of androgens and suppresses hepatic SHBG production, leading to an increase in free androgens and clinically apparent as the hyperandrogenic phenotype typical of women with PCOS. Due to this phenomenon, treatment with weight loss and insulin sensitizers (such as metformin, thiazolidinediones) are often used in women with PCOS to decrease insulin resistance, decrease androgen levels, and improve ovarian function.

The metabolic syndrome has been linked to an increased risk of vascular disease (including myocardial infarction and stroke) and diabetes [4]. Therefore the link between PCOS and the metabolic syndrome has significant health implications. Thus many professional organizations recommend screening women with PCOS for the metabolic syndrome including impaired glucose tolerance with a baseline 2-h 75-g OGTT, prior to treatment and if a diagnosis is made every year or 2 thereafter.

The patient in our clinical vignette has impaired glucose tolerance as reflected by a 2 h OGTT glucose between 140 and 200 mg/dL (greater than 200 mg/dL is a sign of diabetes mellitus). The Rotterdam consensus meeting recommended *against* specific testing for insulin resistance given that tests for insulin resistance are not necessary to diagnose PCOS nor identify treatment. They did recommend screening all obese women with PCOS for components of the metabolic syndrome [assess waist circumference, measure blood pressure, fasting lipids and perform a 2-h oral glucose tolerance test (OGTT)]. The 2 h 75-g OGTT is recommended as normal fasting glucose levels do not identify women with impaired glucose tolerance who are at highest risk for future development of diabetes.

The 2009 Consensus statement from the Androgen Excess-Polycystic Ovary Syndrome (AE-PCOS) Society [10] recommends a 75-g OGTT in PCOS women with a BMI > 30 kg/m$^2$ or in lean PCOS women with age >40 years old, history of GDM, or family history of T2DM. The AE-PCOS statement recommends women with normal glucose tolerance be rescreened at least every 2 years, and IGT screened annually, and endorses a Hemoglobin A1c > 6.5 % as a criterion for risk assessment for diabetes.

There is a high prevalence of dyslipidemia in women with PCOS, as noted above in the clinical vignette. Women with PCOS are more likely to have hypertriglyceridemia and an increase in small dense LDL particles; strongly associated with an increased risk of coronary heart disease. The prevalence of nonalcoholic fatty liver disease (NAFLD) may be increased in women with PCOS, as reflected in our patient by an abnormal ALT level and abnormal liver sonographic characteristics.

A waist circumference of at least 35 in. in Caucasian/African-American women or 31.5 in. in Hispanic, Native American, Asian, and European women establishes the presence of abdominal obesity. Increased weight around the abdominal region ("apple shape") is associated with a greater risk of heart disease and diabetes, compared with around the hips ("pear" shape). The ranges for low, moderate, and high risk are listed below. The patient in the clinical vignette is of moderate risk.

| Female | Health risk based on waist to hip ratio |
|---|---|
| 0.80 or below | Low risk |
| 0.81–0.85 | Moderate risk |
| 0.85+ | High risk |

## Treatment

In order to determine the appropriate treatment for a patient with PCOS, it is essential to consider the patient's major manifestations of the syndrome and her goals of treatment. Potential treatment goals include improving fertility by inducing ovulation, reducing unwanted cosmetic effects such as hirsutism and alopecia and improving metabolic disturbances such as insulin resistance and obesity. It is also important to consider protection of the endometrium as a goal of therapy. The anovulation that is often associated with PCOS leads to a lack of progesterone production. This is associated with dysfunctional bleeding, endometrial hyperplasia, and an increased risk of endometrial cancer.

In obese women, weight loss can be very effective in reversing many of the symptoms of PCOS. A 5–10 % weight reduction can lead to a significant decrease in insulin resistance and in some patients, resumption of normal ovarian function and fertility. Weight loss can be accomplished with diet and exercise, medications, or bariatric surgery (in cases of morbid obesity). There is presently no evidence that one particular diet is better than another, but the choice of diet should likely be based upon a consideration of what the individual patient is able to follow over the long term. Lifestyle modification to induce weight loss is generally considered the first-line therapy for obese women with PCOS who desire fertility as it will lead to improvements in ovulation in a significant number of women and will likely lead to improved pregnancy outcomes and a reduced risk of gestational diabetes. It will often also lead to a reduction in symptoms of hyperandrogenism and will improve many of the metabolic abnormalities.

In women with a preponderance of hyperandrogenic symptoms (such as hirsutism, acne, and/or alopecia) who do not desire pregnancy, oral contraceptive pills should be the first-line therapy. If oral contraceptives alone are not effective, then spironolactone can be added. The most widely used form of the oral contraceptive pill consists of two components, an estrogen and a progestin. It is this combination oral contraceptive pill that is most useful in the treatment of PCOS and will be referred to as OCP in this text. The estrogen component of the pill (generally ethinyl estradiol) serves two main functions. First, it helps to inhibit pituitary production of LH, thereby decreasing ovarian androgen production. And second, estrogen stimulates hepatic production of SHBG, thus decreasing the amount of free androgen that is available to bind to its receptor. Both of these actions help to decrease the androgenic symptoms of the disorder. Many of the newer oral contraceptives contain a lower dose of ethinyl estradiol (20 mcg). This dose seems to be as effective as the higher doses of 30–35 mcg in reducing acne, but it has not been as effective for the treatment of hirsutism. Therefore, if a lower estradiol dose contraceptive is ineffective, it is reasonable to try one containing a higher dose.

The progestin component allows the resumption of regular menses and protects the endometrium from the adverse effects of unopposed estrogen (including dysfunctional bleeding and probably endometrial cancer). It is important to note that the synthetic progestins used in OCPs have varying degrees of androgenicity. Some progestins, such as levonorgestrel have a pro-androgenic effect. Others, such as norgestimate (found in Ortho-Cyclen, Ortho Tri-Cyclen, and Ortho Tri-Cyclen Lo) and desogestrel (found in Mircette, Ortho-Cept, Cyclessa, Apri, Desogen, and Kariva) are essentially nonandrogenic. Finally, progestins such as drospirenone (found in Yasmin and Yaz) are actually antiandrogenic. Because of its antiandrogenic effects, drospirenone would seem to be the ideal progestin for the treatment of PCOS; however, there is no evidence from controlled trials to support this. In fact, the evidence to date would suggest that there is no appreciable difference between the synthetic progestins when used to treat PCOS. Therefore, there is no recommendation to use any particular OCP at this time. Remember that when using an OCP containing drospirenone, potassium levels must be monitored because of its anti-mineralocorticoid effects.

Spironolactone is an antagonist of the mineralocorticoid receptor (potassium sparing diuretic) that is also able to antagonize the androgen receptor, furnishing it with utility in the treatment of PCOS. It is generally used as a second line agent, after an adequate trial of an OCP (6 months minimum) has failed to produce sufficient symptom improvement. While it does not directly lead to increased fertility, it is teratogenic to a male fetus and should be discontinued for 3–6 months prior to attempts at conception. Therefore, it is important to ensure that any female patient of reproductive age who is treated with spironolactone is placed on an effective form of contraception. This is often accomplished by using the oral contraceptive pill, because OCPs and spironolactone have synergistic antiandrogenic effects. However, any effective form of contraception would be acceptable and spironolactone can be used as first-line therapy in patients with a contraindication to OCPs. It is also essential to monitor potassium levels when using spironolactone. Cyproterone acetate is a more potent antiandrogen that is widely used in Europe for the treatment of hirsutism, but is not available in the USA at this time.

In women with the metabolic syndrome, impaired glucose tolerance or overt diabetes, and those desiring fertility, insulin sensitizers can be very useful therapies. The biguanide metformin helps to improve insulin resistance mainly by decreasing hepatic gluconeogenesis. This leads to decreased insulin levels and therefore decreased ovarian androgen production and increased hepatic SHBG production (as discussed in the prior section). In some patients, that is enough to allow the resumption of normal menses and fertility. In addition, metformin has the added benefit of promoting mild weight loss in some insulin resistant patients as well as potentially delaying or even preventing the onset of overt diabetes. There is some evidence that metformin may also reduce the frequency of first trimester miscarriages in patients with PCOS, but this evidence is limited so routine use of metformin for this purpose is not recommended in some guidelines and publications.

The thiazolidinediones (pioglitazone and rosiglitazone) are PPAR gamma receptor agonists that work primarily on the adipose tissue to improve insulin sensitivity. Initial studies with troglitazone and later with rosiglitazone and pioglitazone in women with PCOS have demonstrated a significant increase in ovulation, decrease in androgen levels, and increase in SHBG. However, the safety of these medications in pregnancy is unknown, limiting their use in women desiring fertility (pregnancy risk category C). In addition, the cardiovascular safety of rosiglitazone has recently been called into question making its use in this population potentially harmful. Thiazolidinediones also have the generally unwanted side effect of weight gain, limiting their utility in treating women with PCOS.

Finally, the natural history of PCOS is such that after the age of 35, many women notice a decrease in androgenic symptoms as well as a reduction of serum testosterone without any treatment. This may be due to age-related decreases in ovarian function leading to decreased efficiency of androgen production.

## Long-Term Complications

Because women with PCOS frequently have oligo-ovulation or anovulation, they are chronically exposed to the effects of estrogen without progesterone. Recall that in women with normally functioning ovaries, estrogen produced during the first half of the cycle causes proliferation of the endometrium. After ovulation occurs, progesterone is made by the corpus luteum, decreasing proliferation and leading to differentiation of the endometrium in preparation for implantation. However, in a patient with PCOS who fails to ovulate, the endometrium is chronically exposed to the effects of estrogen without progesterone, causing a continued stimulus for proliferation and thereby an increased risk of endometrial cancer. This risk can be reduced by re-introducing the effects of progesterone, either through the use of combination oral contraceptive pills or insulin sensitizing medications that cause the resumption of spontaneous ovulation. In women with a contraindication to estrogen, progesterone alone can be administered for 5–7 days of every month to induce menstrual bleeding and decrease the risk of endometrial cancer; but, this approach will not provide contraception.

There is also evidence that women with PCOS are at increased risk for nonalcoholic fatty liver disease (NAFLD) [8, 9]. This condition consists of a spectrum of diseases ranging from hepatic steatosis to steatosis with inflammation and steatosis with fibrosis (also known as NASH—non alcoholic steatohepatitis). As it is one of the leading causes of cryptogenic cirrhosis and is potentially reversible if found early in its course, making the diagnosis of nonalcoholic fatty liver disease before it is clinically evident may greatly decrease its morbidity and mortality. It is therefore especially important to pay close attention to high risk populations. Evidence from three retrospective studies indicates an increased incidence of fatty liver disease in women with PCOS. It may be recognized by the presence of elevated liver chemistries on routine lab screening, but normal liver chemistries do not rule out NAFLD. In fact, one study demonstrated ultrasound evidence of fatty liver disease in over half of all women with PCOS, with only one in six of these women demonstrating elevated transaminases. Therefore, some physicians have advocated abdominal ultrasounds in most women with PCOS. It remains unclear whether the women with evidence of fatty liver on ultrasound, but without elevated liver chemistries will progress from simple fatty liver to NASH.

## Lessons Learned

1. Patients with PCOS typically present with oligo- or amenorrhea and evidence of hyperandrogenism. Other causes of these symptoms must be excluded prior to making the diagnosis. The official diagnostic criteria remain controversial, particularly regarding the inclusion of the presence of typical PCO ovarian cysts on ultrasound.
2. PCOS patients may be obese or lean and they may even have normal menses.
3. The metabolic syndrome is common in women with PCOS, and because of its health implications many (if not all) affected women should be screened for its components as well as with a 2 h oral glucose tolerance test.
4. The treatment of PCOS should be guided by the patient's symptoms and individual goals and should always include a discussion on family planning and the use of birth control.
5. Women with PCOS are at risk for developing many complications in addition to the metabolic syndrome, including vascular endothelial dysfunction, endometrial cancer, obstructive sleep apnea, and nonalcoholic fatty liver disease. They should be screened for these conditions in a proactive and aggressive manner.

M. Magnotti et al.

## Questions

1. Which of the following is true about the diagnosis of PCOS in this patient?

   A. This patient cannot have PCOS because she had normal menses for several years (prior to her current episode of amenorrhea)
   B. Because of the presence of amenorrhea and clinical evidence of hyperandrogenism, this patient most likely has PCOS
   C. This patient cannot have PCOS because she has a BMI of less than 30 and is therefore not obese
   D. The diagnosis of PCOS cannot be definitively made in this patient without a pelvic ultrasound to confirm the presence of ovarian cysts

2. Which of the following is true about the diagnosis of the metabolic syndrome in this patient?

   A. This patient has the metabolic syndrome because she has an elevated LDL, a low HDL, and a waist circumference greater than 35 in.
   B. This patient can not have the metabolic syndrome because her BMI is not greater than 30
   C. This patient has the metabolic syndrome because she has elevated triglycerides, a low HDL, and a waist circumference of greater than 35 in.
   D. This patient can not have the metabolic syndrome because her fasting blood glucose is normal.

3. Which of the following treatment options would be reasonable for this patient, assuming she is sexually active, but does not desire pregnancy at this time?

   A. Rosiglitazone alone
   B. Metformin alone
   C. Spironolactone alone
   D. Oral contraceptive pill plus metformin
   E. Any of the above

4. Because she has PCOS, which of the following conditions is this patient at risk of developing?

   A. Vascular endothelial dysfunction
   B. Endometrial cancer
   C. Obstructive sleep apnea
   D. Fatty liver and/or nonalcoholic steatohepatitis
   E. All of the above

## Answers to Questions

1. B.

**Discussion:** The various diagnostic criteria for PCOS are reviewed above. However, no matter which set of criteria you utilize, it is clear that polycystic ovaries are not required to make the diagnosis of PCOS and therefore choice D is incorrect.

Choice C is incorrect because none of the proposed diagnostic criteria require the presence of obesity. Although obesity is often associated with PCOS (at least 50 % of women with PCOS are obese, particularly in the USA), there are clearly a significant number of lean women who meet the criteria for PCOS. Choice A is also incorrect because the presence of normal menses earlier in this patient's life certainly does not exclude the diagnosis of PCOS at the present time. The onset of PCOS is commonly either at the time of menarche or after a period of significant weight gain postmenarcheally.

2. C.

**Discussion:** Using the NCEP (National Cholesterol Education Program) ATPIII (Adult Treatment Panel III) criteria, the metabolic syndrome is defined as the presence of three of the following five criteria:

1. Waist circumference of greater than 35 in. in females or 40 in. in males
2. Triglycerides greater than 150 mg/dL or present drug therapy for hypertriglyceridemia
3. HDL less than 50 mg/dL in women or 40 mg/dL in men or present drug therapy for low HDL
4. Blood pressure greater than 130/85 mmHg or present drug therapy for hypertension
5. Fasting plasma glucose of greater than 100 or the presence of diabetes

Based on these criteria, the patient described does have the metabolic syndrome and only answer choice C is correct. Neither BMI nor LDL levels are included in the current definition of the metabolic syndrome, so answers A and B are incorrect. Although fasting plasma glucose is included in the criteria, it is not required to make the diagnosis if three of the other criteria are present (as in this case). Therefore answer D is incorrect.

3. D.

**Discussion:** Although all of the choices are reasonable options for the treatment of select patients with the polycystic ovarian syndrome, because this patient does not desire pregnancy, her treatment should include some form of contraception. It is important to remember that treatment of the insulin resistance of PCOS with metformin or a TZD (rosiglitazone or pioglitazone) may result in the resumption of normal ovarian function, normal ovulation, and therefore fertility. Thus, it is essential to discuss family planning with these patients prior to initiating treatment in order to prevent unwanted pregnancies. Because she does not desire pregnancy, choices A, B, and E are incorrect. Choice C is incorrect because spironolactone is teratogenic and therefore must never be given without an effective form of contraception.

4. E.

**Discussion:** Patients with PCOS are at risk for a number of conditions, including all of those listed in the question and therefore choice E is correct. Several studies have demonstrated the presence of disorders of endothelial function and vascular compliance in women with PCOS. The degree of dysfunction is not fully accounted for by obesity alone and there is evidence that it can be partially reversed by treatment with insulin sensitizers. There is also evidence to suggest a higher incidence of obstructive sleep apnea in patients with PCOS than can be explained by obesity alone. The reason for this remains unclear, but may also be related to insulin resistance.

# References

1. Dunaif A, Green G, Futterweit W, et al. Profound peripheral insulin resistance, independent of obesity, in polycystic ovary syndrome. Diabetes. 1989;38(9):1165–74.
2. Legro RS, Driscoll D, Strauss III JF, Fox J, Dunaif A. Evidence for a genetic basis for hyperandrogenemia in polycystic ovary syndrome. Proc Natl Acad Sci U S A. 1998;95(25):14956.
3. Goodarzi MO, Jones MR, Li X, Chua AK, Garcia OA, Chen YD, Krauss RM, Rotter JI, Ankener W, Legro RS, Azziz R, Strauss III JF, Dunaif A, Urbanek M. Replication of association of DENND1A and THADA variants with polycystic ovary syndrome in European cohorts. J Med Genet. 2012;49(2):90.
4. Wild RA, Carmina E, Diamanti-Kandarakis E, Dokras A, Escobar-Morreale HF, Futterweit W, Lobo R, Norman RJ, Talbot E, Dumesic DA. Assessment of cardiovascular risk and prevention of cardiovascular disease in women with the polycystic ovary syndrome: a consensus statement by the Androgen Excess and Polycystic Ovary Syndrome (AE-PCOS) Society. J Clin Endocrinol Metab. 2010;95(5):2038.
5. Ehrmann DA. Polycystic ovary syndrome. N Engl J Med. 2005;352(12):1223–36.
6. The Rotterdam ESHRE/ASRM-sponsored PCOS consensus workshop group. Revised 2003 consensus on diagnostic criteria and longterm health risks related to polycystic ovary syndrome (PCOS). Hum Reprod. 2004;19(1):41–7.
7. Azziz R, Carmina E, Dewailly D, et al. Position statement: criteria for defining polycystic ovary syndrome as a predominantly hyperandrogenic syndrome: an Androgen Excess Society guideline. J Clin Endocrinol Metab. 2006;91(11):4237–45.
8. Setji TL, Holland ND, Sanders LL, et al. Nonalcoholic steatohepatitis and nonalcoholic fatty liver disease in young women with polycystic ovary syndrome. J Clin Endocrinol Metab. 2006;91(5):1741–7.
9. Gambarin-Gelwan M, Kinkhabwala SV, Schiano TD, et al. Prevalence of nonalcoholic liver disease in women with polycystic ovary syndrome. Clin Gastroenterol Hepatol. 2007;5(4):496–501.
10. Azziz R, Carmina E, Dewailly D, Diamanti-Kandarakis E, Escobar-Morreale HF, Futterweit W, Janssen OE, Legro RS, Norman RJ, Taylor AE, Witchel SF, Task Force on the Phenotype of the Polycystic Ovary Syndrome of The Androgen Excess and PCOS Society. The Androgen Excess and PCOS Society criteria for the polycystic ovary syndrome: the complete task force report. Fertil Steril. 2009;91(2):456–88.

# Chapter 52
# Bariatric Surgery

**Robert T. Yanagisawa, Daniel Herron, David W. Lam, and Derek LeRoith**

## Objectives

1. To review the appropriate patient criteria for weight loss surgery.
2. To understand the appropriate diabetes management of patients undergoing bariatric surgery.
3. To discuss the effect of gastric bypass surgery on insulin resistance and long-term postoperative medical management.

## Case

A 45-year-old white male presented with morbid obesity. After his brother suffered a myocardial infarction, the patient realized he needed to take control of his health. His weight history revealed that he had gradually gained over 40 lbs over the last 10 years. He had lost 10–15 lbs on several attempts with diet and exercise programs, but he was unable to maintain his weight loss for more than 6 months. He was diagnosed with type-2 diabetes 2 years ago and he has been treated with a combination of glimepride, rosiglitazone, and metformin. He also suffers from a mixed dyslipidemia for which he takes simvastatin 40 mg daily.

R.T. Yanagisawa, M.D. (✉) • D.W. Lam, M.D. • D. LeRoith, M.D., Ph.D.
Division of Endocrinology, Diabetes, and Bone Diseases,
Icahn School of Medicine at Mount Sinai, One Gustave Levy Place,
Box 1055, New York, NY 10029-6574, USA
e-mail: Robert.yanagisawa@mssm.edu

D. Herron, M.D.
Professor of Surgery, Chief of Laparoscopic and Bariatric Surgery,
Icahn School of Medicine at Mount Sinai, New York, NY, USA

© Springer Science+Business Media New York 2015
T.F. Davies (ed.), *A Case-Based Guide to Clinical Endocrinology*,
DOI 10.1007/978-1-4939-2059-4_52

On a physical examination, he was morbidly obese. At 5′8″ tall and 290 lbs, he had a BMI of 44 kg/m² with an android body weight distribution and a waist circumference of 48″. He had no hepatosplenomegaly or any significant peripheral edema. His fasting glucoses ranged from 145 to 225 mg/dL and Hgb A1C was 8.9 %.

He was evaluated and considered as an appropriate candidate for surgical weigh loss by the multidisciplinary team consisting of bariatric surgeons, endocrinologists, nutritionists, and psychiatrists who are all experts with a variety of bariatric procedures. The patient was well informed regarding bariatric surgery and understood the importance of his lifelong adherence to nutritional management. His diabetes control was optimized preoperatively by starting a combination of basal and bolus insulin.

He underwent Roux-en-Y Gastric Bypass (RYGB) surgery and his diabetes was controlled with a reduced basal insulin dose during his immediate postoperative period. Within 2 weeks of discharge from the hospital, he was able to discontinue all his insulin and maintained on rosiglitazone and metformin for his diabetes. Three months after surgery, his diabetes demonstrates remarkable improvement with a Hgb A1C of 6.0 %. His diabetes medications were discontinued. He takes nutritional supplements including calcium citrate with vitamin D, iron, and multivitamins.

## Review of the Diagnosis

### Roux-en-Y Gastric Bypass

The best operations reduce body weight by 35–40 % with most of this effect is maintained for more than 10 years. According to NIH guidelines for bariatric surgery is indicated for patients with BMI > 40 kg/m² or those with BMI > 35 kg/m² plus one or more obesity associated comorbidities such as diabetes or hypertension [1]. Among the variety of bariatric surgery procedures, Roux-en-Y gastric bypass (RYGB) appears to offer the best balance of effectiveness vs. risk, and it is the most widely used surgery for the morbidly obese people in the USA.

**Roux-en-Y Gastric Bypass Surgery** is currently considered to be the "Gold Standard" bariatric operation. Performed most commonly though a laparoscopic approach, the surgery involves creation of a small gastric pouch with a Y-shaped intestinal reconstruction. It is a restrictive and mildly malabsorptive procedure (Fig. 52.1).

### Optimizing Glycemic Control Prior to Surgery

An appropriate preoperative screening includes prior history of failure to lose weight despite proper medical therapy. Patients must be educated regarding the bariatric procedure and the need for lifelong adherence to nutritional management. Glycemic

**Fig. 52.1** Roux-en-Y gastric
bypass (RYGB) surgery.
Diagram courtesy of Dr.
Daniel Herron

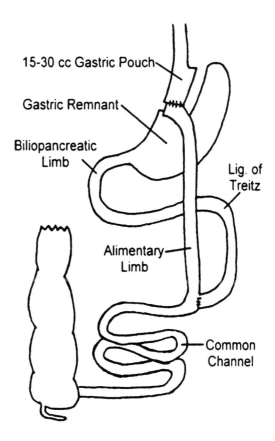

control must be optimized in patients with diabetes prior to surgery in order to minimize the perioperative complications. Preoperatively, patients are more motivated to optimize their medical condition and endocrinologists can help manage their diabetes aggressively. Starting an insulin regimen is appropriate in order to optimize the glycemic control even in a relatively short period of time for patients preparing for the surgery. Perioperative tight glycemic control often requires some insulin coverage, but it must be adjusted accordingly to their insulin requirement (see discussion 2 below). Successful outcome after a surgical weight loss procedure depends on extensive patient counseling and multidisciplinary support postoperatively.

## Long-Term Outcomes of Bariatric Surgery

Bariatric surgery appears to be an effective option for the treatment of severe obesity, resulting in a long-term weight loss, an improved lifestyle, and, an amelioration in risk factors associated with obesity (Fig. 52.2).

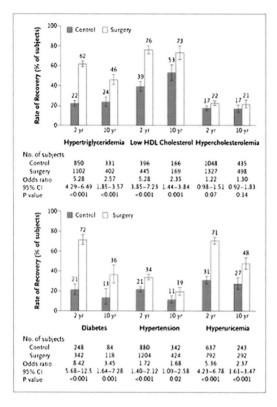

Recovery from diabetes, lipid disturbances, hypertension, and hyperuricemia over 2 and 10 years in surgically treated subjects and their obese controls.

Adapted from Sjöström et al. Lifestyle, Diabetes, and Cardiovascular Risk Factors 10 Years after Bariatric Surgery. NEJM 2004 351 (26): 2683

**Fig. 52.2** Recovery from diabetes, lipid disturbances, hypertension, and hyperuricemia over 2 and 10 years in surgically treated subjects and their obese controls. Adapted from Sjöström et al. Lifestyle, Diabetes, and Cardiovascular Risk Factors 10 years After Bariatric Surgery. NEJM 2004; 351 (26): 2683

The prospective controlled Swedish Obese Subjects Study involved obese subjects who underwent gastric surgery and contemporaneously matched, conventionally treated obese control subjects. One of the largest series, with 4,047 subjects, it demonstrates the benefit of bariatric surgery for morbid obesity [2]. Significant number of patients with diabetes can recover with surgical weight loss, based on either the cutoff values or use of medication to treat diabetes. The mean changes in weight and risk factors were also more favorable among the subjects treated by gastric bypass than among those treated by banding or other form of surgical procedures.

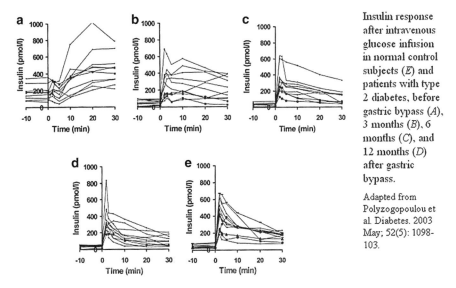

**Fig. 52.3** Insulin response after intravenous glucose infusion in normal control subjects (**e**) and patients with type 2 diabetes , before gastric bypass (**a**), 3 months (**b**), 6 months (**c**), and 12 months (**d**) after gastric bypass. Adapted from Polyzogopoulou et al. Diabetes. 2003 May; 52(5): 1098–103

## *Diabetes Resolution with RYGB Surgery*

The duration of diabetes since diagnosis seems to predict successful improvement of glycemic control postsurgery. The first phase insulin response is typically disrupted early in the course of diabetes and it improves to a near-normal level in patients who undergo gastric bypass surgery with diabetes of less than 3–5 years duration [3]. Recovery of the first-phase insulin response may be the best indicator of diabetes resolution in patients who have had gastric bypass surgery (Fig. 52.3).

The mechanisms underlying the effects of RYGB on body weight and glucose metabolism are still not completely understood, but we can predict the course of diabetes outcome with surgery. In the immediate postoperative period, patients are essentially fasting and resulting in the fast-induced alleviation of diabetes. Patients who are on significant doses of insulin preoperatively often only require a minimal basal insulin. Patients gradually tolerate their oral intake, but they continue to be in a state of negative energy balance, a condition that decreases glucose toxicity and improves ß-cell function. Eventually, a marked weight reduction with baritaric surgery allows patients to increase their level of physical activity. Increased physical activity coupled with decreased glucose load from small quantity of each meal after gastric bypass surgery leads to a dramatically improved diabetes control.

**Table 52.1** Preoperative predictors of improvement in type-2 diabetes

| Factors | Improvement | Resolution |
|---|---|---|
| Duration of T2 DM | <10 years | <4 years |
| HbA1C | <8.8 % | <8.0 % |
| Waist circumference | <53 in. | <48 in. |

In the majority of studies, resolution is defined as some combination of returning to a fasting blood glucose <110 mg/dL or a glycated hemoglobin $A_{1c}$ (HbA$_{1c}$) <7 % without diabetic medications. Improvement is defined as approaching these values or reaching these targets with less medication

Adapted from Stohmayer, E, Via, M, Yanagisawa, R 2010 "Metabolic Management Following Bariatric Surgery" MSJM Vol 77, No 5

## Incretin Effects of RYGB Surgery

Cummings hypothesizes more interesting possibilities of RYGB effect on glucose metabolism [4]. Alterations in gut hormones release after RYGB may act in concert with the above mechanism to improve insulin secretion or action. Ghrelin, secreted by the stomach, exerts several diabetogenic effects including increased levels of GH, cortisol, and epinephrine—three of the four classical counter regulatory hormones. Ghrelin levels are decreased after gastric bypass, resulting in an antidiabetogenic effect. The other effect of surgery is increased GLP-1 secretion from bypassing part of the foregut and facilitated delivery of nutrients directly to the hindgut. GLP-1 is an incretin that stimulates insulin secretion in response to enteral nutrients. GLP-1 and PYY also suppress gastrointestinal motility, gastric emptying, small intestinal transit, and food intake.

Patients with a relatively short duration of diabetes since diagnosis seem to have a better improvement of glycemic control post-RYGB [6]. While there are no standardized guidelines for the optimal timing to recommend patient with diabetes and obesity for bariatric surgery, these findings may call for an earlier referral of morbidly obese patients with diabetes to a surgical weight loss (Table 52.1).

## Long-Term Post Operative Medical Management

On the other hand, we must also understand nutritional consequences of surgical intervention for morbid obesity. While RYGB surgery should not cause severe malabsorptive problems postsurgery, patients will have a decreased absorption of protein, iron, calcium, and fat-soluble vitamins. Postoperatively, patients who have had RYGB surgery need to be periodically monitored for nutritional deficiency for the rest of their life. The Endocrine Society clinical practice guidelines recommend to monitor iron, ferritin, Vitamin B12, folate, calcium, intact parathyroid hormone, 25(OH) Vitamin D, albumin, and pre-albumin on a regular basis. Monitoring of vitamin A, zinc, and thiamine is considered optional [5].

Patients are instructed to eat at least 60 g of protein daily. Due to their limited gastric capacity, they usually require protein supplementation initially to be able to meet their nutritional goal. Chewable multivitamin and calcium supplementation is started on discharge from the surgery.

After RYGB surgery, patients tend to have an increased PTH values, and one must avoid the development of overt secondary hyperparathyroidism from vitamin D deficiency. They need to be consistent with calcium with vitamin D. The goal is to maintain 25OH vitamin D level above 25 and PTH level below 80–90. The amount required varies with extent of malabsorption, but typically 1,000–1,200 IU/day of vitamin D are required to maintain an adequate level.

While this patient may not require any hypoglycemic agents to control his diabetes, he must continue to avoid excess glucose and carbohydrate load. His small gastric pouch is likely to prevent him from eating large meals and hence creating a significant caloric deficit. However, despite RYGB surgery, he will be able to absorb simple sugars and still have a tendency for hyperglycemia. His success in ameliorating his diabetes depends on his success with his weight loss and his behavioral modification.

## Sleeve Gastrectomy

Sleeve gastrectomy is a more recently developed bariatric operation that has rapidly been gaining popularity in the United States. In this procedures, the greater curvature (left side) of the stomach is surgically resected, leaving a banana-shaped stomach of roughly 150 ml volume (Fig. 52.4). Since no intestine is surgically bypassed, intestinal absorption remains unaffected. This procedure results in weight loss that is comparable to that observed after RYGB with a lower complication rate. However, improvement of T2DM may not be as significant with this procedure [7].

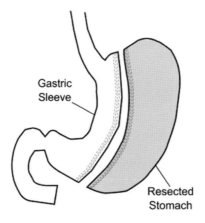

Gastric
Sleeve

Resected
Stomach

**Fig. 52.4** Sleeve gastrectomy. The greater curvature, or left side, of the stomach is resected, leaving a 150 ml banana-shaped stomach pouch (image courtesy of Daniel M. Herron, MD)

## Lessons Learned

1. Bariatric surgery is an effective option for the treatment of severe obesity and obesity related metabolic risks for patients with BMI>40 kg/m$^2$ or those with BMI>35 kg/m$^2$ plus one or more obesity associated comorbidities.
2. Successful outcome of surgical weight loss depends on patient education and teamwork with the multidisciplinary team supporting the patient.
3. The duration of diabetes and strict behavioral modification predict successful improvement of the glycemic control postsurgery. Recovery of the first-phase insulin response improves to a near-normal level in patients who undergo gastric bypass surgery with diabetes of less than 3–5 years duration.
4. Sleeve gastrectomy is a new procedure that provides weight loss nearly equal to that of gastric bypass. Resolution of T2DM, however, may be less pronounced after this procedure.

## Questions

1. What makes him an appropriate candidate for bariatric surgery?

   A. BMI>40 kg/m$^2$
   B. Diabetes and other metabolic risk factors
   C. Failed prior medical management to control his obesity
   D. Ability to comply with his lifelong adherence to nutritional management
   E. All of the above

2. What factors increase his likelihood of achieving his glycemic control postsurgery?

   A. Duration of his diabetes
   B. Patient's ability to exercise with weight loss
   C. Avoidance of his glucose toxicity
   D. Decreased visceral adiposity
   E. All of the above

3. Postoperatively, what are the nutritional concerns for this patient?

   A. Supplemental protein only if they develop signs of malabsorption.
   B. Iron replacement only if they develop anemia.
   C. Any excess calorie will not be absorbed so patients can eat ad lib and lose weight.
   D. Calcium with vitamin D to prevent secondary hyperparathyroidism.
   E. Patient does not need to follow his blood glucose any more.

## Answers to Questions

1. E.

**Discussion:** According to NIH guidelines for bariatric surgery, this patient meets BMI criteria (BMI > 40 kg/m$^2$), but we should further evaluate him to see if he is an appropriate candidate for bariatric surgery. Choices B–D make him an appropriate surgical candidate.

2. D.

**Discussion:** Short duration of his diabetes is important indicator for improving his diabetes. The first-phase insulin response improves to a near-normal level in patients who undergo gastric bypass surgery with diabetes of less than 3–5 years duration. Choices B–D all help to improve his insulin resistance. See diabetes resolution section.

3. D.

**Discussion:** After RYGB surgery, patients will have a decreased absorption of protein, iron, calcium, and fat-soluble vitamins. Choices A and B are incorrect as he will require these supplements to prevent malabsorptive complications. Choices C and E are incorrect as he will be able to absorb simple sugars and still have a tendency for hyperglycemia. Choice D is correct and he needs his calcium, vitamin D, and PTH levels needs to be monitored. See long-term postoperative medical management section.

## References

1. NIH Consensus Development Panel. Gastrointestinal surgery for severe obesity. Ann Intern Med. 1991;115:956–61.
2. Sjöström L, et al. Lifestyle, diabetes, and cardiovascular risk factors 10 years after bariatric surgery. NEJM. 2004;351(26):2683.
3. Polyzogopoulou EV, et al. Restoration of euglycemia and normal acute insulin response to glucose in obese subjects with type 2 diabetes following bariatric surgery. Diabetes. 2003;52(5):1098–103.
4. Cummings D, et al. Gastric bypass for obesity: mechanisms of weight loss and diabetes resolution. JCEM. 2004;89:2608–15.
5. Heber D, et al. Endocrine and nutritional management of the post-bariatric surgery patient: an Endocrine Society Clinical Practice Guideline. J Clin Endocrinol Metab. 2010;95(11): 4823–42.
6. Buchwald H, Estok R, Fahrbach K, Banel D, Jensen MD, Pories WJ, et al. Weight and type 2 diabetes after bariatric surgery: systematic review and meta-analysis. Am J Med. 2009;122(3):248–56.
7. Chouillard EK, Karaa A, Elkhoury M, et al. Laparoscopic Roux-en-Y gastric bypass versus laparoscopic sleeve gastrectomy for morbid obesity: case-control study. Surg Obes Relat Dis. 2011;7(4):500–5.

# Index

**A**

Abdomen
   CT, 187, 208
   MRI of, 165
Abdominal pain, hypertriglyceridemia,
      397–399
ACC. *See* Adrenocortical carcinoma
      (ACC)
ACEi. *See* Angiotensin-conting enzyme
      inhibitors (ACEi)
Acne, 18, 420, 425
Acromegaly, 5–6
   cardiac disease, 23
   complications, 23–24
   cosmetic procedures, 18
   diastema, 18
   growth hormone, 17–19
   hormonal evaluation, 18
   hypertension, 16, 23
   immunostaining, 20
   laboratory results, 19
   mandible, 17
   MR imaging, 16, 17
   orthodenture, 18
   pre-cancerous/malignant polyps, 24
   prolactin, 19
   radiotherapy, 21
   sleep apnea syndrome, 24
   SSAs, 21–23
   surgery, 20–21
   VF testing, 16
   vision symptoms, 16
ACTH. *See* Adrenocorticotropic hormone
      (ACTH)
Actonel, 260

Acute blood loss, 348
Adenomas
   adrenal, 30
   aldosterone-producing adenomas, 190
   corticotroph, 8
   pituitary (*See* Pituitary adenomas)
   somatotroph, 17
   TSH-secreting pituitary adenoma, 12
      abdominal exam, 59
      alpha-subunit, 61–62
      cardiovascular exam, 59
      differential diagnosis, 63
      Graves' disease, 61
      immunoassays, 60
      levothyroxine, 57, 58
      macroadenomas, 62
      medical therapy, 62
      methimazole, 58
      mild diffuse enlargement, 58
      somatostatin receptors, 62
Adipokines, 406
Adjunctive therapy, 175–177
Adrenal adenomas, 30
Adrenal hormones, 203
Adrenalectomy
   bilateral adrenalectomy, 32, 63, 188
   unilateral, 191–193, 212
Adrenal hypercortisolism, 201
Adrenal hypoplasia congenital (AHC), 289
Adrenal incidentaloma, 203, 199–204
Adrenal mass, 199, 200, 202
Adrenal nodule
   follow-up, 202
   hormonally active, 201–202
   malignant, 200–201